Cancer Care

Cancer Care

A PERSONAL GUIDE

Harold Glucksberg, M.D.

Jack W. Singer, M.D.

THE JOHNS HOPKINS UNIVERSITY PRESS
Baltimore and London

Copyright © 1980 by The Johns Hopkins University Press

All rights reserved. No part of this book may be
reproduced or transmitted in any form or by any means,
electronic or mechanical, including photocopying,
recording, xerography, or any information storage and
retrieval system, without permission in writing
from the publisher.

Manufactured in the United States of America

The Johns Hopkins University Press, Baltimore, Maryland 21218
The Johns Hopkins Press Ltd., London

Library of Congress Catalog Card Number 79–16930
ISBN 0–8018–2255–6

Library of Congress Cataloging in Publication data
will be found on the last printed page of this book.

We dedicate this book to our patients, who have taught us about the emotional as well as physical aspects of cancer and who provided criticisms and encouragement. We hope it will help other cancer patients and their families acquire enough knowledge to become intelligent health care consumers and to secure the best care available.

We also dedicate this book to Sonia, Ari, Costa, and Mordecai.

Contents

TABLES

Acknowledgments

We would like to express our appreciation to the following people for their critical reviews of sections of this book: Sandy Barckley; John Blasko, M.D.; Warren Chapman, M.D.; Martin Cheever, M.D.; Phyllis De Friese; David Figge, M.D.; Karen Glucksberg; Sam Glucksberg; Philip Greenberg, M.D.; Theodore Greenlee, M.D.; Jack Hartman, M.D.; Mary Ann Hays; Leonard Johnson, M.D.; Robert Jones, M.D.; Bernice Hodgen; William Kelly, M.D.; George McDonald, M.D.; Kristopher Mikami; Roger Moe, M.D.; Thomas Rudd, M.D.; Thalia Singer; Hope Smulan; Wayne Smulan; Kathryn Spike; Mary Suders; and Roger Tigelaar, M.D.

We would also like to express our appreciation to Sandra Barckley and Grace Skoogs for their expert secretarial assistance.

Cancer Care

Introduction

Cancer is a frightening disease, arousing fear of prolonged suffering and death in all of us. It probably evokes more anxiety than any other ailment in our society. The word *cancer* provokes strong feelings in both physicians and patients. Numerous euphemisms have been used as a substitute: words such as *tumor, growth,* and *spot* are often used instead of the word *cancer.* Unfortunately, there is a rational basis for these quiet and often unspoken fears. Cancer can strike at any age. It is the second most common cause of death in the Western world. About seven hundred thousand Americans yearly develop cancer; one in four develops at least one cancer in his or her lifetime. Only heart disease claims more lives.

In the past, cancer was invariably fatal. To be told you had cancer was a death sentence. Today, however, treatment can cure many people. In fact, one in three—over 200,000 Americans each year—is cured. Most of the other people with cancer either live longer or more comfortably with treatment. Many people, though, do not realize that modern treatment can help. They still think that cancer means suffering and certain death. Others think that cancer has been conquered—that it is almost always curable. The media, unfortunately, unrealistically report progress—giant steps in cancer diagnosis and treatment that are seldom borne out by reality. The facts support neither misconception. Many cancer patients are helped and some are cured with modern treatment, but many still die. Medical progress has been made and is continuing, but giant strides are rare. Most progress is slow. We have written this book in the conviction that the facts will be reassuring and will help you cope with cancer better than the myths, half-truths, and misconceptions that most people believe and that the available lay literature reinforces.

1

Modern treatment cures many and helps most people with cancer. To do this, it has become increasingly complex and specialized. We feel it is important that people receive the best available treatment for their cancer; inadequate treatment causes increased suffering and unnecessary deaths. We believe that people are more likely to receive good treatment if they understand the behavior of their disease and how and by whom it should be treated. To get the best care, people must be knowledgeable, aware health care consumers. This book is written with the aim of providing people who have cancer with enough information for them to evaluate the quality of their medical care.

What Is Cancer?

The word *cancer* is derived from the Old French word *cancre*, which became *canker* in England and was used to describe both infections and malignancies until 1700. We operationally define cancer as *the uncontrolled growth of cells that if unchecked will kill its host.*

Cancer develops from changes or mutations in the genetic material in a single cell. This change results in cell growth that does not respond to normal controls, and it is this characteristic that differentiates cancer, a malignant growth, from benign, nonmalignant growths and from normal tissues. Normal cells respond to signals that limit or control their growth. When you cut your finger, the skin cells receive signals to divide to repair the injury. When the injury has been repaired, signals are sent to stop cell growth. The cancer cell is an outlaw: it does not obey the laws of normal cellular biology. Cancer cells not only grow uncontrollably but also spread to other parts of the body, through the lymph vessels to lymph nodes and through the bloodstream to other organs. Deposits of cancer cells in other organs are called metastases. It is these metastases that usually cause death from cancer. Cancers that are still localized can usually be cured with modern treatment. However, chemotherapy, the only therapy that can eradicate metastatic cancer, cannot cure most people at the present time.

How This Book Can Help You If You Have Cancer

People who get cancer are frightened. Many fantasize an early death with severe pain. Usually fantasies are far worse than the reality. For example, it is commonly believed that most people dying from cancer suffer intolerable pain. Although this may have been true decades ago, with new and more effective approaches to pain control, most pain is now treated quite effectively.

Both living and dying with cancer are crises for the victim and the family. In this book we talk about the common fears and problems of cancer patients and their families. We provide information that can help people to face their illnesses. Many problems common to cancer patients are illustrated by case histories. We also suggest other sources of help, such as the volunteer organizations composed of former cancer patients. We hope what we say will help people both accept and fight against their disease.

Only You Can Make Sure You Get Good Care

To discover you have cancer is a lonely and terrifying experience. Panic is probably a universal reaction. The diagnosis of cancer brings forth fears of toxic treatment, of suffering, and of death. People have no ready source of information about cancer or its treatment. They are in a poor position to assess the qualifications of their physician and his recommendations about treatment. Most place total confidence in their doctors. Blind faith is reassuring but does not assure good care.

The premise of this book is that not all doctors can offer equally good treatment. Doctors differ in their training, experience, common sense, and personality. We will explain how to find out whether your doctor is adequately qualified to treat your cancer, and we will discuss what you should expect from your doctor as a human being. Two extremely important issues relate to who should treat you and where treatment should be done. For example, should a person be treated by his family physician, by a local surgeon, by a surgeon in a large clinic, or by a surgeon in a cancer center five hundred miles away? For each of the common cancers we will suggest what cancer specialists or teams of specialists should be consulted.

Our main purpose is to assist people with cancer and their families by providing a source of information about cancer and its treatment. We feel people have a better chance of receiving good treatment for cancer if they understand the disease, so we will discuss how specific cancers should be evaluated and treated. Knowledgeable, active patients are more likely to do well and less likely to get severely depressed than passive ones. They can become active participants in their care, active partners with their physicians, rather than remaining passive consumers. We will try to give you enough information to decide whether the medical care you are getting is adequate and to do so before major treatments are started.

How to Use This Book

This book should give you enough information about most cancers, their current treatment, and the types of specialists needed for you to decide whether your medical care is adequate. The best chance and often the only chance for cure occurs with the first treatment. When cancer is diagnosed, treatment should begin as soon as possible. People can read the relevant sections in this book and assess their care in a matter of days. We recommend that this book be used in the following way:

1. Read the chapter on your specific cancer. This will tell you how your cancer should be evaluated and treated. It will also discuss who is best qualified to treat you.
2. Read the chapter on the treatment of cancer. Chapter 7 gives an overview of cancer evaluation and treatment.
3. Read about the treatments that apply to your specific cancer. Surgery, radiation, and chemotherapy are the techniques used to combat cancer. Some cancers are treated with only one type of therapy and some with all three. Chapters 8 through 10 explain how the different methods are used. They also describe the background and experience of the doctors who should treat you.
4. Read the chapter on who should treat you and where you should be treated. Chapter 4 will help you decide whether you should be treated in your own community or travel to a larger medical facility.
5. Read the chapter on the doctor-patient relationship. Chapter 5 explores what the patient should expect and needs from a physician as a human being. You will want a doctor who is supportive, with whom you can discuss your feelings and fears. This chapter may help you switch physicians if your doctor does not meet your emotional needs.
6. Read the chapter on experimental therapy. Many people are offered experimental approaches. Chapter 24 can help you understand the benefits and risks of different types of experimental treatment.

By reading only these few chapters, it is possible to get a clear picture of how a specific cancer should be evaluated and treated, who should treat it, and what to expect from the treatment. You will also find out whether it pays to go to a larger center or to try experimental therapy.

Some treatments may have changed by the time you read this book. Use the information here as a basis for asking your physician questions that will help you assess your situation. By using the facts in this book and asking questions, you should be able to have more control over your treatment and to be sure of its adequacy.

About Cancer "Quackery"

Cancer "quackery" has been with us for centuries and will be with us as long as cancer is a dread and often fatal disease. It has become almost a fad in the United States. Many people with cancer are advised by friends, neighbors, or relatives to try treatments that the medical profession considers useless or that are outright quackery. Often, this only further confuses a frightened patient. Recommended treatments are imperfect; cures are never guaranteed and there are side effects. The advocates of Laetrile, diet therapy, megavitamin treatment, and a variety of other unproven cancer treatments seem to promise either a sure cure or improvement without any of the other drawbacks or side effects of standard cancer treatments. The newly diagnosed cancer patient may be vulnerable to these claims. He or she wants to believe they are true. It's only natural to want things to turn out all right. Because of intense public pressure, some of these unproven treatments are currently legal in many states.

We will discuss what we know about cancer quackery and how to recognize when a treatment is unsound. The use of unsound treatments on a patient who is curable by standard treatment costs lives. Quack treatments for the incurable patient cost thousands of dollars, money most families need after the patient dies. We want people to be able to recognize quack treatments and the so-called physicians who use them. We give some simple guidelines for this.

What Is in This Book for People Who Do Not Have Cancer?

Regular Checkups Can Save Your Life

Cancer usually begins in one area and is highly curable until it spreads to other parts of the body. Currently, one in three Americans with cancer is cured. Many more could be cured if all Americans had regular checkups to detect early cancer. Regular checkups will not conqer cancer. There is no simple single test to detect cancer early, and many cancers are inaccessible to the physician's examination or to laboratory tests.

Several very common cancers, however, can be easily detected before they cause problems. Regular checkups for these cancers increase the chance for cure. The best example of this is the halving of the death rate from cancer of the cervix in the past decade because of the widespread use of Pap smears. Regular checkups can detect several common cancers, including cancers of the cervix, uterus, breast, colon and rectum, skin, and mouth. Everyone should be examined for these. In the chapter on early detection of cancer, we present guidelines for cancer screening: Who should be tested? How often? What tests are needed?

Some people are likely to develop a particular cancer either because of exposure to a carcinogen or an inherited disposition. These people need special cancer testing. For example, millions of Americans have had radiation to the neck in the past for trivial conditions. Because their thyroid glands were radiated, they have an increased chance of developing thyroid cancer. Thyroid cancer is rare in the general population but common in people with radiation exposure. They should have a thyroid examination on a yearly basis.

Perhaps there is a strong history of cancer in your family. Most cancers do not run in families but some do. For example, a woman whose mother developed cancer in both breasts before age fifty has a 30–40 percent chance of developing breast cancer. She should begin a screening program for breast cancer in her twenties. Not only is she at high risk of developing cancer, but she is likely to do so at an earlier age than other women.

Most doctors do not screen for cancer as thoroughly as they should.

We list the tests your doctor should be performing and at what age they should be started. Many doctors do not routinely check stool bloods (a simple test for colon cancer), do breast exams, etc. It is up to you to be sure your doctor screens you for cancer.

In chapter 1, we discuss the more common hereditary cancers and give specific recommendations as to what to do about each. In chapter 2, we identify several carcinogens that affect many Americans and place them at a high risk of developing cancer, and we suggest appropriate testing. We have tried to give people the information they need to have cancer found early and increase the chance for cure.

Can You Decrease Your Chances of Developing Cancer?
Is It Possible to Avoid the Carcinogens in Our Environment?

Cancer is becoming more common. This is partly because we now live much longer but also because we are exposed to an ever-increasing number of carcinogens. A carcinogen is a chemical that promotes or causes cancer. It has been estimated that up to 80 percent of all cancers are caused or influenced by carcinogens. Until recently, man lived and evolved in a relatively stable and natural environment. This is no longer true. Since the industrial revolution, a dazzling variety of new synthetic products, the effects of which are at best unknown, have been introduced into the environment. We have altered our environment more in the past decade than in the previous millennium.

Carcinogens produced by industry escape into the air and water around factories. That is why states like New Jersey, dotted with petrochemical plants, have the highest cancer rates in the country. While all of us are exposed to new chemicals, the greatest risks occur in people who work directly with them. In chapter 2, we identify the carcinogens and the jobs where exposure to these carcinogens occurs. Most workers do not know they are in danger, and neither their companies nor the government warns them. We want people to know. Then they can decide what to do.

Many products on our store shelves contain suspected or known carcinogens. For example, polyvinyl chloride, a plastic that has caused liver cancer in exposed workers, is still widely used as a plastic wrapper for meat and fish in large markets. All of us are exposed to low levels of this potent carcinogen. Asbestos, which is known to cause cancer and lung diseases, is present in many talcs produced by the cosmetics industry. The baby powder you use probably contains asbestos.

Food producers like their products to look appealing, which is equated with colorful. Therefore, many products contain food color dyes. Most of these are coal tar derivatives. These dyes are closely related to known carcinogens and are highly suspect themselves. Americans consume large amounts of these probably dangerous valueless substances.

In this book we give the facts about substances in consumer products that worry us as oncologists. We also make several simple recommendations on how to cut down your exposure to these carcinogens. You don't have to retreat to the hills and grow your own food to avoid many of the more common carcinogens.

How to Avoid Financial Ruin If Someone in Your Family Develops Cancer

Cancer treatment is expensive. Few Americans have adequate health insurance for serious, chronic illnesses such as cancer. The problem is compounded if the victim is the family breadwinner and cannot continue to work. In more than 50 percent of American families, both the husband and wife work. Therefore, if either gets cancer, income drops. If the health insurance is not adequate, bills mount up. It is not uncommon for a fairly solid family with "adequate health insurance" to face financial ruin because of cancer. The problem doesn't end when the treatment has been completed. The patient may be cured, but finding a new job may be impossible due to uninsurability.

In this book we describe what we feel are the criteria for adequate health insurance. For the person with cancer who does not have adequate insurance, we make some suggestions about how to cut the costs of treatment and we list some places where high-quality, free treatment is available.

SUMMARY

This book was written because we know of too many people who died when they might have lived if they had been more knowledgeable. It was also written to answer pleas from many of our patients for information about their cancers and their treatments that is not available anywhere except in medical literature.

In effect, this book tries to give the cancer victim some control over his treatment and his fate. It will enable the patient to evaluate his physician's qualifications as a cancer doctor and his recommendations for treatment. We feel this is very important. Many Americans do not receive good treatment for their cancer. This book will make it possible for people with cancer to have some control over the quality of their care. For those who do not have cancer, this book gives important information concerning screening for cancer, avoiding carcinogens, and protecting themselves financially.

Although the facts about cancer may be disturbing, we believe they will help people who have cancer get better care and help those who may develop cancer, a group that includes everyone, take simple steps to discover it at an early, curable stage.

1

Heredity and Cancer

DOES CANCER RUN IN YOUR FAMILY?

Cancer is a common disease in the United States. Approximately one American in four gets cancer at some time in his or her life. Merely because someone in your family has had cancer does not mean you are more likely to have cancer than other people. However, cancer can run in families. You may have a hereditary disposition to develop either a particular cancer or any cancer. Familial cancers tend to occur at an earlier age and are often multiple. It is important that you and your physician know about any hereditary disposition to cancer. Some of these cancers can be prevented; others can be diagnosed early by regular checkups that will give a better chance for their cure.

In this chapter we will discuss the more common hereditary cancers. If you think cancer runs in your family, you should tell your doctor. By taking a careful family history for cancer, by examining you carefully, and sometimes by blood tests, he may be able to determine if cancer does run in your family. If any of the diseases mentioned in this chapter has occurred in any blood relative, you should go to your doctor to see if you are also prone to develop cancer.

You should be suspicious that you have a hereditary disposition to cancer if there have been many cancers in your family, especially if they have developed at a relatively early age. Most cancer develops in older people—usually over the age of fifty. If there have been several cancers in young people in your family, you should check with your doctor. If you have any doubts at all, go to your doctor and tell your story. It may save not only your life but also the lives of other members of your family.

8

CANCER OF THE LARGE BOWEL

Cancer of the large intestine is very common in this country. Most cases are not hereditary but are caused by diet (see chapter 13, "Cancers of the Gastrointestinal Tract"). However, there are several hereditary conditions that predispose a person to large bowel cancer. The more common are polyposis coli, Gardner's syndrome, gastric and colonic polyps, and Peutz-Jegher syndrome. In all these conditions, many polyps develop in the large bowel at an early age (in some of these diseases polyps also develop in the small bowel and stomach). These polyps tend to become cancerous, often before age thirty.

The danger that these polyps may become cancerous varies with the condition. With polyposis coli and Gardner's syndrome, polyps usually develop before age twenty and the chances of their becoming cancerous are extremely high. There are too many polyps to remove and it is impossible with so many to diagnose cancer early. Therefore, for both these conditions, we recommend removal of the colon (a colectomy) to prevent the development of multiple and usually fatal large bowel cancer. It is extremely difficult for a young person to accept the removal of the large bowel and a colostomy, but the alternative is an 80 percent chance of death by age forty. The following case illustrates the type of family history that should alert you to these diseases.

H.B., a high school student, went to see his doctor because of rectal bleeding. The physician examined his rectum but found no hemorrhoids. (Hemorrhoids are the most common cause of rectal bleeding in young adults.) He therefore performed a sigmoidoscopy. This involves the insertion of a tube inside the bowel, allowing the doctor to look at and biopsy the inside of the rectum and large bowel. He saw many polyps in H.B.'s rectum and colon. The physician then asked H.B. about cancer in his family. Three of H.B.'s close relatives had died of colon cancer before age thirty-five.

The physician knew that H.B. probably had familial polyposis because of the many polyps and a strong family history of colon cancer in young relatives. He asked H.B. to come with his parents for the next visit. The physician then explained polyposis coli to H.B. and his parents. They were, understandably, extremely upset. The doctor recommended that each member of the family have a sigmoidoscopy and a barium enema, an x-ray study of the large bowel. He also told them that all those with polyps should have a colectomy with a colostomy. The family was very distressed but all of them agreed to the tests. H.B.'s sister and two uncles were found to have multiple polyps. The physician talked to all four young adults about the need for colectomy. They all thought about it and eventually had surgery. Seven years have now passed and all four are well. No doubt, remembering the illnesses of the three relatives who died of colon cancer made the adjustment easier.

In summary, people with polyposis coli and Gardner's syndrome have a very high risk of developing large bowel cancer. Once polyps develop with either of these syndromes, the colon should be removed, as the risk of colon cancer is too great. (See the chapter on gastrointestinal cancer for more details on colectomy, colostomies, and colon cancer.)

Multiple polyps also develop in another hereditary condition, Peutz-Jegher syndrome. However, only 5 percent of the people with this disease develop colon cancer. Most of the polyps remain benign. Therefore, we do not recommend a colectomy to prevent colon cancer in this disease, but we do recommend careful, regular examinations to diagnose colon cancer early. People with this disorder should have their stools regularly checked for blood and have a colonoscopy and a barium enema every year. They should also have x-rays of their stomach yearly, since cancer may also develop there.

There are several hereditary conditions in which cancer of the gastro-intestinal tract develops without preceding polyps. These include hereditary colonic adenocarcinoma, hereditary gastrocolonic carcinoma, and hereditary adenocarcinomatosis. If anyone in your family has one of these conditions, you should be examined on a regular basis to detect cancer early. By age thirty you should be having stools checked for blood and a colonoscopy and a barium enema yearly.

STOMACH CANCER

Stomach cancer may be familial about 5–10 percent of the time. It usually occurs after age fifty. You should suspect you are prone to stomach cancer if anyone in your family has developed it before age fifty or if more than one member of your family in the preceding generations has had stomach cancer. It is somewhat more common in people with Type A blood. People with pernicious anemia, a disease most common in older Northern Europeans and treatable with vitamin B_{12}, have a higher than normal risk for stomach cancer.

By the time symptoms appear, stomach cancer can only rarely be cured. Therefore, if you have pernicious anemia or a strong family history of stomach cancer, we recommend that you be checked on a yearly basis by a qualified gastroenterologist. He or she may want you to have an upper GI series (x-rays of your stomach) or an endoscopy (see the chapter on gastrointestinal cancer for a description of this procedure). If cancer of the stomach is found early, the chances for cure are greatly increased.

BREAST CANCER

Breast cancer is the most common cancer in American women. Seven percent of American women develop breast cancer and more women die from it than from any other cancer. If there is a family history of breast cancer, your risk is even higher. A family history of breast cancer before menopause or of bilateral breast cancer is extremely worrisome. For example, if a mother develops breast cancer at age forty, her daughter's risk increases threefold; her daughter has a 20 percent chance of developing breast cancer. If a mother develops breast cancer at age forty and at age forty-five a cancer is found in the other breast, her daughter's risk is now increased eight to nine times—the risk is 50 percent. The risk is lower if aunts or other relatives have had breast cancer and also if a mother or sister develops breast cancer after menopause.

Because breast cancer is so common, we recommend that all American women start to examine their own breasts on a monthly basis and have a physician examine their breasts each year once they approach age thirty-five. With a family history of breast cancer, you should begin regular checkups earlier. We recommend that women with a family history of breast cancer start monthly self-examinations and yearly or biyearly physician breast examinations by their early twenties. They also should have yearly xerograms or mammograms by age thirty or thirty-five. This is normally not recommended until women are over fifty.

SKIN CANCER

Cancer of the skin is the most common cancer in this country. There are several dozen rare, hereditary conditions associated with an increased risk of skin cancer. We will not name all of these rare conditions. However, we do want you to know that if there is a family history of skin cancer, you are probably prone to develop skin cancer yourself. Cancer of the skin is easily curable if diagnosed early. If you have a family history of skin cancer, see your doctor on a regular basis. Ask him whether you need protection (sunscreen ointments) from strong sunlight.

Xeroderma Pigmentosum

Xeroderma pigmentosum is an extremely rare condition in which multiple skin cancers develop because there is a defect in the skin cells' ability to repair damage from the sun's rays. Most people with this condition die before age thirty from multiple skin cancers. Recently, children with this condition have been diagnosed early in life and have been protected from the sun by wearing appropriate clothing, dark glasses, and sunscreen ointments (see the chapter on skin cancers). Those children who have been protected since early childhood have not developed multiple skin cancers. This illustrates how a hereditary condition interacts with an environmental factor (in this case sunlight, a carcinogen) and produces cancer. People with this disease only develop skin cancers if they are exposed to the sun's radiation. Simple protective measures against the sun prevent skin cancer.

Neurofibromatosis

Neurofibromatosis is another rare hereditary condition associated with cancer. People with this disease have many brownish colored spots that are most prominent over the back and chest. They also develop soft tumors under the skin that can become cancerous about 5–10 percent of the time. If you have this disease, you should see your doctor if any of these usually soft tumors become harder or change in size.

Albinism

In this condition there is a total lack of skin pigmentation. No matter what racial background, the person is pale and has no coloring of the iris of his eyes. These people are very sensitive to sunlight and develop skin cancer frequently. They should be protected from the sun's rays by appropriate clothing, sunglasses, and sunscreen ointments (see the chapter on skin cancer). With protection, these people can live a normal life span. Without it, they die young from multiple skin cancers.

Malignant Melanoma

Malignant melanoma is a very malignant type of skin cancer. About 5 percent of the people with melanoma have a family history of the disease. If there is a history of malignant melanoma in your family, and especially if more than one relative has had this somewhat rare cancer, you should tell your doctor. He should examine your entire body at least twice a year to detect suspicious lesions early. These should be removed. Malignant melanoma is curable if caught early but fatal if detected late.

RETINOBLASTOMA

Retinoblastoma is a rare cancer of the retina of the eye. It usually develops in infancy or childhood. Almost one-half of the children who develop this cancer have inherited it. The hereditary form tends to occur in both eyes but can occur in only one. If there is a family history of retinoblastoma, children should be examined on a regular basis by the pediatrician. He, or she, does this simply by looking into the eye with an ophthalmoscope. Early detection of retinoblastoma can save your child's life.

ENDOCRINE CANCERS

Cancers of the endocrine glands, with the exception of thyroid cancer, are rare. However, there are several inherited conditions in which both cancer and benign tumors occur in multiple endocrine glands. These are called the multiple endocrine neoplasia syndromes. If you have family members with benign or malignant tumors of the pituitary, parathyroid, adrenal, or thyroid glands, tell your doctor. Ask if there is a possibility that you are likely to develop these tumors. If anyone in your family has had more than one of these cancers (for example, pituitary and parathyroid tumors) or more than one member of your family has had tumors of the endocrine glands, you and your physician should be very suspicious of a hereditary disposition to endocrine cancer.

If your physician thinks you are predisposed to endocrine cancer or tumors, he or she will make sure to look for them by taking a careful history, examining you, and doing the appropriate tests each year. In addition, there are blood tests that can diagnose medullary thyroid cancer, one of the tumors that may occur with these hereditary syndromes. Once such a cancer is diagnosed, it should be removed.

The Cured Cancer Patient

Anyone who develops one cancer is prone to develop more cancers. If you have had one cured cancer, it is very important that you be checked carefully on a regular basis for the development of other cancers. With several particular cancers the risk of a second cancer occurring in the same organ is very high. For example, people with one skin cancer have a 30–40 percent chance of developing a second skin cancer. Likewise, a person with one bladder cancer has at least a 30 percent chance of developing more bladder cancers. The risk is somewhat lower but very real with cancer of the breast and colon. It is very important for people with these cancers to be checked for the possible development of another cancer in the same organ.

There are several associations between development of one cancer and development of another: (1) women with breast cancer have an increased risk of developing cancer of the colon, uterus, and ovary; (2) people with cancer of the colon get cancer of the breast, uterus, cervix, and bladder more frequently; (3) women with cancer of the ovary have an increased risk of developing cancer of the colon; and (4) women with cancer of the uterus have an increased risk of developing cancer of the colon, rectum, and breast. We recommend that if you have had one cancer you be checked at least once a year and possibly more often to detect cancer early.

SUMMARY

1. Most cancers arise in people without a family history or hereditary disposition to cancer. Nevertheless, it is important to know if you have a hereditary disposition to a particular cancer or to cancer in general. If you are afraid that cancer is unusually common in your family, talk to your doctor about it. Let your physician know of your family history of

cancer. This is important; it pays to find out if you have a hereditary disposition to cancer.

2. Regular checkups are indicated starting at a relatively early age in people with a hereditary disposition. These people tend to develop cancer at an earlier age and in multiple sites. Early diagnosis of cancer can save your life.

3. In some cases, cancer can be prevented. For example, removal of the colon in people with polyposis coli will prevent colon cancer, and protection against the sun will prevent skin cancer in people with xeroderma pigmentosum.

4. Any person who has had one cancer is more prone to develop a second cancer, either in the same organ or in a different site. Anyone who has had cancer should have regular, periodic checkups to detect further cancer early.

2

Carcinogens in
Our Environment

EATING, DRINKING, WORKING,
AND BREATHING CAN BE DANGEROUS

M.N. had worked for twenty years in a plastics manufacturing plant. He was forty-three years old and after many years of hard work had at last achieved some financial security. He and his family could look forward to the economic benefits of his steady employment. He had always been healthy and did not make an appointment with their family physician when he started to feel tired and developed a heavy sensation in his upper right abdomen. However, when his symptoms became worse, he went to his doctor. M.N. had an enlarged and hard liver. His doctor suspected cancer and tests showed abnormalities suggestive of liver cancer. M.N. had a very rare type of liver cancer—an angiosarcoma. He died fourteen months later despite treatment. The cancer was caused by exposure to polyvinyl chloride, a plastic that was used in the plant where he worked.

H.L. was a forty-one-year-old man who had been employed in a chemical manufacturing plant for eighteen years. He smoked one pack of cigarettes daily. He had always been in good health and there was no history of cancer in his family. One day he noticed some chest pain and went to see his family physician. A chest x-ray showed a lung tumor. He had oat cell cancer of the lung. It was incurable; it was already widespread in his body, and he died seven months later. His wife and four children were "awarded" a $240 monthly workmen's compensation pension for H.L.'s early death. The cancer was caused by exposure to a chemical in his factory. Several other young workers died of oat cell cancer of the lung before the company took steps to decrease the exposure of workers to the carcinogen in the plant.

In a small New Jersey town, a medical oncologist has seen several dozen people with mesothelioma. This is a rare tumor that develops in the linings of the lungs or abdomen. It is almost never curable. The physician has used radiation and chemotherapy, but all his patients have died. When he meets his colleagues at national meetings, he finds that few of them have seen even one case of this cancer. There is a large asbestos plant in this town. Asbestos exposure causes mesothelioma and lung cancer. Most of his patients have been workers in the plant but several were not. Asbestos escapes beyond the factory walls. People living near asbestos plants are also exposed. They get mesotheliomas as well as other lung cancers.

H.W., a nineteen-year-old girl, noticed pain on sexual intercourse and went to see her gynecologist. He found a hard red area in the vagina and suspected cancer. He was very surprised because cancer of the female reproductive organs is very rare in young women. However, a biopsy showed vaginal adenocarcinoma. The young girl had radical surgery and is doing well two years later. The cancer was caused by exposure to estrogens. Her mother had been given estrogens (DES) while pregnant to prevent a threatened abortion.

All these seemingly isolated and tragic incidents have one thing in common—exposure to a substance that promotes or causes cancer, a carcinogen. Carcinogens are substances or chemicals that cause or promote the development of cancer. The young factory workers who developed cancer, the people in the New Jersey town who developed mesothelioma, and the young girl who developed vaginal cancer were all exposed to high levels of carcinogens.

If these tragic examples were only isolated accidents we would not be so concerned. However, millions of blue-collar workers are exposed to suspected and known carcinogens daily in the United States. Moreover, all of us are exposed to carcinogens merely by living in an industrial society. The air we breathe, the water we use, and the food and drinks we consume often contain suspected or known carcinogens. A polyvinyl chloride wrapper covers the meat we buy. The artificial color additive in sodas and many other foods is probably a coal tar derivative—a probable carcinogen.

Since the industrial revolution, mankind has increasingly tampered with the environment. An amazing number of new chemicals are developed and used each year, but it may take twenty or more years before it is possible to prove that a chemical causes cancer in humans. We live amid a sea of chemicals; many of these are safe but others are dangerous—they cause cancer.

In this chapter, we introduce the reader to the problem of cancer-causing substances in the environment. We do so from the point of view of oncologists who care for people who develop these cancers. People need to be more aware of carcinogens. It is estimated that up to 80 percent of all cancer is related to exposure to them. We want the millions of Americans who are exposed to carcinogens at work to know about it.

Then they can decide what to do. They may wish to change their jobs or, if they continue in their jobs, at least to take some precautions—to wear a mask or protective clothing. We hope people in general and especially workers will push for more protection. We also want consumers to be more aware of the many suspected and known carcinogens on the shelves of stores in the United States. Then they can determine whether it is better to use them or substitute safer products. We hope that with increased awareness, there will be a public outcry so that more safeguards are instituted by the government. We need stricter laws to protect both industrial workers and everyone else from suspected and known carcinogens. It is obvious that carcinogen producers will not voluntarily control themselves. We feel the government isn't doing enough to protect us.

What Is a Carcinogen?

Carcinogens are substances that cause or promote the development of cancer. They act by altering DNA. DNA contains the cell's genetic material and directs cell function on a daily basis. It carries the genetic material from one generation to the next. DNA makes us what we are. Not all alterations of DNA result in cancer. The defect depends on how the DNA is changed. Substances can interact with DNA and have no effect, cause birth defects several generations hence, kill the cell, or induce or promote the development of cancer.

In the past century many substances have been proven to cause cancer. Many others are highly suspect because they structurally resemble known carcinogens or because scientists know from their structure that they will interact with DNA. In the following section we will briefly review the problem of carcinogen exposure and suggest ways for people to protect themselves.

Carcinogens Work Silently

Most people try to avoid dangerous situations or substances. But we can only do this if we know what is dangerous. For example, we avoid or move away from fire because we know it can burn us. Likewise, we do not eat food that smells spoiled because we know it might make us sick. The problem with carcinogens is that there is no signal warning of danger—they act silently. Although they may cause irreparable harm to the DNA in our cells, one feels nothing. Even precancerous cells may look and function normally for years. However, someone exposed to carcinogens lives with an internal time bomb. After five, ten, or even thirty years cancer may develop. The lack of symptoms upon exposure to carcinogens and the very long latent period (the time between exposure and the development of cancer) make it necessary to protect people from these substances. People cannot protect themselves. Millions of people can be unknowingly exposed to a carcinogen for years before cancer starts developing. By the time society recognizes the carcinogen, it is years too late. In this situation people need help; they need protection. It seems most sensible to avoid even potential carcinogens unless the benefits far outweigh the risks.

The government does not do enough to protect us. Several government agencies are charged with protecting us from carcinogens. The Occupational Safety and Health Administration (OSHA) and the National Institute of Occupational Safety (NIOS) are directed to protect workers. The Food and Drug Administration (FDA) is supposed to protect the general public from drugs and food additives that may cause cancer. Finally, the Environmental Protection Agency (EPA) is supposed to control exposure to carcinogens in the air and the water. These agencies have not acted often enough on the side of the consumer or the exposed worker. They do not have enough money, staff, or authority to do the things they should to protect us. We hope that, with the recently increased awareness of carcinogen risks, the government will do more to protect us.

Can We Predict Which Substances May Be Carcinogenic?

We may now be able to predict which chemicals cause or promote the development of cancer. Simple, quick, and inexpensive tests can show if a substance can interact with or alter DNA. Such substances are called mutagens. Not all mutagens are carcinogens, but many are. Many also can cause birth defects if taken during pregnancy. We think that all new and old untested substances should be tested. If they are mutagenic, they should then be tested on mice to see if they are carcinogenic. Animal testing should be done before workers and everyone else are exposed to possible carcinogens. We have little to gain from these new substances and a lot to lose—many lives. In the past, except for drugs and food additives, chemicals were not tested on animals before workers were exposed to them.

Substances that closely resemble known carcinogens are also suspect as carcinogens themselves. Therefore, we think that these substances should also be tested on animals before people are exposed. We don't think an insecticide that is closely related structurally to DDT should be put on the market until it is very extensively tested on animals to be sure that it is not also dangerous.

What we're saying quite simply is that a lot of new chemicals are introduced into the environment daily. Many of these are mutagenic or are closely related in structure to known carcinogens. Few of these substances really enrich our lives; mankind has lived without them for thousands of years. We believe that these new substances should be tested on animals before humans are exposed. We don't think workers and consumers should be the guinea pigs.

If a Substance Causes Cancer in Animals,
Avoid It When Possible

The Saccharin Controversy   The carcinogenic potential of a substance is tested by exposing animals (usually rodents such as mice or rats) to the substance. Usually a relatively small number of animals are exposed to high doses or concentrations of the substance. The aim is to detect *any* cancer-causing or cancer-promoting properties. Rats exposed to high doses of saccharin develop cancer. Some people have argued that these tests are not valid because the animals are exposed to such large quantities of saccharin, equivalent in humans to thousands of pounds of the substance. Critics of the saccharin ban say that any substance in large enough amounts will cause cancer in animals. However, the evidence points the other way. Very few chemicals, even in very large doses, cause cancer in animals. In one study, only 11 of 120 substances given to animals in very large amounts caused cancer. It seems wiser to assume that any substance that causes cancer in animals might also cause cancer in man.

We feel that animal carcinogen testing errs on the side of proclaiming products safe. Small animals live a short period of time compared to humans, and relatively few animals are exposed to carcinogens compared to the potential human exposure. Thus, a low-potency carcinogen with a long latency period could easily be missed on animal testing. However, after it is widely used by humans, cancer could result.

Most experts feel there is no safe dosage for a carcinogen. A large dose may cause more cancer but even lower doses are dangerous. The potential damage from a carcinogen depends on its potency and the degree of exposure. In the case of saccharin, millions will be exposed to relatively low doses. This might result in thousands of cases of cancer. Most people who took saccharin probably will not develop cancer, but so many have been exposed that even if only a small percentage develop cancer, the result will still be many thousands of cases of unnecessary malignancies.

Critics of the saccharin ban have also argued that no human cancer has resulted from its use. However, you must remember that if saccharin caused a 5 percent increase in bladder cancer, a relatively common cancer also influenced by smoking, it would be almost impossible to relate the increase to intake of saccharin.

The decision to use a chemical or substance that is highly suspect as a carcinogen depends on the relative risks and benefits. Some suspected and even known carcinogens are necessary in our society. Individuals or the society as a whole may be willing to take the risk. But if the substance is not necessary or if a safer substance can be substituted, it seems foolish to expose ourselves. Most people do not need saccharin. People with diabetes, however, do need sugar substitutes, and for the diabetic the slight risk of bladder cancer might be a small price to pay for a palatable artificial sweetener.

Carcinogens in the Work Place

Many human carcinogens were discovered after workers in a particular factory or industry developed an unusual type of cancer or a common cancer at an unusually young age or much more frequently than the rest of the population. The first connection between occupation and cancer was noted by Percival Pott in 1775. He found that chimney sweeps had a high incident of scrotal cancer. They were exposed to coal soot, which contains benzopyrenes. These same chemicals are in cigarette smoke and in the air of industrialized cities. Since this first association between a particular job and a cancer, many other occupational carcinogens have been discovered. As increased numbers of new chemicals are manufactured, we can expect to see more occupational carcinogens in the future. Unfortunately, there is a long interval between exposure to a carcinogen and the development of cancer. Thus, the number of occupation-related cancers will undoubtedly increase in the future unless more care is directed at detecting possible carcinogens by testing them in animals before exposing workers.

Most Workers Do Not Know They Are Being Exposed to Carcinogens

There has been no outcry by workers or the public concerning occupational exposure to carcinogens. Most workers are not aware they are being exposed to cancer-causing agents. The companies and even some unions involved often belittle the danger. Corporate management has been lax about instituting safety measures to protect workers and has fought government-mandated worker protection. It costs money to protect workers. The government agencies charged with protecting workers have been remiss in informing workers of risks and in forcing companies to protect the worker from carcinogen exposure.

Workers are not aware of their carcinogen exposure for two important reasons. First, many people develop cancer years after occupational exposure. Often cancer develops after the worker retires. Current employees in the factory do not see these retired people with cancer. And second, most people exposed to carcinogens do not get cancer; only a few do. For example, perhaps eight or nine of several hundred employees in a factory exposed to a carcinogen developed cancer. How are other workers to know that these eight or nine cancers were caused by exposure? There is also a natural tendency to deny that you will be one of the 5 or 10 percent who develop cancer. For example, few workers will wear masks to prevent breathing asbestos even when told of the risk. It is hard for a young, vigorous worker who is supporting a family to see enough damage in carcinogen exposure to change an often well-paying job or put up with the discomfort of taking simple precautions.

Millions of Workers Are Being Exposed to Carcinogens

The facts about carcinogens in the work place are frightening. Millions of American workers are exposed to suspected and known carcinogens daily. The exact number of cancers caused by such exposure has not been accurately determined. Certainly thousands of workers develop cancer yearly because of carcinogen exposure. A partial list of known carcinogens in the work place includes uranium, asbestos, nickel, chromate, arsenic, aromatic amines, benzoyl chloride, chloromethyl ether, chloroprine, benzopyrene, and benzene. By very conservative estimates, at least 20 million Americans are currently working with known carcinogens. Many millions of others are being exposed to suspected carcinogens. Occupational exposure to carcinogens is not a minor health problem in the United States. Often workers' families are exposed as well, through contact with contaminated workclothes.

Is the Government Protecting American Workers?

The Occupational Safety and Health Administration and the National Institute of Occupational Safety both are charged with protecting workers from exposure to carcinogens. These agencies have not done enough. Their budgets are too small. They certainly are not fully protecting workers who are exposed to carcinogens. Often they are not even warning them. For example, workers were allowed to be exposed to polyvinyl chloride for several years after it was shown to be a potent carcinogen in animal studies. They were not warned and the factories were not directed to decrease or to prevent worker exposure. Only after workers started to develop angiosarcoma of the liver was exposure limited. Another example is that of chloromethyl ether. Workers were exposed to this carcinogen after it had been shown to cause cancer in animals. Again, only after workers began developing a high incidence of lung cancer were protective steps taken. Thus, we feel government agencies have not adequately informed or protected workers.

Advice to the Worker

We want workers to know if they are being exposed to suspected or known carcinogens at work. We think people should know of the risks involved. Then they can decide if they want to keep their job or switch to a safer one. We want people to have the opportunity to protect themselves if they stay at a dangerous job (by wearing a mask or adequate protective clothing). This is certainly a difficult problem. Many people cannot afford to change jobs. However, if workers continue the same job after they are informed of their risks, at least they have made their own choice.

We advise workers to find out about possible exposure to carcinogens at their job by asking their union or their union doctor. The employee can even ask his company about it. Many companies will not volunteer information but will answer questions if asked. Perhaps your family physician can help you. If you know what chemicals or substances you work with, you can go to the library and find out.

Table 1 lists the more common occupations in which workers are exposed to carcinogens and some of the more common carcinogens or cancer-causing agents. This list is not complete; it includes only the most common known carcinogens.

If you work in one of the industries mentioned or with one of the substances mentioned, we advise the following:

(a) Change jobs if possible.

(b) If you cannot change jobs, protect yourself by wearing protective clothing and/or a mask.

(c) Do not smoke. Exposure to a carcinogen increases your risk for cancer. Exposure to two carcinogens increases the risk dramatically. Workers exposed to carcinogens who also smoke have a far greater likelihood of developing cancer than either smokers or workers just exposed to the one carcinogen.

Carcinogens Get Beyond the Factory Walls

Workers certainly have the highest exposure to occupational carcinogens. However, carcinogens get beyond the factory walls. Carcinogens from the factory or mines often escape into the air or the water around the site. For example, polyvinyl chloride, nitrosamines, and arsenic have been found in air around factories. Likewise, carcinogens often enter rivers and lakes near the work place. For instance, asbestos has been detected in Lake Superior near Duluth, Minnesota. It got there from nearby mines. Other carcinogens have been detected in many rivers in industrial areas of the United States.

We do not know how many people develop cancer because of such industry-related exposure. We do know, however, that the cancer rates in the United States roughly mirror the degree of industrialization in the area. For example, New Jersey, with one of the highest cancer rates, is heavily dotted with petrochemical plants. These plants work with many known carcinogens. In the far west, cancer rates are generally lower. However, in towns or areas with factories or mines that work with known carcinogens, the cancer rates are higher. For example, residents near mines or smelting plants have a much higher incidence of cancer than the rest of the population in the far west. We think the evidence is quite strong that people who live near plants or mines involved with carcinogens have a higher incidence of cancer. They share the workers' risk.

Workers may also bring carcinogenic substances back into their homes.

TABLE 1. OCCUPATIONAL CANCERS

Agent	Site of Cancer	Occupation
inorganic substance		
metal		
arsenic	lung, skin, liver	oil refiner, smelter, miner, insecticide maker and sprayer, chemical worker, tanner
chromium	nasal passages, lung, larynx	glass and linoleum worker, potter, acetylene and aniline worker, bleacher, battery maker
iron oxide	lung, larynx	iron foundry worker, iron ore miner, silver finisher, metal grinder and polisher
nickel	lung, nasal passages	nickel smelter and mixer, electrolysis worker
dust		
leather	nasal passages, bladder, urinary tract	leather worker, shoemaker
wood	nasal passages	woodworker
fiber		
asbestos	lung, pleura and peritoneum (mesothelioma), gastrointestinal tract	textile and insulation worker, shipyard worker, brake and clutch repairer, miner, miller
organic substance		
petroleum	lung, larynx, skin, scrotum	textile weaver; diesel jet tester; worker in contact with lubricating, paraffin or wax oils, or coke; rubber filler
wax		
creosote		
paraffin		
anthacene		
shale		
mineral oils		
coal soot	lung, larynx, skin, scrotum, urinary tract, bladder	asphalt, coal tar, and pitch worker; gashouse worker, stoker, and producer; chimney sweep; coke oven worker; miner
coal tar		
other products of coal combustion		
benzene	bone marrow (leukemia)	dye user; painter; shoemaker; explosive, benzene, and rubber cement worker
benzidine	bladder	dyestuffs producer and user, rubber worker (laborer, filterer, presser), textile dyer, paint manufacturer
α-naphthylamine		
β-naphthylamine		
4-aminodiphenyl		

TABLE 1. (CONTINUED)

Agent	Site of Cancer	Occupation
vinyl chloride	liver (angiosarcoma), brain	plastics worker
bis (chloro- methyl) ether chloromethyl methyl ether	lung (oat cell carci- noma)	chemical worker
radioactive sub- stance		
nonionizing radiation		
ultraviolet rays	skin	sailor, farmer, construction worker, lifeguard
ionizing radia- tion		
x-rays	skin, bone marrow	radiologist, medical personnel
uranium radium radon mesothorium	skin, lung, bone, bone marrow	radiologist, radium dial painter, radium chemist, miner

For example, asbestos workers often carry asbestos fibers on their dirty clothes. X-rays of the wives and children of asbestos workers often show asbestos-related lung changes. We think workers should know this. If you work with dangerous substances, you should change your clothes before going home. You should not bring the carcinogens home.

We think that occupational exposure to carcinogens in the United States is a major health problem. Thousands of workers will develop cancer because of such exposure. We hope that with increased awareness, there will be political pressure on the government to do a better job of protecting us.

Carcinogens in the Marketplace

In this section we will mention the more common suspected and known carcinogens present in or on products currently sold to American consumers. Americans unknowingly consume many products we consider dangerous. The government is not protecting us. Suspected and known carcinogens are allowed in our foods and drinks. Furthermore, often there is nothing on the label that tells us a dangerous substance has been added. We hope the following information will not only alter some of your dietary habits but will also upset you or anger you enough to make you write companies and your representatives in the government. Each individual can avoid some carcinogens, but we need more protection and help from the government.

Asbestos

Exposure to asbestos causes mesothelioma and lung cancer in workers; there is no question that it is a potent carcinogen. Despite this, it is present in some products used by millions of Americans. Talc, which contains asbestos, is present in many cosmetic products. For example, 30 of 100 cosmetic powders tested had asbestos particles. Therefore, when you use talcum powders after bathing or on your baby's body, you probably are exposing yourself and your baby to asbestos. When you use these powders, you can smell them. There is no doubt that some is getting into your lungs. The exposure may be less than that of an employee in a powder factory, but it may be dangerous nevertheless.

About 2–3 percent of white polished rice also contains asbestos. The rice has been coated merely to make it look better, to make it more marketable. The consumer is not informed of this. We think that any product containing asbestos should be so labeled. Then people can make a choice. We also think that there should be stricter regulations. Rice coated with asbestos-containing powders should not be allowed in stores. Likewise, talcum powders containing asbestos, especially those for children, should be taken off the market.

Color Additives

Many of the foods and drinks we consume contain color additives. Only 20 percent of these are safe, natural products; 80 percent are suspected carcinogens, produced from aromatic amines derived from coal tars. Coal tars contain many potent carcinogens. In fact, the first known occupational carcinogen in chimney soot was a coal tar derivative. Likewise, the carcinogens in cigarettes are coal tar derivatives. Look on the labels of foods and drinks on your store shelves. You will be amazed. For example, butter and margarine often have color additives to make them look nicer. So do most soft drinks. So do processed meat products. The list is endless. Why are these added? Merely to make the foods look better, so that products will be more marketable. They have no other function. They have no nutritional value and are not important as preservatives. They are not essential but are potentially dangerous.

The Food and Drug Administration is charged with protecting the public from dangerous food additives. Food additives must be of proven safety before they are used. In reality, products sometimes must be proven unsafe before the FDA removes them from the marketplace. All coal tar derivative color additives are closely related to known potent carcinogens. Only three have been declared unsafe after years of use. Red dye no. 1, red dye no. 32, and butter yellow have been removed by the FDA because they are proven carcinogens. Millions of people consumed these dyes before they were prohibited. This should tell you enough about the inadequacies of the present regulations. At the present time many coal tar derivative color additives are being used, including citrus red dye no.

2, blue dye no. 1, orange dye B, red dye no. 3, red dye no. 4, and yellow dye no. 5. They have not been proven safe. In fact, many are suspect as carcinogens.

The quantity of color additives in each product is very small; often there is only a trace amount in each product. However, color additives are present in an unbelievably large number of products. Therefore, Americans consume large quantities of these suspected carcinogens over the years. For example, it has been estimated that in 1976, 4 million American children had each eaten at least 4 pounds of coal tar dyes by the time they reached age twelve. It seems society is trying to test carcinogens in humans by high-dose, lifelong exposure.

We see no reason to allow these suspected carcinogens to be added to our foods and drinks. They have no real value and are added merely to increase sales. If they were removed from all the products in the marketplace, no single manufacturer would have an unfair advantage. Sales would not change. We think unnecessary food additives such as coloring should be prohibited. But until that time, products should at least be accurately labeled. At present, the label merely states that a color additive has been used. It does not tell the consumer whether it is a natural product or a coal tar derivative. People should know what they are eating. We advise people to avoid artificial food coloring additives as much as possible. This is especially important for children. Unfortunately, this is very hard to do, as so many food products contain such additives.

Nitrites and Nitrates

Nitrites and nitrates by themselves are not carcinogens. They are added to luncheon meats to improve color and also as preservatives. Nitrates, however, readily transform into nitrites, which may react with other compounds or foods in the stomach to form nitrosamines. Nitrosamines are among the most potent carcinogens known. We think it is wise to avoid these compounds as much as possible, and this can be done without much change in diet. They are only used in a limited number of products. Moreover, foods containing these are accurately labeled. Nitrates are present in dry-cured meats such as sausages, fermented sausages, luncheon meats, bacon, etc. It would not take a drastic change in eating habits to avoid them. It would be possible but expensive for manufacturers of these products not to use nitrates.

We believe that adults should avoid or decrease their consumption of products containing nitrites and nitrates as much as possible. We feel even more strongly about exposing children: children should not be fed these substances. Unfortunately, millions of children are regularly given hot dogs, bacon, and luncheon meats on a daily basis. Remember, cancer from carcinogens is related both to dose and length of time of exposure. Thus, children have a far greater cancer risk from nitrates than adults.

Polyvinyl Chloride

The plastic polyvinyl chloride is a known potent carcinogen. It causes cancer in animals and exposed workers. But it is still being produced in huge quantities. This plastic is used to wrap foods: hot dogs and luncheon meats are wrapped in semirigid polyvinyl chloride containers, while meat, fish, and cheese are wrapped in polyvinyl chloride soft wrappers. Products wrapped with polyvinyl chloride become contaminated to some extent. A very small amount of the plastic leaches out into the foods. Polyvinyl chloride is a very potent carcinogen—there is no safe dosage. Millions of Americans are being exposed to very small amounts of polyvinyl chloride. Although convenient, it is not essential to the economy. Other, safer plastics can be substituted. We should not wait ten or twenty years for cancers from polyvinyl chloride to appear before we remove this dangerous product from the marketplace.

We urge people to avoid polyvinyl chloride as much as possible. Ask your butcher or fish vendor to wrap your food in wax paper. If you do buy products wrapped in plastic, when you get home unwrap them and rewrap them in safer containers.

Pesticides: Wash Your Fruits and Vegetables Very Carefully

DDT was banned because it was a carcinogen. However, other insecticides structurally closely related to DDT (the chlorinated hydrocarbon insecticides) are still used. Farm workers are frequently exposed to high concentrations of these dangerous products. The general consumer does not need to be exposed. You should wash the insecticides off your fruits and vegetables to rid them of highly suspected carcinogens.

If You Are Pregnant Be Extremely Careful

Many substances pass freely from the mother's circulation into the placenta and the fetus. Therefore, we think that pregnant women should be extra careful to avoid dangerous products. They should avoid all suspected carcinogens and they should not smoke. The carcinogens that are inhaled might get into the circulation and affect the child. Women who smoke also have lower birthweight children. Lastly, pregnant women should avoid taking medicines or pills unless absolutely necessary. We don't know all the effects of drugs on the fetus. Only recently, some commonly used tranquilizers have been linked to birth defects. It is safest to avoid all but essential drugs. Always tell your doctor if you think you might be pregnant when he gives you a drug.

How Can People Decrease Exposure to Carcinogens?

It is important to minimize exposure to carcinogens. Living in an industrialized society such as ours means that you will be exposed to some carcinogens no matter what you do. Therefore, we feel strongly that when you have a choice you should avoid additional exposure. The more carcinogens you are exposed to, the greater your risk of developing cancer. We recommend the following common-sense measures. These do not entail a radical change in life style; they only involve some simple measures that are not that hard to do.

—Wash fresh fruits and vegetables carefully to remove insecticides.

—Ask the butcher or fish vendor to use wax paper or paper wrapping for fresh meat and fish.

—If the meat, fish, or cheese you buy is wrapped in plastic, this plastic is probably polyvinyl chloride, a carcinogen. Remove the food when you get home and rewrap it.

—Avoid luncheon meats such as salami, bologna, and frankfurters as much as possible. Do not encourage your children to develop a taste for these. They contain nitrates and nitrites and may cause cancer.

—Avoid color additives as much as possible. This is very difficult because so many products contain them. If you must use a product, write the company and find out whether the color additive is natural or a coal tar derivative.

We hope this brief review of common carcinogens will make you more aware of the problem. Workers should find out if they are being exposed to carcinogens. Does it pay to risk your life for your job? We hope all Americans become more concerned about carcinogens in their food and drink. Both corporations interested in profit and a government dependent on your support respond. We hope you will write to corporations and to your government representatives. Demand more safeguards in the work place and in the marketplace. Carcinogen-caused cancer is a growing problem in our society. We feel that if more safeguards are not instituted soon, cancer will be even more prevalent by the year 2000 and will occur increasingly in younger people.

SUMMARY

1. Carcinogens are substances that cause or promote the development of cancer. They are responsible for up to 80 percent of cancers in industrialized countries.

2. All of us are exposed to carcinogens in the air we breathe, the food we eat, and the water we drink.

3. In this chapter we make several commonsense recommendations that will minimize carcinogen exposure for you and your family.

4. Many workers are unknowingly exposed to carcinogens. We advise workers to find out if they are being exposed at their jobs. Some of the common industrial carcinogens, along with the occupations where exposure occurs, are listed in table 1.

3

Early Cancer Detection
Can Save Your Life

You are more likely to be cured of a cancer if it is found and treated early, when it is still small. For example, three of four women with small, ½-inch diameter breast cancers are cured, but only one in four with 2-inch cancers. Likewise, four of five people are cured of early carcinoma of the larynx, but only one in four with advanced disease. Smaller cancers also may need less treatment. When cancer is detected early, it is less likely to require radical or disfiguring surgery or extensive radiation. In this chapter we give you the information you need to know what to do to have cancer diagnosed early. We will discuss the cancers that can be detected with regular checkups and make specific recommendations as to what age cancer checkups should begin and what tests are needed.

Why Regular Checkups for Cancer Can Save Your Life

Most cancers start in a single spot from a single cell. They grow and sooner or later spread (metastasize) through the lymphatics to nearby lymph nodes or through the blood to other parts of the body. The smaller the cancer, the greater the chance that it is still localized. Your chances for cure are best if the cancer is still confined to the original site, such as the breast or the tongue. The cure rate decreases if cancer spreads to nearby lymph nodes and usually vanishes if it has spread through the blood to other parts of the body. Surgery and radiation can cure localized cancer; few cancers that have spread through the bloodstream can be cured. Only chemotherapy can eradicate widespread cancer and unfortunately at present it can do so only for a few cancers. Regular checkups will increase your chance for cure if smaller, still localized cancers can be found.

Early diagnosis with regular checkups is feasible for several but not all common cancers. Breast cancer can be diagnosed early because lumps can be felt. Cancer of organs in the abdomen, like the pancreas, cannot be diagnosed early. At the present time early diagnosis by regular check-ups is feasible for several very common cancers: cancer of the breast, cervix, uterus, mouth, skin, colon, rectum, and prostate. Approximately three hundred thousand Americans get and one hundred thousand die yearly from these cancers. Regular checkups can prevent many of these deaths.

CANCER OF THE CERVIX

Deaths from cancer of the cervix have decreased 50 percent in the past two decades because of the widespread use of Pap smears. A Pap smear is done by scraping the surface of the cervix to obtain cells that are then examined under the microscope. Very early cancer of the cervix can be detected. Most cervical cancers found by Pap smears are still localized to the very surface of the cervix—so-called *in situ* cancer—and more than 95 percent of these are curable. If you wait for symptoms, such as bleeding between periods, your chance for cure will drop to 40–50 percent. Pap smears are simple and may save your life.

Currently only one in three American women has a yearly Pap smear taken. We strongly recommend that all women start getting yearly Pap smears by age twenty-one. More information about Pap smears is included in chapter 14, "Cancers of the Female Reproductive Organs."

UTERINE CANCER

Cancer of the uterus cannot be diagnosed reliably by a Pap smear. Early detection of this cancer is not as easy as cervical cancer but is still possible. It can be detected by a uterine scraping (D&C), by multiple biopsies of the uterus, or by jet washings. The last procedure is done in a gynecologist's office by inserting a small tube through the cervix into the uterus. Fluid is then instilled into the uterus and collected. It contains some of the lining cells from the uterus that can be examined. These tests are expensive and somewhat uncomfortable, and if a uterine scraping is done a short hospitalization is required.

It is not feasible at present to screen all women for uterine cancer. The disease is rare before menopause. Taking estrogens after menopause increases your risk for getting this cancer. We recommend, therefore, that women who have gone through menopause and are taking estrogens have a yearly screening test for uterine cancer. Also, any bleeding after menopause may signal endometrial cancer. A uterine scraping, or D&C, is needed to be sure that the bleeding is not caused by uterine cancer.

BREAST CANCER

Breast cancer kills more women than any other cancer in this country: it is the No. 1 cause of death in American women between ages forty and forty-five, killing more than 30,000 women yearly. The breast is on the surface of the body; it is accessible. Breast cancer can be detected early by self-examination, by examinations done by nurses or physicians, and by x-rays of the breast, called mammograms. More information about early detection of breast cancer is included in chapter 12, "Breast Cancer."

We strongly recommend that all women over age thirty-five have yearly breast examinations by a trained nurse or doctor and that they learn how to do monthly self-examinations. Women should be trained to examine their breasts properly by a nurse or doctor. Women over the age of fifty should also have yearly mammograms. If you have a family history of breast cancer, the examinations and mammography should start at a younger age. More detailed recommendations for early breast cancer detection for those whose mother or sisters have breast cancer are discussed in chapter 12.

COLON AND RECTAL CANCERS

Approximately one hundred thousand people develop and almost fifty thousand die yearly from cancer of the colon and rectum. Thousands of lives could be spared if the disease were caught early. Colon and rectal cancer can be diagnosed early with rectal examinations, with sigmoidoscopy, and by testing stools for small amounts of blood. Rectal examinations by your physician will detect about 15 percent of these cancers. One-half of all colon or rectal cancer can be found with a sigmoidoscope (see chapter 13, "Cancers of the Gastrointestinal Tract"). More than 90 percent of all people with these cancers have microscopic traces of blood in their stool. It is simple to have your stool checked for blood. Three or more stool samples are placed on a specially prepared paper disk. These are brought to your doctor, who chemically tests them for blood. Checking stools for blood is painless and inexpensive, and if negative means it is highly unlike that even early colon cancer is present.

We recommend that all people over the age of forty have a yearly rectal examination and several samples of stool examined for blood. Both of these tests are simple and inexpensive. Sigmoidoscopy is also valuable in early cancer detection but is more expensive and uncomfortable. However, we think it is worthwhile if stools show traces of blood. We also strongly recommend an annual sigmoidoscopy if you have a family history of colon or rectal cancer. Some physicians feel a yearly sigmoidoscopy is indicated for everyone over age fifty.

HEAD AND NECK CANCERS

Many cancers of the head and neck (including cancers of the mouth and throat) can be seen during an examination. Most people see their dentist yearly. Your dentist is in an ideal position to detect these cancers early by carefully examining your mouth. Although they should, not all dentists do this. We strongly recommend that you go to a dentist who spends several minutes carefully looking at and feeling in your mouth for early cancer. If you don't go to a dentist, ask your doctor to do this during your annual examination.

PROSTATE CANCER

The prostate can be felt during a rectal examination. If prostate cancer is present, a lump or nodule may be detected. Cancer of the prostate becomes increasingly common after age fifty. We strongly urge that all men have a rectal examination to detect this cancer as well as cancer of the rectum.

LUNG CANCER

Lung cancer cannot usually be detected early. Chest x-rays are too insensitive. By the time a shadow appears on the x-ray, the cancer has often spread and is incurable. However, despite the shortcomings of x-rays, we feel that heavy smokers should have a chest x-ray every six months after age forty-five. Occasionally a cancer will be found when it is curable.

We recommend that all people who have smoked more than one pack of cigarettes per day for twenty years or more have a chest x-ray twice a year. There is a small chance that this will save your life.

People with One Cancer Must Be Even More Careful: Their Risk Is Greater for Second and Third Cancers

People who have had one cancer are more likely to get additional cancers than the average person. We urge people who have had one cancer to follow the recommendations in the previous section about screening very carefully. In addition, people who have had cancer of the breast, skin, head and neck, bladder, or colon and rectum may get a second or even a third cancer of the same organ. For example, a person with one cancer of the bladder has a 40 percent chance of developing at least one other bladder cancer. Likewise, a person who has had one cancer in the mouth has a 15–20 percent chance of developing a second cancer of the mouth. These people obviously must be checked more carefully than others. We recommend the following:

—People who have had bladder cancer should have a cystoscopy on a regular basis—at least every six months and possibly more often.

—People who have had skin cancer should have their skin examined every six months by a physician.

—Women who have had breast cancer should examine themselves every month, have a physician or trained nurse examine them every six months, and have yearly mammography.

—People who have had colon or rectal cancer should have a rectal examination, sigmoidoscopy, and several stools examined for occult blood each year.

Some People Are at High Risk for Certain Cancers because of Exposure to Carcinogens

People who have been exposed to cancer-causing substances (carcinogens) must take special precautions. Three examples should make the point.

Cancer of the thyroid is extremely uncommon unless a person has been exposed to radiation. However, millions of Americans have been exposed to radiation in the past several decades. (More information on this is included in chapter 20, "Thyroid Cancer.") People who think or know they have been exposed to radiation in the area of the neck should have their thyroid examined on a yearly basis. This merely involves seeing your doctor each year and having him feel your thyroid for any enlargement or lumps. This is not an important part of an annual examination for most people, but it is for those who have been exposed to radiation.

Workers in the aniline dye industry are quite likely to get bladder cancer. We recommend that these workers have a cystoscopy annually. The procedure is expensive, uncomfortable, and not useful for screening a low-risk population. However, it is the best method of detecting early bladder cancer for aniline workers, a high-risk group.

Women who were exposed to estrogens in utero may get vaginal adenocarcinoma at a young age. These young women should be examined by a gynecologist every six months once they begin menstruating. Cancer of the female reproductive organs is almost unheard of in teenagers except in this group. (Additional information is included in chapter 14, "Cancers of the Female Reproductive Organs.")

In summary, some people have a high risk of developing otherwise rare cancers because they were exposed to carcinogens. These people should be checked very closely by physicians.

People with a Hereditary Disposition to Cancer Need to Take Special Precautions

People with a hereditary predisposition to cancer not only have an increased risk of developing cancer but also tend to develop cancer at an earlier age. Therefore, regular checkups are extremely important for these people and should be started at an early age. For example, women with a family history of breast cancer should begin monthly self-examinations and yearly physician's examinations while in their twenties instead of their thirties. Yearly mammograms should start at age thirty instead of age fifty. Breast cancer in the general population is uncommon before age forty. However, in women with a marked family history, it is common by age thirty. Further information about the inherited cancers can be found in chapter 1, "Heredity and Cancer."

SUMMARY

1. Regular checkups for several cancers (cancer of the breast, colon and rectum, head and neck, cervix, and uterus) increase the chance for

early detection and cure. With regular checkups, some cancers can be detected when they are small and more likely to be localized; they can then be cured.

2. Table 2 summarizes the schedule of checkups we recommend for the general population in this country.

3. People exposed to carcinogens need special attention. For example, people who have had radiation to the area of the neck should have their thyroid examined each year.

4. People with a strong family history of cancer also need very close observation. Regular examinations should start at an earlier age for these people than for the rest of the population.

5. People who have had one cancer are more likely to get additional cancers than the average person. They especially should have regular checkups as outlined in table 2.

6. People who have had certain cancers have a high risk of developing other cancers in the same organ. People with cancer of the bladder, breast, colon, skin, or mouth need careful follow-up to catch additional tumors in these same organs at an early stage.

TABLE 2. RECOMMENDED CHECKUPS FOR EARLY CANCER DETECTION

Cancer Site	Age Regular Screening Should Begin	Indicated Procedures
Breast	35	monthly self-examinations of the breast
	35	yearly breast examinations by a physician
	50	yearly xerography or mammography
Cervix	21	yearly Pap smears
Head and neck	40	yearly careful examinations of the mouth by a dentist or doctor
Prostate	40	yearly rectal examination
Colon and rectum	40	yearly rectal examination
	40	yearly evaluations of several stools for blood
	50	sigmoidoscopy
Uterus	50 and taking estrogens	jet-washer aspiration of the uterus for cytologies and if necessary four quadrant uterine biopsies or a D&C
	postmenopausal women with vaginal bleeding	D&C

4

Who Should Treat You?
Where Should You Be Treated?

One American in four will develop cancer in his or her lifetime. The treatment of cancer is far from perfect, but it is improving. As of 1979 one in four cancer patients could be cured. Many others live longer or feel better with treatment. It is important that cancer victims receive the benefits of recent progress in treatment.

One premise of this book is that not all doctors or all hospitals can offer you the best treatment for cancer. Physicians differ in training, knowledge, experience, common sense, and personality. The person with cancer needs specialists in the treatment of cancer. Many patients need a team of specialists, since surgery, radiation, and chemotherapy are now being used together to treat cancer more often than in the past. Your family physician almost certainly does not have the knowledge and experience to offer you the best care for your cancer.

The benefits and the complexity of cancer treatment vary with different cancers. Thus, the need for a team of specialists depends on your type of cancer. For example, a small basal cell or squamous cell cancer of the skin can be treated adequately by a board-certified dermatologist. However, with a large basal cell or squamous cell skin cancer, a team approach is better. The dermatologist, radiation oncologist, and plastic surgeon should work together to offer the best chance for cure with a good cosmetic result. All children with cancer should be evaluated and treated at cancer centers or larger children's hospitals. The team of specialists needed to offer children the best care (specialists in surgery, radiation, chemotherapy, and psychological support for the child and the family) are usually available only at these large centers.

The aim of this chapter is to help you be sure that you see the cancer specialist or specialists who can offer you the best treatment for your cancer. It should be read with the chapters on the treatment of cancer (surgery, radiation, and chemotherapy), with the chapter on the doctor-patient relationship, and with the chapter on your particular cancer. This chapter in conjunction with these others will help you decide which specialists should treat you.

A person with cancer needs doctors who will provide both emotional support and the best modern care. He needs a close, supportive relationship to help him face his disease. He also needs one or more specialists who are trained, knowledgeable, and experienced in cancer therapy to give him the best treatment for his cancer.

The Cancer Specialist

This book was written because we feel that someone with cancer is more apt to receive good treatment if he finds out about his cancer, how it should be treated, and some aspects of quality medical care. When someone is told he has cancer, he may panic. What should he do? To whom should he turn? By far the best and most reassuring thing to do is to find out about your cancer: how should it be treated? by whom? Then you will be more likely to receive good care than if you go on faith alone.

Unfortunately, there is no assurance that the doctor you trust, like, and can communicate with personally has the training, knowledge, and experience in the field of cancer to offer you the best treatment. You must find out if your physician is qualified to treat you for cancer. Is he a specialist in cancer care? Finding a specialist to care for you is only the beginning. You should find out before treatment is started whether there are alternative courses of action. For example, if your doctor is a surgeon and wants to operate, can your cancer be treated better by radiation? For some cancers, a team of doctors is best. The aim of this chapter is to help you find the cancer specialist or team of specialists you need.

How Do You Find Cancer Specialists?

If you have cancer, you should be treated by doctors with special training and experience in cancer surgery, radiation, and chemotherapy. How do you find these specialists?

The Role of the Family Doctor

Many Americans have a family doctor, the doctor whom they see for the flu, aches and pains, pregnancy, and immunizations. The family physician may be either a general practitioner, an internist, or, for some women, a gynecologist, and he is usually the doctor who first sees you when you develop cancer. You go to him because you're not feeling well or for a routine checkup. If he finds a lump or other symptoms that lead him to suspect that you have cancer, he should send you to a specialist (most often a surgeon or surgical subspecialist) for a biopsy of the suspicious lesion.

Although the family physician is usually ideal for emotional support, unfortunately he isn't an expert in cancer treatment. Well-qualified, competent family doctors who are interested in their patients' welfare usually refer patients to specialists who are also well trained. Some general characteristics of any good physician follow.

—He spends enough time with you. The doctor who has a sincere interest in his patients takes time to listen to and talk with them. He wants to know about the people he cares for.

—On the first visit, your doctor should take a careful, complete medical history. This includes your present problem, your past medical history, your family history, a review of how different parts of your body are working, and a review of your personal habits. He will also want to know about your work history and your family life. Physicians often learn more from the history than the physical examination.

—He will examine you carefully and thoroughly.

—He or a "covering" physician is always available.

These characteristics are basic to any good physician, from a family physician to a cardiac surgeon.

Do You Have a Friend Who Is a Doctor?

If you have a friend who is a doctor, regardless of his specialty, it is probably worth asking him what he thinks of your cancer doctor. No matter what your friend's specialty, he will probably know your cancer doctor, at least by reputation in the medical community. He also may know whether you can receive adequate treatment in your community or should travel to a larger medical center for care. Although in general, doctors should not treat their family or friends, a doctor who is your friend can give you valuable advice about who are the best doctors in your community.

The National Cancer Institute, Regional Cancer Centers, and the American Cancer Society Can Help

The National Cancer Institute in Bethesda, Maryland, has an office of cancer communications to help patients and doctors find the names and addresses of cancer specialists in their communities. You can call this office and obtain the names of qualified specialists to treat your cancer. The telephone number is in the reference section at the back of this book.

There are presently eighteen comprehensive cancer centers in the United States. These centers give patients or doctors the names of qualified specialists in cancer treatment. You can call the cancer center nearest your community and find out the names and addresses of these doctors. These cancer centers are also listed in the reference section.

The American Cancer Society has offices in most middle-sized and large communities. This society will often help patients and doctors find qualified specialists.

Who Are the Specialists in the Treatment of Cancer?

What Is a Specialist?

Specialists are doctors who have trained in and restrict their practice to a limited area of medicine. The family physician, the internist, and the pediatrician are generalists. They must take care of many different problems. The specialist, by contrast, concentrates on and knows a lot about a limited area of medicine. The treatment of cancer is complex, and doctors with training and experience in the use of surgery, radiation, and chemotherapy for cancer are needed.

It may surprise you that any physician can call himself a "specialist." For example, a doctor with no special training in heart disease can call himself a cardiologist. Likewise, if a doctor wants to do surgery, he can hang out a shingle and call himself a surgeon. We feel this is unfortunate and very misleading to the public. When we refer to specialist, we mean a doctor who has had specialized training in a restricted area.

What Is a Board-Certified Specialist?

There are formal training programs in many areas of medicine. Physicians who complete the formal training and pass an examination become board certified in a specific area of medicine. This certification assures you that the specialist actually has had special training and that he is knowledgeable and experienced. Not every board-certified specialist is better than the self-trained physician who specializes. However, most are. You can find out if your physician is board certified by asking him, by looking on his wall for a board certificate, or by looking in the *Directory of Medical Specialists* or the AMA *Directory of Physicians*, both of which list all board-certified specialists. These are available in large public libraries and in county medical society libraries.

We stress board certification, not because all board-certified specialists are excellent physicians, but because your chances are better that the board-certified doctor will offer "state of the art" care. However, we caution you not to trust a physician blindly merely because he is a board-certified specialist.

Who Are the Specialists in Cancer Therapy?

The three proven treatments for cancer are surgery, radiation, and chemotherapy. It is not very difficult to find a well-trained and experienced specialist in radiation or chemotherapy. There are formal training programs, examinations, and board certifications in these two specialties.

The Board-Certified Radiation Oncologist

We recommend finding out whether the physician who is to give you radiation is a board-certified radiation oncologist. This is extremely important when radiation is being used to treat localized, and potentially curable, cancers because if you do not receive proper radiation you may lose your chance for cure. The board-certified radiation oncologist has had three or more years of formal training in evaluating patients for, planning, and administering radiation to treat cancer. He or she is best qualified to evaluate you and to give radiation if you have cancer.

Radiation oncology is a fairly new specialty. In many areas of the country, radiation is still given by radiologists. Radiologists have had several years of training in diagnostic radiology and usually only nine months of training in the use of radiation to treat cancer. Most radiologists received their training ten or fifteen years ago. There have been dramatic improvements in radiation since then. Most radiologists don't have the training or the experience of radiation oncologists.

Many radiologists do both diagnostic radiology and radiation treatments for cancer. We advise against being evaluated and treated by radiologists who do both. However, some radiologists devote themselves exclusively to the treatment of cancer. These doctors belong to the American Society of Therapeutic Radiologists, and many of them are excellent. However, we still recommend that a person with cancer be seen by a board-certified radiation oncologist if possible. You are more assured of excellent care with a board-certified radiation oncologist than a radiologist.

The Board-Certified Medical Oncologist

The medical oncologist is a board-certified internist with two additional years of training in evaluating and treating cancer patients with chemotherapy and hormones. If you need chemotherapy, you should at least be evaluated by a board-certified medical oncologist. He or she should also administer the chemotherapy if it is toxic and difficult to give. Low-dose, nontoxic chemotherapy can often be given by nonspecialists. A board-certified pediatric oncologist is the equivalent of the board-certified medical oncologist for children with cancer.

Board-certified hematologists are internists who have done two additional years of training in hematology. They are qualified to treat people with lymphomas, leukemias, and multiple myeloma. They are not formally trained and may not be qualified to treat you for other cancers.

Board-Certified Surgical Oncologists: There Are None

Most people with suspected cancer are sent first to a surgeon. He is the one who usually performs the biopsy to find out if you have cancer. He is often the first doctor to treat you. Since your best chance for cure is with the initial treatment, it is very important that your surgeon know what he is doing.

It is very difficult to assess a surgeon's qualification to perform cancer surgery. There are no board-certified surgical oncologists or surgical subspecialty oncologists, with the exception of the gynecologic oncologist. There are board-certified general surgeons and surgical subspecialists, who have been trained and have passed an examination in general surgery or in a special area of surgery. They have had an unknown amount of training and experience in evaluating and treating cancer patients.

In the chapter on surgery in this book, we suggest how to find out if your surgeon has the background—the knowledge and experience—to offer you good care for your cancer. Some of the questions you need to ask are: has he had any training in cancer hospitals? is he a member of the Society of Surgical Oncology? does he often operate for cancer? does he often operate for the cancer you have? do board-certified radiation and medical oncologists refer cancer patients to him for surgery or evaluation?

The Board-Certified Gynecologic Oncologist

Gynecologists are physicians with three years of training in the diseases of female reproductive organs. The board-certified gynecologist who has two or more years of formal training and passes an examination in the treatment of cancers of the female organs becomes a board-certified gynecologic oncologist. Unfortunately, there are only about one hundred such physicians in the United States, so not every woman with cancer of the ovaries, uterus, or cervix can be treated by a gynecologic oncologist. However, soon there will be more of these specialists. More information about the gynecologic oncologist and his place in the treatment of cancer of the female organs is included in chapter 14.

In summary, the board-certified radiation oncologist, the board-certified medical oncologist, and the board-certified surgeon or surgical subspecialist experienced in cancer surgery are the specialists you need to evaluate, plan, and administer treatment for your cancer. Other specialists, such as plastic surgeons, dental surgeons, and rehabilitation doctors, may also be needed.

Not All Board-Certified Specialists Are Equal

Specialized experience and training does not ensure competence in a doctor, nor does it make him a compassionate person. You want and deserve a physician who is competent and concerned—who cares about you. You probably will decide on a gut level if your doctor meets these standards. Your specialist should meet all the qualifications we listed earlier in this chapter that apply to all physicians, but in addition to these, cancer specialists should have several other qualities.

—Competent and secure physicians will be open with you. A good specialist wants his patients to be knowledgeable. He will welcome questions, because interested people are easier to care for. They are more cooperative. If you are reading this book, you probably want and need a doctor who is open with you. You want to know what's going on and to share in the decisions concerning you.

—The competent and confident specialist is not unhappy if you want a second opinion. He knows that your peace of mind is very important. He will not be offended if you question his judgment. The doctor who is offended when you ask for a second opinion is more concerned about his feelings than yours.

—The well-qualified specialist who cares for cancer patients is open to a multidisciplinary, team approach to cancer treatment. If you question whether other specialists should evaluate you, he will usually agree. He may tell you that for your particular cancer, there is no advantage in a team approach. However, he will not be offended. He will probably say that for many cancers a team approach is essential.

Most cancer specialists at the very least will discuss their patients at conferences ("tumor boards") even if they are caring for the patient by themselves. Specialists and physicians interested in cancer attend these tumor boards. If your physician presents his patients' histories at tumor boards, it means he wants his patients to receive the benefit of other doctors' training and experience. It also means that he is open to advice from others. This is a most important quality in a physician. Tumor boards tend to minimize mistakes.

Do You Need a Team of Specialists for Your Cancer?

Surgery, radiation, and chemotherapy are used together to treat cancer now more than in the past. For many cancers either surgery or radiation or both are accepted treatments. The more complicated the treatment decisions are, the more there is a need for more than one specialist to be involved. For many cancers, a team of specialists is needed to plan and administer treatment. A team approach to cancer leads to fewer mistakes in treatment.

You should read about whether there is a need for a team approach for a particular cancer in the specific disease chapters. For each cancer, the type of specialists needed and the currently accepted treatments are discussed in detail. In general, a team approach is called for if there are treatment alternatives or if more than one type of therapy is needed. For example, if either radiation or surgery can treat a cancer, the patient should be seen by both a radiation oncologist and a surgeon. Likewise, if the treatment for a cancer is radiation and chemotherapy, the two appropriate specialists must work together to plan and coordinate the therapy.

A few specific examples about when one or more specialists are required to treat a specific cancer may be helpful. For instance, small squamous cell or basal cell cancers of the skin can be treated by one specialist, the board-certified dermatologist. He is a specialist in the treatment of skin diseases and can cure most people with small skin cancers by himself. (See chapter 16, "Skin Cancers.") However, large squamous cell or basal cell cancers of the skin should be treated by a team consisting of a board-certified dermatologist, a board-certified radiation oncologist, and a plastic surgeon. (See chapter 16.)

A small superficial bladder cancer can be adequately treated by a board-certified urologist (see chapter 15, "Cancers of the Urinary Tract and Male Reproductive Organs"), whereas a large invasive bladder cancer should be evaluated by a board-certified urologist and a board-certified radiation oncologist. Large bladder cancers can be treated by either surgery or radiation or both. The patient needs to see both specialists and to decide with both of them which treatment is better. (See chapter 15.)

Cancer of the colon can be treated by a board-certified general surgeon or board-certified colon and rectal surgeon. There is little advantage to seeing additional specialists during the initial evaluation and care for colon cancer. (See chapter 13, "Cancers of the Gastrointestinal Tract.")

Acute nonlymphocytic leukemia, chronic leukemias, or multiple myeloma can be treated by one specialist, a board-certified hematologist or board-certified medical oncologist. A surgeon or radiation oncologist may be needed at some time, but the initial evaluation and treatment can be done well by one specialist. (See chapter 18, "Cancers of the Blood Cells and Lymph Glands.")

Children with cancer should always be seen by a team of specialists in childhood cancer. Most childhood cancers are treated with combinations of surgery, radiation, and chemotherapy. Therefore, several medical specialists should be involved. Also, social workers and psychologists are needed to help the patient and his family face this terrible crisis. (See chapter 23, "Cancer in Children.")

Head and neck cancers can be cured by either surgery or radiation. Some need both. Chemotherapy is used for advanced cancers. Therefore, a surgeon experienced in head and neck cancer surgery, a radiation oncologist, and, in some cases, a medical oncologist should plan the treatment. In head and neck surgery the cosmetic result is almost as important to the patient as a cure; a plastic surgeon and a dental surgeon are needed on the team. Many clinics that treat people with head and neck cancer routinely use a team approach. No single specialist is as good as a team of experts for these cancers. (See chapter 19, "Head and Neck Cancers.")

Thus, some people with cancer can receive excellent care from one specialist. However, for many cancers more than one specialist is needed. We recommend that you read the chapter about your cancer. If you find that a team approach is often used, ask your physician about its advantages.

The Role of a Nonspecialist in the Care of a Cancer Patient

We recommend that people with cancer be evaluated and have treatment planned and usually begun by specialists. Surgery and radiation must be done by specialists. Chemotherapy can be given either by the medical oncologist or by a family physician if it is not complex or toxic. But, for example, high-dose combination chemotherapy for Hodgkin's disease, which can cure people, should be given only by a medical oncologist.

Many cancers are not very responsive to chemotherapy. In these cases chemotherapy offers only temporary relief from symptoms such as pain, and it often involves a single drug in relatively low doses. The family physician can give single-drug therapy. He often lives closer to his patient, knows him well, and is less expensive. So if you are getting 5-Fluorouracil for colon cancer, this can be given by an interested family practitioner. You do not need to travel to a specialist if your family doctor is willing to treat you under the direction of a medical oncologist.

The family physician, internist, or pediatrician may care for people with cancer after the treatment has been planned and begun. The generalist should consult the specialist for advice if problems arise.

In summary, the types of specialists and the need for a team of specialists vary with the type of cancer. The best chance for cure is always with the first treatment. You want physicians who are trained and experienced in the use of radiation, chemotherapy, and surgery. These are board-certified specialists. Many cancers require a team approach because of complex treatment programs. You should find out whether a team will help you. Although the treatment for cancer should not be delayed, it is not an emergency. You should take the time to find out about the qualifications of your specialist and whether you need a team of specialists to give you the best care.

Where Should You Be Treated for Your Cancer?

People with cancer often travel to famous medical or cancer centers for treatment. The large center has cancer specialists, the latest technologic advances, and experimental therapy. However, for many cancers, treatment in smaller communities is as good as that at the larger centers. Communities that have board-certified radiation oncologists, medical oncologists, and board-certified surgeons and surgical subspecialists experienced in cancer surgery can offer good treatment for many cancers. It pays for some but not all cancer patients to travel to large university hospitals or cancer centers for care.

You need to know whether a large medical center, a large clinic, a university hospital, or a cancer center can offer you better care than that available in your own community. Will your chances for cure improve? Will you live longer? Will you be more comfortable? The benefits of a larger center compared to treatment in your own community depend upon several factors. (1) What resources are available in your community? What cancer specialists and hospital facilities are available in your community? (2) What resources do you need for optimal treatment of your cancer? What specialists or team of specialists are needed to offer you the best care for your cancer? (3) What can the best treatment do for your particular cancer? For some cancers, there is no effective therapy, even at famous cancer centers. For others, treatment offers a high chance for cure. When the benefits of treatment are great, you should make sure you receive them.

Where you should be treated is closely linked to who should treat you. You need to see well-trained specialists to evaluate you and plan and give treatment. Many people think that a university hospital or a cancer center can offer miracles. They may offer better treatment for some diseases, including cancer. However, it all depends on the type of cancer. For many cancers, good treatment is available in most large communities. Experimental programs, though, which are promising for some cancers, are only available at certain cancer centers or university hospitals.

In this section, we will help you decide whether you should remain in your own community, travel to a nearby larger town or city, or travel even further to a cancer center or university hospital for cancer treatment.

If You Can Receive Good Care in Your Community, Stay There

If the specialists and other resources you need are available in your own community, you should be treated there. The advantages of treatment near your home are obvious. First, you do not need to travel and leave your family and friends. When you have cancer, you need their support. Therefore, it is better if you can be treated in your own community.

Second, cancer centers are strange and often frightening. Many rural and small-town people are uncomfortable in larger cities. The person with cancer should be in as familiar an environment as is compatible with good treatment.

Finally, you save money if you are treated near your home. Travel and living expenses for you and any accompanying family members are not covered by medical insurance. It can cost up to several thousand dollars extra to be treated away from your community.

The type and number of specialists and the size of the medical center you need depend upon your cancer. Most middle-sized and large communities now have trained surgeons, radiation therapists, and medical oncologists. Many people with cancer can receive adequate treatment in their own communities. Others cannot. For example, if you have a head or neck cancer that should be treated by a large team of physicians, you may need to travel to a large medical center. Most smaller communities do not have all the specialists needed to best treat this type of cancer.

The treatment of Hodgkin's disease requires a board-certified radiation oncologist, a medical oncologist, and often a board-certified surgeon. Treatment can cure most people with Hodgkin's disease. Although many small- and middle-sized communities have these specialists, we think it pays to go to a large medical center where many people with Hodgkin's disease are evaluated and treated. It can mean the difference between cure and death.

Childhood cancers are usually highly malignant but can often be cured by the use of surgery, radiation, and chemotherapy together. A team approach is always needed, and all children with cancer should be referred to major children's hospitals or cancer centers for children.

The need for various specialists or a team of specialists depends upon your cancer. You can find out what specialists you need and whether a team approach is best ·by reading the chapter on your cancer and by asking your doctor. Then you have to find out if the specialists are available in your community. If they are not available, you should go to a larger medical facility. But if you are traveling to a larger medical facility for the treatment, you should make sure the specialists you need are available at that facility. You don't want to travel four hundred miles and not get good care.

If Good Treatment Is Not Available in Your Community,
Where Should You Go?

If you must go to another community for treatment, you will be either seeing a specialist in private practice or going to a large clinic, university hospital, cancer center, or children's hospital. Before you accept a referral to a larger medical facility, find out what specialists you need and make sure they are available. We generally recommend going where more than one specialist practices. Most larger medical facilities have several board-certified radiation oncologists, board-certified medical oncologists, surgeons, and surgical subspecialists. Although you may need only one specialist to direct your care, you want the benefit of the advice of a team of specialists.

Some advantages and disadvantages of different types of medical facilities for cancer treatment will be briefly reviewed.

Cancer Specialists in Individual Private Practice   The specialist in private practice has only one job, to care for his patients. He offers personalized care; he himself will take care of you in his office and in the hospital. He or his partners will always be available. Many specialists in solo or small group practices give excellent care. Often, they can even offer experimental therapy. We feel more comfortable, however, with groups of specialists who practice together. This enables the physicians to review patients together and thereby exchange ideas and knowledge. It also minimizes error because more than one doctor is thinking about your case. Finally, it allows the specialist more time to keep abreast of new developments in the field by reading and by attending scientific meetings where new developments are presented.

The Large Medical Clinic   There are many large clinics in the United States. Some well-known examples are the Mayo Clinic, the Cleveland Clinic, Virginia Mason, and the Lahey Clinic. These usually have several board-certified radiation oncologists, medical oncologists, surgeons, and surgical subspecialists. The doctors spend most or all their time caring for patients, so they offer personalized and usually expert care. Such clinics are also often involved in research, and many offer experimental treatment for cancers. Thus, large clinics, particularly the well-known ones, generally offer good care for people with cancer.

The University Hospital   University hospitals usually give good cancer treatment. Most medical schools have departments of radiation and medical oncology, and surgical specialists who are experienced in the treatment of cancer. Experimental treatment programs are often available. Thus, university centers usually have an abundance of well-trained specialists in cancer treatment.

The care at university hospitals may be less personalized than elsewhere. One important function of university hospitals is to train students and young doctors. Therefore, you will have students or residents caring for you under the direction of an older, experienced "staff doctor." In addition, you may not see the same doctors each time. This disturbs many people. Most university physicians do not devote their full time to patient care; they are also involved in research and teaching. Your staff doctor may not be available. He may be teaching or out of town. If he is away, in an emergency, you may need to use a doctor who does not know you. Despite these disadvantages, in some areas, the university hospital is the best place to be treated.

Whether you will be satisfied at a university hospital depends upon which one you go to and what your needs are. Some people are disturbed at the less personalized care, but others are reassured by the many doctors whom they see and by the fact that their staff doctor is good enough to be on a medical faculty.

The Cancer Center   The cancer center offers many of the same advantages and disadvantages as the university hospital. There are many cancer specialists, many of whom subspecialize and are true experts on a single type of cancer. At some large centers, there are teams of specialists who treat each type of cancer. For example, breast cancer may be treated by one group of surgeons, radiation oncologists, and medical oncologists. Another group of specialists treats head and neck cancers. Thus, you will see a very experienced team of specialists. However, as with the university hospital, you may be treated by residents or other physicians in training and get less personalized care.

Much of the treatment at cancer centers is experimental. One of their functions is to make advances in the treatment of cancer. This may or may not be to your benefit. If you have a cancer in which experimental treatment is promising, it is to your benefit to receive it. However, for many cancers the standard treatment is as good or better than newer treatments. Unproven experimental therapy offers hope but can have undesirable side effects. (See chapter 24, "Experimental Treatment for Cancer.")

The Large Children's Hospital   The large children's hospital is the only place for the child with cancer. Only at these hospitals are the teams of specialists and support personnel available to offer the child with cancer the best treatment. Often treatment can be planned and started at a large center and then completed in your own community by your pediatrician.

If you cannot receive the treatment you need in your own community, you should go to one of the facilities discussed above. We cannot give more specific guidelines because there are many factors that enter into the decision of where you should go. For example, let us consider two people with the same cancer. One lives in a small town and one lives in New York City. The person in New York can go to a cancer center without traveling. The person in the small town may be able to receive as good treatment a hundred miles away in a large clinic as in a cancer center five hundred miles away. These two people should be treated at different facilities.

Will You Have Problems Paying for Your Care?

If you have little or no insurance to pay for your treatments, you should consider obtaining care free of charge. Cancer treatment is expensive. In addition, if you are the breadwinner, you will have to use your savings just to live. Good quality free care is available for many people.

Veterans Administration and Public Health Hospitals

Both the Veterans Administration (VA) and the Public Health hospitals treat people free of charge. You should find out if you are qualified to go to either of these facilities. All people who have been in the armed forces are qualified to go to a Veterans Administration hospital. Eskimos,

Native Americans or Indians, merchant marines, and some civil servants are qualified to go to Public Health hospitals. There are VA and Public Health hospitals all over the country. Many of these are quite large, are affiliated with medical schools, and offer excellent care. Qualified cancer specialists are available in many of the larger VA and Public Health hospitals. If you are having financial problems, consider going to one of these facilities. However, you should apply the same guidelines to the quality of your doctors and your care at these hospitals as elsewhere. Do they have the board-certified specialists you need? Is there a tumor board? Etc.

The Cancer Center

Many cancer centers (such as Roswell Park Hospital in Buffalo, New York; M.D. Anderson in Houston, Texas; and Memorial Hospital in New York City) offer some treatment free of charge. The National Cancer Institute in Bethesda, Maryland, also treats people free of charge. One reason to go to a cancer center, then, is to receive free treatment. We do not suggest that you take experimental therapy because you cannot pay for standard treatment. However, at the larger cancer hospitals, people are treated with standard treatments in addition to experimental ones. Therefore, if you do not have insurance and are not eligible for Veterans Administration hospitals, you may be able to receive treatment at a cancer center.

Even if you do not live in a large city, you can still be treated in your own community if the physician or physicians you need (board-certified radiation oncologist, board-certified medical oncologist, and/or board-certified surgeon) are available. If you have to travel to receive care for your cancer, there are both personal and medical factors to consider. You should go to the most convenient medical facility that has the specialists and equipment to treat you. For some cancers, you should go to a hospital that offers promising experimental treatments. These facilities may be large children's hospitals, cancer centers, or university hospitals. Read about the treatment of your cancer in the appropriate chapter in this book. It will help you decide who should treat you and where you should be treated.

SUMMARY

1. One in three cancer patients is cured, many live longer, and many feel better because of modern treatment. Thus, it is important to receive the best treatment. People with cancer should be evaluated and treated by specialists—doctors with formal training and experience in the treatment of cancer.

2. Any doctor can call himself a specialist. This is misleading but legal.

For example, a doctor with no training can call himself a cardiologist or a medical oncologist. He can also list himself in the telephone directory as a specialist without specialized training or experience. Therefore, you cannot assume that a specialist has had the training and experience you want.

3. A board-certified specialist has had formal training and passed an examination assessing his skill in a particular area. You can find out whether your specialist is board certified by asking him, looking on his office wall for his certificate, or looking in the *Director of Medical Specialists* or the AMA *Directory of Physicians* (available in many public libraries and county medical society libraries).

4. You can find out which specialist or specialists are needed to treat your cancer in the chapter on your cancer in this book. Then find out whether a team approach is helpful. You should be treated in your own community if the specialists and facilities you need are available. Travel to a larger medical center if the specialists you need are not available in your community.

5. The more likely you are to be cured or helped by therapy, the more you have to lose by not getting the best treatment. If, after checking, you are not sure whether adequate treatment is availiable in your community, go to a larger center.

5

The Doctor-Patient Relationship

DOES YOUR PHYSICIAN MEET YOUR EMOTIONAL NEEDS?

In other chapters of this book, the professional qualifications of physicians who specialize in cancer care (such as board certification) are discussed. In this chapter, we will explore some very important but less tangible aspects of the good physician. These cannot be measured by prestigious certificates; they are measured best by how you react to him. Good medical care involves more than treating a disease the correct way. It is more than applied technology. A good physician deals with the whole person and his family, not a disease. He is concerned for his patients and helps them deal with their illnesses. Especially if you have cancer, a caring physician to whom you can relate can help ease the emotional as well as physical burdens of your illness. A person with cancer faces frightening treatment and the possibility of death. A close, supportive relationship with your doctor can make a world of difference.

People tend to hold physicians in awe. Even the most critical and sophisticated patient views the physician as a powerful figure. It is difficult for the patient to think of his rights or needs, especially when he has cancer and is crying out for help. However, you—the patient—need to have some control over this relationship. Doctors do not treat all people alike. They will react and often accommodate your needs. But if the relationship is not satisfactory, you always have the option of changing physicians. The aim of this book is to help you, the patient, gain more control over your own care. The aim of this chapter is to give you a better idea of what you can reasonably expect from your doctor as a human being, someone who should help you through the many emotional crises you and your family must face.

The person with cancer needs a close relationship with his physician.

50

The physician must not only be able to provide quality medical care for cancer but also must help his patient and family face emotional crises. Cancer is the most frightening illness in our culture. People's reactions to it vary, but fear, anxiety, depression, anger, and guilt are universal. When people find out they have cancer they and their families are usually stunned by the news. They need a caring physician with whom they can communicate. This will not solve any problems by itself, but it is extremely helpful.

People with cancer face a series of psychological crises. They especially need help when they are told the diagnosis, when frightening treatments are begun, and if the cancer recurs. Your physician should help you and your family deal with your fears. You and your family will fare better if you can share your troubles and become closer rather than facing your problems alone. If someone dies from cancer, the spouse and children will accept the death better if they feel "good" about how they reacted during the illness. If they helped and shared feelings, they will not feel guilt, and they will accept the loss better than if they were unable to share the illness. The caring physician realizes that helping his patient and family is as important as choosing the right treatment. He also realizes that additional professional help may be needed. He will not hesitate to call upon a social worker, psychiatrist, psychologist, hospice, or another doctor if he feels he is not able to help the family by himself.

You, the patient, can best decide whether your doctor is meeting your emotional needs. To help you, we list some of the qualities we think are desirable in a doctor caring for a person with cancer or any other serious chronic disease.

—He spends enough time with you. He gives you time to talk about what is on your mind. A person with cancer has many fears, and he can face them better if he shares them rather than holding them in. Your doctor should allow you enough time for such conversations.

—He will spend time with other members of your family. The spouse or other members of the family should be almost as involved as a patient with cancer. The doctor should help the family come to terms with their fears and anxieties about the cancer, the treatment, and what might happen in the future. They will then be better able to help the patient emotionally weather this crisis.

—He should be able to listen to your fears about suffering and death. Many physicians do not want to hear about a patient's fears, especially those about death. Until recently, death has been taboo in our culture. It is too frightening for some doctors to handle except on a very intellectual level. If you feel your doctor does not want to hear about your fears, you will not want to talk about them.

—He or his partner should be available around the clock. People with cancer need a doctor they can call and see day and night. They can become desperately ill in a matter of hours. Patients undergoing chemotherapy can develop life-threatening infections that need immediate treatment. Your physician should give you a phone number at which he can be reached at any hour. If he or his partner is not available on a twenty-four hour basis, we advise you to change physicians.

—Your physician should encourage you to learn about your illness. The patient who understands his disease and its treatment is better able to participate in his own care. He will anticipate problems, and will know when to call his doctor for help. For example, he will understand that chemotherapy may lower his white count and a fever or chill may signal a very serious infection. The good physician realizes this and spends time educating his patients. He will discuss and explain the treatment, expected side effects, and other potential problems. He will also educate his patient's family. One of the purposes of this book is to help you understand your disease and its treatment. If you are reading this book you probably want a doctor who wants you to understand your disease and not blindly accept everything he tells you.

You must decide whether your doctor meets your emotional needs. If you are dissatisfied, we hope that the characteristics we have listed for a supportive physician will help you understand why you are. Perhaps they will help you to ask more of your physician or to change physicians if necessary.

A patient should expect two things from his doctor that form the basis of the doctor-patient relationship: good medical treatment and emotional support. Your physician should realize his responsibility for both of these aspects of good care. Therefore, he must refer his patient to a cancer specialist if he is not qualified to offer the best care. He should also refer his patient to another physician if he cannot or does not want to deal with the patient's psychological problems. The physician may realize that he can meet the patient's needs with the help of others. He may have a social worker, psychiatrist, or psychologist help his patient and the family through emotional difficulties.

A caring, sympathetic physician, regardless of his specialty, can serve the emotional needs of a patient and his family. Often the most emotionally supportive physician is your family doctor. He knows you and your family and does not have many very sick or dying patients. The radiation or medical oncologist may have many dying patients and may become emotionally drained; he may have the time but not the emotional energy to help all his patients. People do not always realize that their physicians become very involved with them. Helping a patient face cancer, its treatment, and especially impending death is very trying. Cancer specialists are needed to provide the best treatment. However, they may not be the right physicians to deal with advancing cancer after treatment has been exhausted. Often the family physician provides the best emotional support. Another alternative to which some cancer specialists are turning is a specially trained nurse or social worker who helps their patients in a crisis.

The following two cases illustrate relationships between one physician and two different patients and their families. In the first case, the doctor-patient relationship was poor. The physician did not help his patient and family deal with the illness and impending death. The second relationship was far more successful. It was supportive and gratifying for the physician, the patient, and his family. No physician is right for every patient. You should not hesitate to change physicians if you cannot communicate satisfactorily with your physician.

D.V., a twenty-nine-year-old married welder, noticed a swelling in his left testicle and went to his family physician. His family physician referred him to a urologist, who suspected cancer and removed the testicle. D.V. had a highly malig..ant form of testicular cancer. Tests showed that the disease was widespread and had spread to his liver and lungs. He was referred to a medical oncologist for chemotherapy.

D.V. came with his wife to his first appointment with the medical oncologist. The medical oncologist had to tell them some unpleasant facts about the side effects of high-dose chemotherapy but also gave them real hope. He told them there was about a 50 percent chance for cure. He also told them that if treatment did not work, D.V. might be dead within a year. Both D.V. and his wife were very quiet during the interview. They did not ask any questions but appeared to approve of the therapy.

Chemotherapy with a toxic combination of anticancer drugs was started several days later. D.V. got very sick from it. He became severely nauseated, vomited often, and had muscle pain for which he required large doses of narcotics. He spent much of the time in the hospital to receive chemotherapy or because of side effects. During the first several months his cancer shrank but he became increasingly depressed over his side effects. The medical oncologist explained that everyone goes through almost the same problems: although D.V. felt badly, it did not mean that the therapy was not working. D.V. listened quietly to the medical oncologist and continued to take therapy. He asked few questions but seemed very depressed.

After several months of improvement, the cancer started to grow again despite therapy. The medical oncologist now told him this and said that although he would change the therapy, D.V. could no longer be cured. A week after this conversation, D.V.'s wife phoned and asked for a referral to another medical oncologist.

The oncologist requested that the patient and his wife visit him to discuss their problems. At this visit for the first time D.V. and his wife showed their true feelings. D.V. expressed great anger at all the doctors who were taking care of him—the urologist, the oncologist, and the interns and residents. He said that he had been lied to. He was led to believe he would be cured and now he was told he would probably die. He felt his doctors had "pulled the rug out from under him." He refused to believe that he would die—that therapy could no longer cure him. Despite a long discussion with the oncologist, D.V. and his wife left the office bitter and angry. They felt he had been treated with very toxic drugs that had not helped him at all, but in fact had made him sicker.

D.V. went to two other oncologists but received the same information. He returned to his original medical oncologist and died four months later despite additional chemotherapy. After D.V. died his wife visited the oncologist several times. She was very depressed and also extremely angry about her husband's treatment. Her husband had died feeling angry. She felt badly that he had not resolved his feelings and she now felt it would take her years, if ever, to get over her experience. At this point she couldn't see putting herself under a doctor's care, no matter what might happen to her. She no longer trusted physicians.

The oncologist felt extremely frustrated and badly about this case. Looking back, he felt he had left the door open for frank discussion throughout the entire period he had been caring for D.V. However, he had to admit that he had not actively tried to find out what was on his mind. During six months of extremely toxic therapy, D.V. had rarely talked, and the medical oncologist did not try to draw him out. Perhaps he was too busy. But in fact D.V. had made him feel uncomfortable. The oncologist could remember other cases where he had the time and energy to help his patients talk about their feelings.

The physician caring for a patient with cancer must initiate communication. Many patients will open up and face their problems more successfully if they can verbalize their fears and anxieties. All we can say about this case is that the patient and his wife did not receive the emotional support that they needed from their medical oncologist. Although this doctor is a caring and compassionate physician, he was the wrong physician for D.V. and his wife. He did not offer sufficient emotional help.

D.V.'s main reaction to cancer was depression. Like many depressed people, he was reluctant to talk about his feelings. A physician may unconsciously welcome avoiding such patients, as they are very difficult to talk to. Perhaps the doctor sensed the deep anger inside of D.V. and did not want to deal with it. It takes a lot of energy and commitment to respond to these difficult problems; often it is easier to withdraw. The physician should recognize what is happening when a patient is quiet and does not communicate. He should try to help the patient himself, refer him to another person (such as a psychologist), or transfer his care to another doctor who might deal with the problem better.

In summary, the inability of D.V. and his wife and their doctor to communicate and resolve their problems made it impossible for D.V. to accept his death and left his wife with many unresolved feelings. No doubt she would have grieved in any case, but chances are she will grieve much longer because of the poor way in which D.V.'s death was handled.

The next case is an example of a patient who reacted differently to his cancer. He was able to confront his problems and his physician, the same medical oncologist who treated D.V. In this case, a supportive physician-patient relationship resulted that was gratifying to both the physician and the patient.

S.R., a twenty-nine-year-old married construction worker with two children, was born with an undescended testicle. It was surgically brought down into his scrotum at age twelve. At age twenty-nine he developed swelling in that testicle, and a very malignant type of testicular cancer was found upon surgery. S.R. was sent to a medical oncologist for chemotherapy because he had widespread disease. The medical oncologist explained the treatment, both the many side effects and the small chance for cure.

S.R. was very upset. On his second office visit, he spent over an hour talking with the doctor about chemotherapy. They discussed the side effects and how sick he would probably be during his year of therapy. The medical oncologist told him that he would probably feel worse before he felt better and would spend much of the time in the hospital. If the treatment failed, he would probably live less than a year.

S.R. was still extremely angry. He did not know why he had been struck down at this young age with a terrible cancer. Nevertheless, he vowed to face therapy and told the oncologist he would be one of the few patients to be cured of his disease.

After three courses of treatment, S.R.'s cancer had shrunk in size so much that it was almost gone. However, S.R. refused to continue to take one of the drugs that made him extremely nauseated. He told the oncologist that he would take all the other drugs—he could stand the mouth sores, the fevers, the loss of appetite, and the muscle pain—but he could not tolerate the four or five days of nausea and vomiting every month. He would rather die than take this drug. The medical oncologist understood how bad the drug was for him but tried to convince S.R. to continue it. His cancer was responding and he might be cured if he stayed with it. However, after frank discussions, the medical oncologist agreed to drop the one drug. S.R. had made his own decision. He was the one who got the nausea and would also be the one either to die or be cured. He had the right to refuse to take a drug.

Few patients have the inner strength to disagree openly with their physicians and argue with them. This is especially true of people with cancer who are extremely frightened and very dependent on their cancer specialists. Fortunately, S.R.'s medical oncologist was not dogmatic. He wanted to give his patient the best treatment but he also respected S.R.'s wishes. He realized that if he insisted, S.R. might refuse all therapy. Some doctors would be so angered that they would refuse S.R. further treatment and refer him to another doctor. We think there are many occasions when you, the patient, need to stand up for your own interests. A caring doctor will respect you for this.

S.R. took one year of high-dose therapy. Four years later, he is alive and free of cancer. Perhaps if his doctor had refused to stop one drug,

S.R. would have discontinued all treatment and would now be dead instead of alive. We hope that S.R. would have gone to another oncologist or even a third oncologist to find someone who would treat him without that one drug. If you feel your doctor is not respecting your opinion or meeting your needs, you should ask for a second opinion or ask to be referred to another doctor for treatment. Most doctors will find you another specialist. If your doctor refuses, you can request referral from the county medical society or find another doctor through one of your friends or relatives.

The medical care industry should be thought of as a service industry. It is up to you to obtain satisfactory service. No physician is capable of giving everyone what he needs, either medically or emotionally. Many patients realize when they are in an unsatisfactory physician-patient relationship, yet they are afraid of antagonizing their physician or of not being able to obtain care elsewhere. So they remain in a bad care relationship. We have been told by many patients that they stayed with their cancer specialist for months or years although they were dissatisfied. They were afraid to ask for a second opinion or to be transferred to another cancer specialist. In this chapter we have outlined what emotional help or support you should expect from your doctor. In other chapters we outline what you should expect from him medically. The cancer patient needs both to cope with his disease.

SUMMARY

1. Cancer patients and their families need a close, supporting relationship with the physician to help them face the disease and its treatment.

2. You, the patient, can best decide whether your doctor is meeting your emotional needs. If you are dissatisfied, we urge you to tell your doctor and either alter your relationship with him or her or else ask for a referral to another physician.

6

Four Problems Common to People with Cancer

PAIN, NUTRITIONAL, PSYCHOLOGICAL, AND FINANCIAL PROBLEMS

This chapter discusses four common problems that afflict people with cancer: physical pain; lack of appetite, weight loss, and the associated fatigue; the emotional consequences of cancer; and monetary problems —the cost of care and of lost wages. We would like to help you face these problems by providing information that will help you make realistic decisions while avoiding ungrounded fears.

Pain

When people have cancer, they fear pain almost as much as they fear death. It is a common misconception that all or almost all people who die from cancer suffer terrible pain. Although pain is common, it is not a universal problem for people with advanced cancer. Only about 40 percent of people with cancer have significant pain. Perhaps you remember family members or friends who died in terrible pain or you have heard stories about people with cancer who had intractable pain. Years ago the ability of medical science to treat or control pain was not good. However, now there are better methods of pain control that can successfully relieve pain in almost everyone. In our combined experience, only ten of several hundred people with end-stage cancer had severe pain that we could not control. Thus, fewer than half of people dying from cancer have pain, and we can almost always control it. In this section, we will tell you how pain can be controlled.

Most pain from cancer is due to one of three mechanisms: pressure or irritation; obstruction of a viscous organ such as the bowel, stomach, or ureters; or metastases to bone. Pain is a signal—a helpful though disturbing signal—that something is wrong. Without pain to warn us, we would continually get into serious trouble. For example, without pain we would not jump away from fire. In the cancer patient it is usually a signal of advancing disease.

Pain from Cancer Has Special Significance

Pain is one of the most subjective symptoms. We cannot measure it. You feel it and tell others about it. For the person with cancer, pain usually means "I'm getting worse and I'm going to suffer a lot." Pain is often not well tolerated in a person with cancer due to its emotional significance— it signals impending death. For example, if two people had equivalent pain, one from a sport injury and the other from cancer, the person with cancer would probably feel worse. The person with a sport injury knows his injury is temporary and he will get well again. To the person with cancer, pain means advancing cancer; it means that he may die soon. Pain with cancer is associated with anxiety and depression, which contribute to the perception of pain. Depressed people feel and react to pain more than other people. Thus, pain from cancer cannot be dealt with by treating only the physical pain. Often emotional support from the doctor, family, and friends coupled with drugs to treat anxiety and depression are necessary to help relieve pain from cancer.

Methods of Controlling Pain in the Person with Cancer

There are two general approaches to pain control in cancer:
—Therapy against the cancer. By controlling the cancer, radiation, surgery, or chemotherapy can often relieve pain. Whenever possible, this approach is preferable.
—Therapy to control the pain without affecting the cancer. There are several ways of controlling pain symptomatically without affecting the growth of the cancer. These consist of pain-killing drugs such as narcotics, neurosurgery (cutting nerves to block pain impulses to the brain), nerve blocks (injecting alcohol or other substances to block nerve impulses that transmit the sensation of pain to the brain), and psychologic support, which includes the use of counseling, hypnosis, and tranquilizers to decrease anxiety and mood elevators to decrease depression.

As a rule, the person with cancer need not suffer pain. It can be controlled in almost all cases by one of the above treatments. We will explain in more detail how each should be used. In general, we try to control pain with as few side effects as possible.

Controlling Pain by Treating the Cancer

It is preferable if possible to treat pain by treating the cancer. The three methods used are radiation, chemotherapy, and surgery.

Surgery   Surgery is used to control pain caused by cancers that obstruct the colon, stomach, small bowel, or ureters. In these organs pain results from pressure that builds up behind an obstruction. Surgery can create a bypass of the obstruction, which often dramatically relieves pain.

Radiation   Radiation causes cancer to shrink and relieves the pain cancer causes. It can usually relieve pain from bone metastases and can often control pain from other local tumor growths. For example, if the liver is tender and enlarged from cancer, radiation to the liver can often relieve the pain. The aim of this type of radiation is not to try to kill all the cancer cells, it is merely to shrink the cancer enough to control the pain. Low doses of radiation to small areas are all that are needed. Therefore, the side effects are minimal. The following case history illustrates how well radiation can control pain.

A.R., a sixty-two-year-old nurse, had a mastectomy for breast cancer. She felt well and had normal checkups for three years. Then she noticed pain in her left hip. She went to her doctor, who took an x-ray. It showed destruction of her left hip bone, almost certainly due to metastatic breast cancer. All other tests were negative. Her surgeon presented her case to other cancer specialists at the tumor board. It was decided that radiation was the treatment of choice, because it could control the pain without side effects.

A.R. was referred to a radiation oncologist. He examined her and explained the radiation treatment, and she readily agreed to it. Ten radiation treatments were given over two weeks. The pain improved after the third treatment and was gone by the end of treatment. Six months later A.R. was working, felt well, and had no pain. She was not given any systemic treatment for her breast cancer.

Radiation almost always controls pain from bone metastases. It is given over two to three weeks, usually without side effects. A.R. no doubt will have future problems from her cancer; however, her short course of nontoxic radiation has taken care of her present pain.

Chemotherapy   Chemotherapy, or for some cancers hormonal therapy, can relieve pain by killing cancer cells. For example, bone pain from prostate cancer is relieved in at least 50 percent of patients with daily tablets of estrogen, a female hormone. Similarly, breast cancer frequently responds to either hormones or chemotherapy. Bone pain and other pains disappear if the cancer responds.

Controlling Pain When the Cancer Can't Be Treated

When radiation, surgery, or chemotherapy are either not likely to help or have been used and have failed to relieve pain, a cancer victim's pain must be controlled nonspecially. The actual method of relief depends upon the location and severity of the pain, how long the cancer victim is likely to live, and what the person wants. The doctor must choose among drugs (both nonnarcotic and narcotic painkillers, tranquilizers, and mood elevators), neurosurgical techniques, and nerve blocks by injection. The doctor should always consider how much his patient's emotional state contributes to the pain. Emotional support, tranquilizers, or antidepressants can help and even sometimes completely relieve "severe cancer pain."

Dealing with the Patient's Anxieties and Fears Can Lessen the Pain   People with cancer fear all pain. Even aches and pains that many of us would ignore can panic a cancer patient, who then turns to his doctor for help and complains of severe pain. A perceptive and experienced physician will understand that the problem isn't physical pain. Talking with and counseling the patient and his family and judiciously using tranquilizers or antidepressants with mild painkillers such as aspirin are sometimes all that is needed. The following case illustrates this point.

V.N., a sixty-four-year-old longshoreman, developed inoperable lung cancer. When his doctor told him the bad news, V.N. became very depressed. He stayed home and lost interest in all of his old activities. Two months later he developed some pain in his chest. He rushed to his doctor, saying he had continuous pain that was so severe that he could not sleep.

His physician sensed V.N.'s anxiety. He discovered that V.N. had been sleeping poorly and had been too depressed to do almost anything since he found out he had lung cancer. V.N. had not talked about his feelings with his wife or anyone else. His doctor spent several hours talking with V.N. and his wife about his illness, about dying, and about the need to share feelings. V.N. and his wife started to talk to each other. Their conversations were painful but good. V.N. was not alone anymore. His doctor assured him that his pain could be controlled. V.N. was given a prescription for an antidepressant and told to take two aspirin tablets every four hours. Three weeks later V.N. was almost painfree. He died three months later, but he needed narcotics only during the last two weeks of his life.

This case is not rare. Many people with cancer cannot tolerate pain because of its emotional significance. Helping the patient emotionally accept advancing cancer often helps more than strong pain-killing drugs.

The Role of the Pain Clinic and Pain Specialist

In many areas of the country there are now doctors available who specialize in relieving pain. They often work in "pain clinics." These doctors treat people with pain from any condition, from cancer to psychosomatic pain. These specialists often can control or relieve pain when other physicians fail. They have more training and experience with different methods of pain control. They are experienced in the use of drugs and are trained to do nerve blocks. They also work with neurosurgeons who can operate and cut nerves to relieve pain. These pain clinics are usually in large clinics or university centers. There is no board certification in this specialty yet but there probably will be soon.

We recommend you ask your physician to refer you to a pain specialist or pain clinic if you are suffering from pain that he cannot control.

Pain-killing Drugs: Analgesics

Analgesics are drugs that decrease pain. Cancer pain can often be well controlled with these drugs. We prescribe the least potent drug that will control the pain, and aim to relieve pain with as few side effects as possible. Often tranquilizers and mood elevators are used with analgesics and can decrease the dosage needed to relieve pain.

Nonnarcotic analgesics   Aspirin, Tylenol, and Darvon often control minor cancer pain. They can be used with tranquilizers, mood elevators, hypnotics, or sleeping medicines to control mild to moderate pain. People with cancer are upset and often have problems sleeping, and a sleepless night can make minor pain feel severe. A mild analgesic and a sleeping medicine are often used together to control pain and work better than either alone. The following case history illustrates this point.

H.R. was a fifty-six-year-old truck driver who had had surgery for colon cancer two years previously. He did well for two years but then he became tired and started to lose weight. He went to his surgeon, who found that the cancer had spread to his liver. The surgeon told him that his cancer had spread and that it was not curable. H.R. was referred to a medical oncologist, who started chemotherapy. The medical oncologist also told him this only offered a possibility of temporary relief.

H.R. became very depressed and anxious. Although he was tired all the time, he could not sleep. He developed some discomfort in the upper right side of his abdomen, in the area of his liver.

The medical oncologist sensed H.R.'s anxiety. He doubted that H.R. was in severe pain, since few people with liver metastases from colon cancer have severe pain. Therefore, he spent several hours over the next week helping H.R. deal with his depression. Instead of prescribing narcotics, he treated him with aspirin, antidepressants, and a sleeping medication. H.R. started sleeping eight hours a night. He felt like a new person. After two weeks he was in better spirits; he even felt stronger. Chemotherapy was not working. H.R.'s tumor was actually growing. However, his pain was no longer troublesome. Once he faced his cancer and was able to sleep, he could stand the pain and needed only aspirin.

Marijuana   Marijuana has helped control pain in some of our patients when used in conjunction with analgesics. For example, it has allowed some of our patients to live comfortably with lesser doses of narcotics.

Narcotics   If your pain is not controlled by nonnarcotic analgesics, neither you nor your doctor should hesitate to use narcotics to control your pain. Many people, especially those who are older, feel guilty about taking narcotics. They feel narcotics are evil and addicting. We know from experience that narcotics are the best drugs for people with severe pain. Although they are addicting, in our experience people with cancer who need temporary pain relief and who have specific treatment to relieve cancer pain have little difficulty discontinuing narcotics. For example, a person may be placed on narcotics for severe pain from bone metastases. Two weeks later, after radiation has relieved the pain, most people stop the narcotics themselves. They no longer need them and do not like the sedation they cause. We urge people with cancer to accept narcotics if they are needed. They should not feel guilty or uneasy about taking these very necessary drugs. Often only narcotics can relieve severe pain.

Weaker narcotics.   Codeine, Talwin, and Percodan are weaker narcotics frequently used to conrtol mild to moderate pain. Their side effects include depression and constipation. A few people actually hallucinate with these milder narcotics, and so cannot take them. All narcotics can be constipating, especially for inactive people who are not eating well. If you are taking narcotics, you may need laxatives, stool softeners, or a change in your diet to avoid suffering severe constipation.

More potent narcotics.   Potent narcotics are used to control severe pain from cancer. Many physicians do not know how to use narcotics properly: they use either too much or too little and on the wrong schedule. Narcotics should be used to relieve pain while leaving people as alert as possible. Most people with advanced cancer and a short time to live want to be alert enough to function. A few people who cannot face their disease should be given enough narcotics to give them peace. If you are not happy about how your pain is being controlled by narcotics, ask your physician to refer you to a pain clinic where you can see a pain specialist. The pain specialist will change either your narcotic or its schedule and will also evaluate you for alternate methods of pain relief.

There are many narcotics used to control severe pain. Demerol, Dilaudid, and methadone are the most common oral narcotics. Demerol and morphine are used either intravenously or intramuscularly. If one narcotic does not work well, your doctor should try another.

Use the narcotic that works best.   We generally first try an oral narcotic such as methadone and then either increase the dosage, give the drug more frequently, or switch to another drug if the first doesn't adequately control the pain. No narcotic works for all patients. We don't know why one is better than another for an individual. It is also important to individualize the dose and schedule. Except for methadone, most of these narcotics work for only two to three hours, and therefore should be given frequently. Since we aim to relieve pain, if the pain persists the drug is not doing its job. Narcotics sometimes work better if used with tranquilizers, mood elevators, or sleeping medicines. Narcotics control pain better in relaxed people who are not depressed.

Methadone is often the best narcotic.   For many people with cancer, methadone, a narcotic that can be taken by mouth, offers good pain control. Its advantage is that it gives more long-lasting control of pain than other narcotics: it is effective for six to eight hours. The other narcotics only relieve pain for three to four hours. They are metabolized quickly by the body. To get four hours of good pain relief from other narcotics, a fairly high dosage must be used. This will make a person very sleepy for the first hour or so. Methadone often controls the pain while allowing a person to be functional. Furthermore, instead of taking pills every two to three hours, methadone is taken every six to twelve hours. We have seen people whose pain was controlled with methadone twice a day who beforehand needed pills or injections every three to four hours.

The "pain cocktail."   Methadone is often used in what we call a "pain cocktail." The make-up of the potion is unknown to the patient, enabling the physician to control the dosage of methadone and add other drugs without the patient's knowledge. This eliminates some of the emotional complications that people often have when they use narcotics to control their pain. The pain cocktail is started at a high enough dosage to control the pain completely. The dosage of methadone is then decreased by diluting the mixture, so the patient always takes the same volume. We have often been able to decrease the pain cocktail's content to minimal amounts of methadone and/or other drugs and still control pain. "Suggestion" plays a large role in pain control. In fact, in one study of pain control in people with cancer, a sugar pill or "placebo" was fully one-third as effective as narcotics.

If you have cancer and are dissatisfied with how narcotics are working to control your pain, ask your doctor about methadone. If you are not almost pain free, or if your narcotics are confusing you or making you too sleepy, or if you have to wake up at night to take additional narcotics, methadone may be of help. It may control the pain and allow you to sleep all night and better continue your daily life. Many cancer specialists such as medical, radiation, and surgical oncologists use pain cocktails with methadone as the mainstay of painkiller therapy. Pain specialists in pain clinics developed this approach and use it frequently.

The following case illustrates how effective methadone can be. W.K., a fifty-year-old school teacher, had an inoperable lung cancer. He did well without any treatment for six months, but then developed pain in several bones. This was controlled by radiation. However, soon he developed pain in almost all his bones. It was impossible to radiate all the areas where he had pain, and his cancer was not responsive to chemotherapy.

He was miserable. Codeine did little to control his pain. He was switched to Dilaudid, which did not work well either. Morphine injections controlled the pain, but the dosage needed made him sleep most of the time. He still wanted to work as a teacher and to finish out the school year.

W.K.'s doctor wisely sent him to a pain clinic at a nearby university hospital. He was seen by specialists, and his case was presented at their conference. It was decided that a pain cocktail consisting of methadone and a mild tranquilizer might do the job. This was started in relatively high doses four times a day. W.K.'s pain was not completely relieved but it became very tolerable. He was able to go back to his town and resume teaching. If he was asked, he would say that he still had some pain, but most of the time he was able to disregard it. He died five months later, but he was able to work until his last month.

Methadone often controls pain effectively when other narcotics do not. It can be taken by mouth. It is long acting and is often as strong as morphine injections.

Blocking Nerves to Control Pain

For some people with localized pain, blocking the nerve impulses that transmit pain sensations helps dramatically. This can be done in two ways: the nerve impulses can be interrupted surgically, or nerve fibers can be deadened by injections of alcohol or phenol. Both methods result in permanent damage to the nerves.

Neurosurgery   A person who has severe pain localized to a small area or even to one side of the body that cannot be relieved by other means can sometimes be helped by surgery. These operations must be done by skilled surgeons, since they can be quite dangerous. Only a board-certified neurosurgeon experienced in this type of surgery should operate on you for pain control. Ask your neurosurgeon if he does pain control operations frequently. If he does not, ask if another neurosurgeon in your community does.

There are several operations used for pain control. We will describe two of them, rhizotomy and cordotomy. A rhizotomy involves cutting nerve tracts outside the spinal cord. This operation is used to relieve localized pain in the face, mouth, throat, and torso, and it is often helpful. More than half the people with severe pain from head and neck cancers get good relief. The main side effect is loss of sensation to the area supplied by the nerves that are cut. This is disturbing, but if the pain is relieved most people feel it was worth it.

A cordotomy is a spinal cord operation. The section of the spinal cord carrying pain fibers is selectively cut or frozen. This is an extremely delicate operation, so it is most important that it be done by a neurosurgeon who is very experienced with cordotomies. If the "cut" is too big, partial paralysis will result. The side effects are quite serious, including weakness or paralysis of lower extremities and loss of bowel and bladder function. These complications can result even if the neurosurgeon is experienced with cordotomies. Obviously, the operation is done only if nothing else works and the pain is very severe. In our experience, not many patients need cordotomies to control pain. However, there is still a place for them with an occasional patient.

The following case illustrates how the neurosurgeon can help control pain in a person with cancer. B.W., a sixty-seven-year-old heavy smoker and drinker, went to his doctor with a large cancer of the tongue. He had ignored the lump for almost a year. It was treated by surgery and radiation, and he did well for two years. Then it recurred and did not respond to chemotherapy. He developed severe pain that could not be controlled with strong narcotics. His otolaryngologist referred him to a neurosurgeon, who explained that cutting the nerves that carry pain impulses might control his pain. B.W. agreed to the operation. The neurosurgeon performed a rhizotomy and B.W. woke up pain free. Although he died seven months later from widespread cancer, he never again required narcotics. About 60 percent of the people with severe pain in the mouth, face, or neck from cancer have good relief from a rhizotomy.

Nerve Block Injections   Nerve blocks can be used in place of a rhizotomy or cordotomy to control localized pain from cancer. Nerves carrying pain impulses can be interrupted by injections of alcohol, phenol, or other toxic substances. Nerve blocks are very often useful to control pain in the face, mouth, neck, ribs, and especially the abdomen. They are performed by neurosurgeons and anesthesiologists who specialize in pain control; they should not be performed by doctors without specialized training and experience. Do not undergo a nerve block without first asking your physician about his or her training and experience. The following case history illustrates the value of abdominal nerve blocks.

J.S., a fifty-one-year-old schoolteacher, went to her doctor because she was tired and had lost twenty pounds. She had some mild pain in the left upper part of her abdomen. Her doctor was worried. J.S. previously had looked very healthy; now she looked ill. He suspected that she had cancer. Tests revealed a mass in the area of her pancreas. He asked her to see a surgeon.

At surgery, a pancreatic cancer was found. The surgeon did only palliative surgery, since the cancer had spread. After surgery J.S. continued to teach, but gradually the abdominal pain became worse. She was treated with narcotics but did not get effective relief. She could no longer teach and was miserable. Her physician wisely referred her to a pain clinic for help.

The pain clinic physicians decided to do a block of the nerve in the abdomen that transmits pain from the pancreatic area, a "celiac-axis" nerve block. The doctor told J.S. that pancreatic pain was often controlled with a nerve block. A needle was inserted through her back to the area of the nerve and an anesthetic was injected. She had temporary relief. She had been told that first a temporary block would be done to determine if a permanent block was worthwhile. Two days later she had an alcohol injection into the same area, and her pain disappeared.

J.S., like more than half the people with severe, localized abdominal pain, had excellent relief with a nerve block. She went home pain free and off narcotics. She died several months later from malnutrition, but did not suffer from pain even at the very end.

If you have severe abdominal pain with cancer, ask your doctor whether a nerve block can help. It will not help everyone with abdominal pain, but for some it is the ideal treatment.

Hypnosis

Fear, anxiety, and depression contribute to the perception and reaction to pain. We have already discussed the use of tranquilizers, antidepressants, and emotional support in helping cancer patients live with pain. We want to mention briefly that some people are helped by hypnosis. People who believe in hypnosis and who have been previously hypnotized are the best candidates. We have seen patients both decrease their need for narcotics and feel better after hypnosis. People can be taught self-hypnosis and can control their pain themselves.

Pain is a problem for almost half of those who die from cancer. It is almost always controllable by one of a variety of methods now available. Specific treatment directed at the cancer, such as radiation, is best. If this is not possible or if it fails, analgesics and nerve blocks usually control cancer pain. Tranquilizers, antidepressants, sleeping medications, and emotional support often help as much as the treatment for the pain itself. Suffering is often related more to fear and anxiety about cancer than to the actual physical pain.

Nutritional Problems

Everyone knows that people with advanced cancer have poor appetites and lose weight. Anxiety and depression, treatment for cancer (such as surgery, radiation, or chemotherapy), and the advancing cancer itself can interfere with eating an adequate diet. We will discuss these three separate but interrelated causes of poor nutrition and weight loss in cancer patients and give some practical suggestions for dealing with them.

Anxiety and Depression

Some people eat more and some less when they are anxious. However, most people lose their appetites when they are depressed. People with cancer often lose their appetites and become nauseated because of anxiety and depression associated with their fears of suffering and death. The sensitive and experienced doctor recognizes these problems and deals with them by: helping the patient face and deal with his fears; administering tranquilizers, antidepressants, or sleeping medications as needed; or suggesting appetite stimulants (such as marijuana) or prescribing antinausea pills (such as compazine). Often helping the patient emotionally and the judicious use of medications will result in a better appetite and will help people to eat.

If you have cancer and your doctor does not recognize that anxiety and depression are the cause of your poor appetite and weight loss, tell him. You need counseling, and medication may also help you. Don't be ashamed to ask for help. No one can face cancer easily.

Nutritional Problems Associated with the Treatment for Cancer

The treatment for cancer can interfere with adequate nutrition in several ways. After major abdominal surgery, you cannot eat normally for one week or more. Surgery always increases your body's need for calories and accelerates weight loss. Sometimes cancer surgery makes it mechanically difficult to eat. For example, surgery for mouth, throat, or esophageal cancer may interfere with your ability to swallow food for months. Radiation and chemotherapy also make it difficult to eat normally by producing a loss of appetite associated with a loss of taste for food, nausea and vomiting, a dry mouth, or sores in the mouth or esophagus.

The nutritional problems from surgery, radiation, or chemotherapy are usually temporary. When the treatment is over, you will be able to eat again if the cancer is controlled and you feel well. Nevertheless, it is important to minimize the weight loss during cancer treatment, for two reasons: people feel better if they don't lose weight, they are stronger, and they function better; and people tolerate surgery, radiation, and chemotherapy better if they are well nourished.

Problems with Surgery and Nutrition Surgery usually interferes with adequate nutrition only for one to two weeks. Therefore, for most people no special steps to safeguard nutrition are needed. However, there are two situations where action to ensure adequate nutrition should be taken.

If a patient with cancer has already lost weight, is malnourished, and needs surgery, he or she may benefit from being fed either by a tube into the stomach or small bowel (enteral nutrition) or through a large vein (parenteral nutrition). A full diet of protein, carbohydrate, fat, and vitamins can be given by either method so that a person will gain weight and become stronger. The patient will now be better able to withstand the surgery. A malnourished person does not do as well with any type of cancer treatment as the well-nourished one.

Intravenous feedings or tube feedings are also needed if surgery will interfere with the ability to eat for more than two weeks. Head and neck cancers and some other cancers require more than one operation. During this time artificial feedings may be needed. With instruction from nutritionists, nurses, or doctors, people can easily feed themselves through a tube into the stomach or small bowel. (Hyperalimentation is discussed in further detail below.)

Radiation, Chemotherapy, and Nutrition   People who receive radiation or chemotherapy frequently have difficulty eating an adequate diet during their treatment. Radiation is usually given for one to two months, but intensive chemotherapy may be given for over a year. Therefore, poor nutrition can be a significant problem for some people who get intensive, long-term chemotherapy.

Radiation and chemotherapy both interfere with nutrition in several ways. This may cause loss of appetite, loss of taste, nausea, and vomiting. They may cause a dry mouth, making it difficult to chew and swallow food. They may also cause mouth and esophagus sores that can make eating or drinking painful. As a result, food and liquids are taken in minimal amounts. We will give some common-sense suggestions that have helped many patients deal with these problems.

Loss of appetite.   People receiving radiation and chemotherapy often do not feel like eating. Radiation is usually given five days a week for four to eight weeks. A normal appetite usually returns several weeks after radiation is finished. The type of chemotherapy that suppresses appetite is usually given intravenously either once a week or, more commonly, once a month.

The loss of appetite with chemotherapy usually starts on the day of therapy and lasts for several days. If you are getting chemotherapy once a month, try to eat a lot for the three and a half weeks that you feel well. Don't force yourself to eat during the two or three days that you lose your appetite and feel nauseated after chemotherapy; make up for it during the other part of the month when you feel well.

If you don't feel like eating, forcing yourself will not help. However, often people can eat small amounts more frequently when they can't face normal meals. We recommend that you try high-calorie snacks, such as milkshakes, desserts, fruit, candy, jam, or honey. Avoid fatty foods, since these are harder to digest and make you feel full. Sugar and carbohydrates give you calories without making you feel full.

Loss of appetite and nausea from chemotherapy and radiation can be decreased or controlled by several drugs. Tranquilizers such as Compazine can decrease nausea and help you tolerate food. If you are having problems with nausea, ask your doctor for an antinausea medication. These can be taken by mouth or by rectal suppository.

Marijuana helps many cancer patients with nausea or a poor appetite associated with radiation and chemotherapy. Their appetite is better and they have less nausea. We urge you to pressure your legislators to pass laws legalizing the use of marijuana for medicinal purposes.

Loss of taste.   Radiation and chemotherapy cause a loss of taste. Until you lose your taste for food, you don't realize how much your appetite depends upon it. By preparing food that looks and smells appealing, a person's appetite can often be stimulated even if he can't taste the food.

Nausea and vomiting.   Nausea and vomiting are often part of the same reaction to chemotherapy and radiation as loss of appetite. If you question people receiving treatment who don't feel like eating, you'll find that they are nauseated and on the verge of vomiting. The same recommendations hold for nausea and vomiting as for loss of appetite. You should avoid greasy or fried foods and you should try antinausea pills such as Compazine. Marijuana may also help. If you are nauseated and vomiting from chemotherapy, eat very little for the few days you feel ill and eat more the rest of the month.

If you get very sick from either radiation or high-dosage chemotherapy, tell your doctor how you feel. Chemotherapy is usually given in a clinic or doctor's office. Most people receiving radiation and chemotherapy do not have to be hospitalized. However, you may feel better if you are hospitalized and given higher dosages of Compazine or other drugs to control your nausea. Intravenous fluids can be given so that you don't have to drink anything for a few days.

Dry mouth.   Radiation to the mouth and some chemotherapy interfere with salivary secretions and cause dry mouths. This can make it difficult to eat meat and other dry foods. Until the salivary glands start to work again, sauces and gravies are very helpful. Sauces over cake and gravy over bread and meat and even dipping toast or cookies into tea or milk all help a person chew and swallow otherwise too dry food.

Mouth and esophageal sores.   Radiation to the mouth and esophagus and some drugs can cause sores in the mouth. This is usually temporary, lasting a matter of days to weeks. You should avoid pepper, chili, nutmeg, and other spices, acid beverages such as citrus juices, and rough foods until your mouth or esophagus heals. Cold foods such as watermelon, grapes, popsicles, and other nonirritating foods and liquids can be soothing.

Hyperalimentation

Hyperalimentation is the administration of nutrients either into a large vein or into the stomach or small bowel. For intravenous feedings, called parenteral nutrition, a tube is inserted into a large vein at the base of the neck under local anesthesia. For feedings called enteral nutrition, a tube is surgically inserted into the stomach or small intestine in a short, safe operation called a gastrostomy or jejunostomy.

Hyperalimentation has a small but defined place in the treatment of people with cancer. We have already mentioned the need for hyper-alimentation when surgery is complicated and protracted. Some cancers can now be cured with chemotherapy. In general, this requires very toxic, high-dose chemotherapy for six months or more. Often radiation is given in addition. Such therapy is used only if there is a chance for cure. Many patients become very ill with this therapy, cannot eat, and lose weight. Obviously, severe weight loss is undesirable. It depresses, weakens, and makes a person less able to tolerate chemotherapy and radiation. If you have lost more than 10 percent of your weight because of high-dose chemotherapy and more high-dose therapy is needed, ask your doctor about the advisability of hyperalimentation. It has been shown that parenteral nutrition in the face of toxic chemotherapy or radiation can help a patient maintain his or her weight and strength. People stop losing weight; in fact, they often gain weight and feel stronger.

Testicular cancer is one of the tumors that is curable by chemotherapy: at least half of all men with widespread testicular cancer can now be cured with chemotherapy. However, the treatment is very toxic. It causes mouth sores, loss of appetite, nausea, and vomiting, and can even stop the bowels from working. Most patients without parenteral nutrition lose twenty to thirty pounds over the six-month period they are treated with chemotherapy. More and more, doctors are turning to hyperalimentation for this type of patient, and the results thus far are very impressive.

Advancing Cancer and Poor Nutrition

Everyone has seen or heard about cancer patients who slowly lose weight and strength until they die. People with advancing cancer lose their appetites, do not eat enough, and thus lose weight. Also, the grow-ing cancer takes needed nutrition from the rest of the body and alters the body's metabolism. Weight loss is a signal of advancing cancer. Un-fortunately, many people feel guilty about not eating. Often relatives and friends pressure a person with cancer to eat. However, both the cancer victim and his family must accept this change in appetite. It is not voluntary; it is part of the disease. We urge that people with cancer accept the lessened and changed appetite but try to eat as much high-quality food as possible.

The loss of appetite from advancing cancer is like that from chemo-therapy or radiation. However, it is not temporary. There are some things that can be done to minimize weight loss.

—People with cancer should be encouraged to eat when and what they want. People with advancing cancer may have altered food preferences and get hungry at odd times. They should eat whatever appeals to them whenever they feel like eating.

—Try to maximize calorie intake without increasing food volume. Sugar and carbohydrates provide many calories without much bulk. Vegetables are bulky but have few calories. Fatty foods have high calorie contents, but are hard to digest. Foods such as milkshakes, ice cream, candy, fruit, jello, jam, or honey give a lot of calories with very little bulk.

—Liquid diet supplements are available in many stores. Try various ones until you find one that tastes good. These provide a lot of calories, protein, and vitamins in small volumes.

—Try to eat small amounts often. Snack between meals. People with cancer may not be able to eat a full meal.

—Make the food as visually appealing as possible. People will often eat more if they are given an attractive plate of food.

—Never put too much on the plate. A person with a decreased appetite is often repulsed by a huge plate of food.

—Try marijuana. It often improves appetite in people with advancing cancer.

—People with cancer often have dry mouths because their salivary glands do not function well. It is difficult for them to swallow and chew dry foods. Use sauces and gravies and dip cookies or toast into tea, cocoa, or milk. This will make it easier to chew and swallow otherwise dry food.

—It pays to see a trained dietitian once or twice to get helpful hints about how to prepare food and what types of foods are best.

—The American Cancer Society has a recipe book that you can get from your local chapter.

A Dietitian Can Help

If you are having problems eating because of chemotherapy, radiation, or advancing cancer, a short visit to a trained dietitian can help. Dietitians are trained in all aspects of nutrition maintenance. They can (a) tell you about high-calorie foods that you can eat, (b) give advice about eating with a sore mouth, (c) give you recipes to prepare appealing foods, (d) give advice about liquid food supplements that contain a total diet in a small volume, (e) teach you to keep a calorie count so that you can see whether you are making progress, (f) give you a book that lists the calories in each food, (g) help you keep track of what you eat (to realize what kinds of foods you should be eating), and (h) make recommendations to your doctor. The dietitian may recommend that you receive hyperalimentation if he or she cannot help you maintain your weight.

Constipation

People with cancer get constipated because they eat less bulk, because they are on narcotics that are constipating, and because they are less active than usual. It is important to prevent severe constipation because it can be very uncomfortable and adds to other cancer-related problems. You can minimize constipation by taking one of several laxatives. Ask your doctor about them. He or she will usually start you with a mild laxative and change to more potent ones if they are needed. Your diet can also make a difference. A high-fiber diet often helps. You should try to eat whole grain cereals and bran, raw fruits and vegetables, nuts, and dried fruits such as prunes and raisins. These foods with laxatives can often correct the problem. Many cancer patients cannot tolerate high-fiber diets and are helped by artificial bulk that is taken like a medicine.

Psychological Problems

Much has been written about how people react to cancer—how to live and die with it. We will not go into any depth in this area. Rather, we will briefly mention some common emotional problems faced by cancer patients. We want you to know that everyone with cancer is frightened, anxious, and depressed. These reactions do not mean that you are weak; they merely mean you are human. To find out you have cancer, to face toxic treatment and possibly suffering and death, is trying for everyone. All are shocked and stunned at first. All are frightened by cancer treatment and by the possibility that it will not work. In this section we will suggest ways of handling emotional reactions to cancer that have helped some of our patients.

You Need a Doctor Who Can Help
You and Your Family Face Cancer

We explain in some detail what we feel are the characteristics of a supportive physician in chapter 5, "The Doctor-Patient Relationship." We will only say here that the patient and family need a close relationship with a doctor to help them face the many psychological problems associated with cancer.

There are four emotional crises that are common to most people with cancer. These occur when (1) they find out they have cancer, (2) they have to face threatening treatment for cancer, (3) they realize they will die, and (4) they are cured by therapy and realize they will live for many years. Although the problems that result from the first three situations overlap, there are important differences and also various ways of helping people adjust.

Our Society and the Person with Cancer

To be told you have cancer is to be reminded of your mortality. Intellectually we all know we will die someday, but our feelings and fears about death are carefully and safely tucked away. People's reactions to death vary, but are conditioned a great deal by the society in which they live.

Our society does not include death as a natural part of life. It does not even accept aging well. Americans feel or are made to feel that they can overcome any obstacle with enough effort. It isn't surprising, then, that most Americans do not easily accept mortality.

Our society values youthfulness, optimism, courage, aggressiveness, independence, and positivity. People with cancer, however, are the opposite. They often feel old, are pessimistic, depressed, afraid, and dependent. They are isolated from the mainstream of American society and are often also isolated from their friends and relatives who see life differently.

Finally, our society doesn't encourage the expression of feelings, especially by men. Strong emotion is not considered polite. However, people with cancer have very strong feelings and usually need to express them. They want to cry, shout, and yell. They are angry and scared. They do not want to express these feelings to a blank wall; they need someone to listen. A doctor can help a lot by listening and offering advice, though it is most natural for the spouse, the children, or other close relatives and friends to listen, to share, and to help the person with cancer face his disease. But frequently friends, relatives, and even the spouse withdraw, isolating the patient just when he most needs supportive, intimate relationships.

There has been some progress in society's attitudes toward death. Even newspapers discuss reactions to death. People are starting to feel freer about expressing their emotion about it.

Reactions to the Diagnosis of Cancer

To be told you have cancer is shocking. People are stunned. They often feel fragmented and divorced from their emotions. They feel that what is happening is unreal; it is not happening to them. Most people are frightened and anxious. Thoughts of a slow death—often with pain, disfigurement, rejection, and loss of love—are extremely common. Surprisingly many people feel guilty when they find out they have cancer; they often think they are paying for some past wrongdoing. In fact, the guilt often reflects the location of the cancer. For example, women with cancer of the reproductive organs often feel they have gotten cancer because of sexual transgressions. Likewise, rectal cancer may arouse guilt of latent homosexual desires.

It is extremely important for a person to be told his diagnosis in a caring and compassionate way. We believe most adults should know they have cancer. Most people can deal with cancer better if their doctor tells them the truth. Fortunately, most doctors are honest with their patients, tell them if they have cancer. Treatments and the prospects for cure are usually discussed frankly. This is a significant change from the past. Ten to twenty years ago, when the family but not the patient was told the diagnosis, it became impossible for the patient and his family to share anything. In our experience, patients who have not been told of their cancer generally are very angry when they find out. The patient needs honesty with compassion and hope from his physician. This does not mean a false promise of cure when it is impossible. Rather, the physician should make the patient feel that he will never be abandoned.

People who have just been told they have cancer cannot think. The experienced physician understands this and does not confuse his patient by talking in detail about the diagnosis, treatment, or prognosis. Most people adjust well enough over the next few days to accept the treatment recommended by cancer specialists. However, some people may need additional time and help before treatment can be started, the help that may come from a variety of sources including physicians, psychologists, psychiatrists, social workers, clergy, family, or friends. Cancer treatment is seldom an emergency. It pays to wait several weeks and give the person a chance to adjust rather than to try to force treatment on someone who is in emotional chaos.

Common Fears about Treatment

Surgery, radiation, and chemotherapy are all frightening treatments. Surgery causes deformities or significant alterations in the body image; radiation and chemotherapy are both thought of as poisons. People think of extreme side effects such as weight loss, hair loss, nausea, and vomiting. They often associate chemotherapy with impending death, thinking it is used only as a "last ditch" measure.

People face treatment better if their physicians explain why the treatment is needed and its side effects. Most patients fantasize worse side effects than those that actually occur. People who are not informed become angry when they get sick from treatment. We feel people need to be told what to expect and to be given some degree of control over their treatment. Powerlessness is a frightening feeling. If people can be made to feel that they participate in treatment decisions, they will feel and do better.

Surgery   People are frightened of disfigurement. They are most frightened of surgery that affects their appearance or their sexual attractiveness. For example, a woman will be more upset about losing her breast than her kidney. We will discuss the types of surgery that cause the most fears of disfigurement and altered body image and suggest ways you can be helped to adjust.

Mastectomy.   The loss of a breast is a severe blow. Especially in our culture, breasts are very important to a woman's self-image. Many women fear that men will no longer be attracted to them or that their husbands will lose sexual interest in them after they have a mastectomy. In our experience, the greatest help for a woman who needs a mastectomy is for her to talk with another woman who has gone through the same experience and done well. Reach to Recovery is a volunteer organization of the American Cancer Society that has chapters all over the country. At the surgeon's request, a volunteer who has undergone a mastectomy will visit and discuss what it was like. She can do more for the patient than doctors or friends. (More information about this service is included in the chapter on breast cancer.)

Laryngectomy. The loss of the voicebox is another severe blow. The patient must learn to talk again, and usually will have a stoma or hole in his or her throat. There are a variety of volunteer organizations made up of laryngectomy patients. At the physician's request, a volunteer will visit. These organizations can usually be contacted by calling the local chapter of the American Cancer Society. (The services offered by these organizations are described more fully in chapter 19, "Head and Neck Cancers.")

Abdominal ostomies. Surgery for lower colon, rectal, and bladder cancer leaves the patient with an artificial opening in the abdominal wall for the collection of feces or urine. People have a difficult time adjusting to this. They often feel dirty or smelly. Many withdraw and cannot adjust. They feel they will be rejected by their spouse, and many spouses do sexually reject their partners. In our experience, a volunteer who has successfully faced life with an ostomy is helpful to such a patient. At the surgeon's request, the volunteer will come and visit the patient in the hospital and offer continued help afterward. These volunteer organizations can be contacted through the American Cancer Society.

Head and neck cancer. Surgery for advanced head and neck cancer is deforming. Our facial appearance is important to us, so the effect of such surgery can be great. There is no national volunteer organization for people with disfiguring head and neck surgery. However, counseling with psychologists, social workers, and physicians and group sessions with other patients with the same problems can help.

Patients with disfiguring surgery all have serious problems adjusting. No one undergoing body-image-altering surgery can adjust successfully alone. Some people cured of their cancers may not be able to face life with an altered appearance or an ostomy. We have seen people after fifteen years still depressed, withdrawn, and not really living. The physician's job is to give these people a chance to adjust. This means helping people face their real fears and getting involved with the patient and his family, especially his spouse.

Not uncommonly the spouse is repulsed by the ostomy or the lost breast. To adjust, both the patient and the spouse may need help. The involved and caring physician, with the help of others including the volunteer organizations we have just mentioned, plays a vital role in helping people adjust. Thousands have adjusted and lead full lives after such surgery.

Radiation   People both rationally and irrationally are afraid of radiation. They fear the real side effects such as skin burns and nausea but also, irrationally, the machinery and the unseen potent rays it generates. In our experience, people do better if the radiation oncologist explains what radiation is, its side effects, and even the machinery used to give it. It often helps to talk to other people who are going through or have gone through radiation.

Chemotherapy   Although people are afraid of the side effects of chemotherapy, they are even more afraid that chemotherapy means that all hope is lost. Many people know of friends who died soon after receiving chemotherapy. You should realize that this is not always true; some people can even be cured with chemotherapy. It is important for the medical oncologist to assuage these fears. Chemotherapy does not mean that you will soon die. It now helps many people to live better. It cures some and prolongs life for many others. We are also using chemotherapy in earlier stages of cancer than ever before. Because your oncologist wants to give you chemotherapy does not mean that you will soon die.

The Dying Patient

Until recently, talk of death or dying was taboo in our culture. Doctors as members of society reflected this taboo. They avoided the subject and ignored dying people when possible. The dying patient found he was alone. Physicians and nurses avoided him or when they had to visit him avoided real contact.

In the past decade the subject has become much more popular. Elizabeth Kubler-Ross and others helped bring about a new era. We owe her a debt. She and others have made death and dying more acceptable in our culture. Now articles and books about this subject flood the market. Kubler-Ross described five stages of dying: denial, anger, bargaining, depression, and acceptance. Some people do go through all these stages but people vary tremendously. Some deny from beginning to end while others accept their impending death very early.

Fewer people now have to face death alone. Many more doctors are trained and willing to help the dying. They have faced some of their own fears about death. In addition, many social workers, nurses, and psychologists are now actively interested and experienced in helping dying people. In many cities there are also groups that help the dying. The hospice movement, which started in England and is now finding acceptance here, is one such group.

The patient with advancing cancer knows he is dying. Death with cancer rarely comes suddenly. A dying person slowly loses strength. The person fears pain and must adjust to his lessening physical abilities. He becomes more and more dependent as his condition weakens. If the dying person and his family can face their fears and trials together, this can be a time of sharing and getting closer. Some of our patients and close friends and relatives have told us that their closest and most intimate moments have occurred in their last few months of life. People who can share their fears and hopes with their families and friends face death better. The family members also feels better after the death because they have helped and feel less guilt.

The physician plays an important role. He can help by listening to his patient, listening to the family, and helping them share feelings and come closer together. The physician can also help by being available and making his patient feel he always has someone to turn to. The physician can call on community resources, such as visiting nurses, that help people stay at home as long as possible. He can help people chose where they want to die. More people now want to die at home. The physician can help by reassuring the family, by making home visits when necessary, and arranging for nurses and homemakers to come in and help.

In summary, the understanding and caring physician can help both his patient and the patient's family cope with dying and death. It is difficult for a physician to enter into the picture at the last moment and help. That is why we strongly suggest that you find a caring and helpful physician early on.

The Cured Patient

One of three people who develop cancer is now cured. The psychological effects of having cancer, being treated for it, and facing the possibility of suffering and death are great. Some people never get over their fears that cancer will recur. Others, who have had disfiguring surgery, focus on problems with their altered self-image. Some people remain depressed and withdrawn for years. These people need help. We strongly urge that you seek psychological help if you have had cancer and are probably cured, but are still depressed and cannot live a full life.

Most people who have had cancer and are cured, however, adjust quite well. In fact, the experience of facing death seems to help many people to enjoy life. They are more relaxed, more confident, more interested in the essentials of life and less bothered by the trivial. It seems that the experience of facing death makes life look better. We know of several people who were extremely unhappy before they had cancer. Afterward, they felt thankful for life and had a greater capacity for joy.

Financial Problems: The Cost of Cancer

Medical care is expensive, and the costs rise yearly. Treatment for cancer is no exception. For example, the initial tests and curative surgery for breast cancer cost between $3,000 and $5,000. If you are not cured, the costs become much higher.

Patients with advancing cancer often live for years. They require constant medical attention, often receive radiation or chemotherapy, and may need to be hospitalized. Much of the time they are too ill to work. The combination of medical bills and loss of income can devastate a family. In more than half of American households, both the husband and wife work. No matter who gets cancer, if he or she is too ill to work, family income drops and expenses rise.

Cancer is an expensive disease. For the ill-prepared family it can be ruinous. With foresight and the means to provide adequate protection against catastrophe, protection against financial ruin is possible. Money problems for the person with catastrophic illness and his family cut across socioeconomic boundaries. They affect the middle class as well as the poor. The purpose of this section is to acquaint you with some of the shortcomings of what many people consider adequate health insurance. We will suggest how to protect your family. Adequate financial preparation for major illness should be part of every family's plans. We will also suggest ways to meet costs if you haven't protected yourself beforehand. With the current system of health care financing, there is no magic solution. However, ignoring the fact that cancer may disastrously hurt you monetarily as well as physically will not make it go away.

The story of R.T. illustrates some of the pitfalls inherent in our present insurance and health care systems. R.T. is a twenty-five-year-old engineer. He married at twenty-two after graduating from college, took a job with an aerospace firm, and has been working toward a master's degree at night. Two years after his marriage his wife had twin boys.

Six months after the twins were born, R.T. felt some enlarged lymph nodes in his neck. His health insurance through his job was excellent. He was enrolled in a plan that completely covered his whole family for all medical bills. He saw his physician, who referred him to a surgeon for a lymph node biopsy. The biopsy showed Hodgkin's disease. Tests, including an exploratory laparotomy, showed that R.T. had disease in his liver. Therefore, his cancer was widespread, or advanced. He was referred to a medical oncologist for chemotherapy.

R.T. was out of work for three weeks after the abdominal surgery and used up his entire sick leave. He started combination chemotherapy and tolerated it poorly. He was too sick to work at least four to five days per month. His work performance faltered, and after three months he was fired. He had a small life insurance policy with a disability clause through his job that was continued and three months of additional health insurance. After that time, he had to pay for his health insurance himself, at a cost of $700 per year. He was ineligible for either more life or disability insurance.

After six months of chemotherapy, R.T. was in complete remission. He began to feel better after treatment was stopped and tried to get another job. His credentials were excellent, but his history of Hodgkin's disease was a major stumbling block even though he had a good chance of being cured. Each time he filled out an employment application and saw a personnel officer, he was denied employment on the basis of his health history. After becoming increasingly discouraged, R.T. decided that he would lie about his health history on his applications. He was finally able to get a job with a small subcontracting firm that did not check his background thoroughly.

R.T. constantly worries about what will happen to his family if he relapses and dies. He cannot provide for them with life insurance, because no life insurance firm will insure him. He also cannot get disability insurance that will cover his Hodgkin's disease. Luckily, the cost of his illness was completely covered by his health insurance, so he had no medical bills. The cost of his initial hospitalization, lymph node biopsy, multiple tests and exploratory surgery, and six months of chemotherapy was about $15,000. Most insurance policies would only adequately cover the inpatient costs. Outpatient costs including the chemotherapy are usually poorly covered: the patient often has to pay 20–40 percent or more. In R.T.'s case, these bills would have amounted to several thousand dollars. Some policies do not cover outpatient radiation therapy. The cost for the drugs alone was more than $100 per month.

Most people do not consider the possibility of catastrophe until it is too late. We would strongly urge that each individual, especially if there is a family dependent on you either as a homemaker or as a breadwinner, consider the following questions: how good is my health insurance? would it cover outpatient costs? will it cover radiation therapy? will my coverage continue at the same level if I am unable to work for more than several months? am I covered by sufficient disability insurance? If you are relying on Medicare disability, you are grossly undercovered.

The aim of this section is to alert you to the enormous costs of treating cancer. Without adequate insurance, the average family faces economic ruin. You have to protect yourself adequately before cancer develops. Every family needs health insurance that will cover a major illness that lasts for years. This is so-called catastrophic insurance. We will outline what we consider to be minimal adequate health insurance. We will also suggest ways of obtaining financial help to pay your bills and/or free medical care if you do not have adequate insurance.

Do You Have Adequate Health Insurance?

Most people do not really think about what their health insurance policy covers. Even most doctors don't know what their policy covers. Many Americans have health coverage from a group policy taken out by their employer. You should read your policy and see what it does and doesn't cover. The specific points to look at concerning coverage for the treatment of cancer are:

—The insurance policy should be noncancelable. This means that the insurance cannot be discontinued unless you do not keep up the payments. The treatment of cancer can stretch over many years, and it is important that your insurance cannot be canceled. If you develop cancer you cannot get other health coverage.

—Coverage for hospitalization. What percentage of your hospital bills is paid by your policy and how many days are covered? Most policies provide fairly good coverage for hospital bills. Many pay 100 percent and most pay 90 percent or more of all hospital costs. This is extremely important because hospitalizations are so expensive. It is not unusual for a week's hospital stay for the treatment to cost $5,000–$10,000. The initial hospital treatment for leukemia costs between $10,000 and $30,000. We recommend 100 percent coverage or as close to that as you can afford so that you are not caught with several thousands of dollars of bills to pay yourself.

You should also see how many days of hospitalization per year the policy covers; it may be 30, 60, or 180 days. If the coverage is only for 30 days, you are liable for all costs after that. Only extremely wealthy people can afford to pay their hospital bills. You need catastrophic coverage or coverage that is unlimited. The unlimited coverage is usually not as complete as the initial coverage. For example, your policy may cover 100 percent of hospital costs for the first 60 days and then 80 percent thereafter. This is reasonable. In any case, you need reasonable catastrophic coverage or you can be ruined by one long hospitalization or several in one year.

—Outpatient coverage. Does your policy cover the costs of clinic or outpatient visits? If so, what percentage of the bill is covered? Current health insurance companies in the United States do not cover outpatient as well as hospital costs. The majority cover between 40 and 80 percent of outpatient bills. The treatment of cancer often involves outpatient visits. Most chemotherapy, for example, is given in a clinic or doctor's office. We recommend 80 percent coverage for outpatient costs, including costs of intravenous drugs. The treatment of cancer with chemotherapy is expensive. It is not unusual for a patient to incur $3,000–$5,000 yearly in outpatient bills. Forty percent coverage would leave the patient $1,800–$3,000 to pay himself. Most people with cancer cannot afford this.

—Coverage for radiation and chemotherapy. Find out if your policy covers radiation and chemotherapy. We recommend a policy that covers 100 percent of radiation and 100 percent of the cost of drugs given in the office.

—Coverage for home services. Most health insurance policies provide poor coverage for home care expenses. The patient with cancer often needs help at home. Twenty percent of all Americans over the age of sixty live alone. Even when they have a spouse or family, people with advancing cancer often need help to stay at home. We think it is a shame that some people have to go to nursing homes or hospitals merely because they can't afford help in their own home. It is especially unfortunate because it costs the taxpayers more to care for someone in a nursing home or a hospital. The sick person with cancer can often stay home if the following is supplied to him: a homemaker, a housekeeper, a nurse, a psychologist or counselor; equipment such as a hospital bed, a walker, or oxygen; and transportation to and from the doctor's office.

Most health insurance policies provide inadequate coverage for these important services. We think you, the consumer, should pressure the government or insurance companies to provide this coverage.

—Is there coverage for psychological help or counseling? People with cancer often need counseling to deal with the many stresses of having cancer. Does your policy pay for psychologists, psychiatrists, or social workers? Most policies do not provide good coverage for such services.

—Does your policy cover rehabilitation and devices such as artificial limbs? People with cancer often need rehabilitation if they are to deal with their cancer, even when they are cured with treatment. Check to see if your policy covers these services.

Many people do not have adequate health insurance. One study from 1973 showed that the average cost of a catastrophic illness such as cancer was $20,000. The average health insurance policy for that year covered approximately $8,000, leaving $12,000 for the patient or family to pay. The average poor or middle-class family in the United States cannot afford such bills. The costs of catastrophic illness are now much higher than in 1973, and although the average policy covers more than it did at that time, it still leaves many thousands of dollars for the patient or his or her family to pay by themselves. See if your policy covers you for cancer or other catastrophic illnesses. If your group policy does not provide such coverage, we advise buying added coverage privately.

Do You Need Disability Insurance?

How will you make ends meet for yourself and your family if you can't work? People with cancer often live for years but may be too sick to work. You should obtain some disability insurance privately or through your employer. This provides you with an income if you are disabled by an illness and cannot work. Remember that the disability insurance will pay you a flat sum that will not increase with inflation. Therefore, you should get as much disability insurance as possible and review your coverage periodically as your income and living expenses rise.

Don't Change Your Health Insurance If Someone in Your Family Is Chronically Ill

When a person changes health insurance, the new policy often excludes preexisting or past illnesses in family members. If you or your dependents have cancer and you change your health insurance, any expenses of treatment for metastatic cancer may not be covered. We know of one man who changed jobs. He was never a day without health insurance. His wife, whose only coverage was under his policy, had had a mastectomy for breast cancer three years before he changed his health policy. One year after changing jobs, she developed recurrent breast cancer. He then found out he had no coverage for his wife's cancer treatments. Over the next five years she received radiation, chemotherapy, and other treatments. She saw her doctor several times a month in a clinic and was hospitalized four times. The total costs of her care amounted to $27,000. She and her husband had to pay all of it.

If a member of your family has a chronic illness such as cancer, don't change your insurance policy without finding out if it will cover for this illness. Whenever you change jobs, your health insurance policy changes. The new job may not be better if it means you will not have medical insurance for a "preexisting" illness.

Life Insurance

The family breadwinner in our society needs life insurance. Americans don't have an extended family or close-knit community to help. We advise you to take out life insurance while you are young. It is cheaper, and you cannot predict when you may develop an illness such as cancer that will make you uninsurable.

Financial Help for the Patient without Health Insurance

Veterans Administration and Public Health Hospitals   If you have poor health insurance and have cancer, we advise finding out if you qualify for free care at a Veterans Administration Hospital or a Public Health Service Hospital. If you have been in any of the armed services, you are eligible to be treated at a Veterans Hospital. Likewise, if you have been in the Merchant Marine or are a native Indian, you can be treated free of charge at a Public Health Service Hospital. Call your nearest facility and find out. It can save you thousands of dollars.

Cancer Centers   At the National Cancer Institute or certain other cancer centers, treatment is completely free. At others, at least part of the cost is paid by the institution. Some cancer hospitals will not accept payments even if you have the money. For example, Rosewell-Park in Buffalo provides free treatment regardless of your financial situation.

We do not advise going to a cancer center for experimental therapy if that is not what you want. However, standard treatment is available for many cancers at these large centers. For other cancers only experimental therapy is available. If you have financial problems, ask your cancer specialist about the chances of getting the same treatment or alternative good treatment free of charge at a cancer center. But never accept treatment merely because it is free.

The American Cancer Society   Financial help from the American Cancer Society varies from community to community. You should call up and find out if your local chapter has an emergency fund to help you pay your medical bills and has money to help you pay for drugs or for home care such as homemakers, housekeepers, or nurses. Most chapters offer free transportation, home equipment such as hospital beds and walkers, and free rehabilitation programs for people with mastectomies, laryngectomies, or ostomies. Call your American Cancer Society and find out what they can help you with.

The Leukemia Society of America   The Leukemia Society of America helps people with Hodgkin's disease, non-Hodgkin's lymphoma, and leukemia. It may pay part or all the costs of chemotherapy, radiation, and blood transfusions and may also help with transportation. Most larger communities have local chapters of this society.

The Government: Medicare, Medicaid, Public Assistance   Federal, state, and local government agencies may be able to help you meet your medical expenses. If you are over sixty-five, you can get Medicare, which will pay for much of your hospital and outpatient costs. Medicare provides totally inadequate coverage for home services. Medicaid offers additional coverage, including free drugs and many home services. However, in many states you must be financially ruined before you qualify for Medicaid.

You should consider whether you qualify for public assistance or welfare. Many people feel guilty or strange going on welfare. We urge you to use this avenue of assistance if others aren't open to you. We feel that every person in the United States deserves good care. Many people have worked all their lives and yet cannot afford good medical care. We do not think that a country as rich as the United States should deny this to anyone. For many people, public assistance is the only way to pay for the huge costs of treating cancer.

We also ask you to consider bankruptcy as an option. Many cancer patients and their families are faced with economic ruin. We do not think that someone who has worked thirty or forty years and who has always had what he thought was adequate health insurance should lose his savings, his house, and his car to pay for medical bills. If you are faced with this, you should go to a financial adviser and find out if bankruptcy can save some of these resources for your family.

A Social Worker Can Help You

If you are having problems meeting your medical expenses, talk to a social worker. He or she can help you find out if you qualify for Medicare,

TABLE 3. AVERAGE COST OF CANCER CARE

Disease	Treatment	Average Cost
Acute leukemia (adult)	one year	$30,000–$50,000
Hodgkin's disease (stages 1–2)	initial evaluation and radiation	$10,000
Breast cancer	initial evaluation and curative surgery	$ 5,000
recurrent		$25,000
Colon or stomach cancer	initial evaluation and surgery	$ 5,000
recurrent		$25,000

Medicaid, or public assistance. Social workers also often know of other resources in the community.

The person with cancer faces enormous medical bills. Table 3 shows a few representative bills to emphasize the enormity of the problem. Obviously, these figures are only rough estimates. The costs of treating your cancer will vary from several thousand to over a hundred thousand dollars, depending upon the type of cancer and whether the first treatment cures you or not. These costs do not include loss of income or the cost of the patient, spouse, or other relatives traveling to another community for treatment.

A surprising number of people are treated by cancer "quackery," and health insurance does not cover these costs. Many people are taken in by the claims of special diets, megavitamins, Laetrile, and other remedies. All these remedies have one thing in common—they make their proponents wealthy. Some patients spend between $3,000 and $5,000 to obtain Laetrile in Mexico, up to $5,000 to obtain psychosurgery in the Philippines, or up to $2,000 to obtain special diets, enemas, and vitamins.

We cannot advocate any single solution to the financial woes of the cancer patient. We do recommend that each person get adequate health insurance, disability insurance, and life insurance. If you find yourself without adequate coverage, try to take advantage of the resources mentioned in this chapter. A federally financed health insurance plan would help. However, at the present time it is up to each family to provide protection against catastrophic illnesses such as cancer.

SUMMARY

Pain

1. About 40 percent of people dying from cancer suffer pain.

2. Cancer pain is often poorly tolerated even if it is not severe because it signifies advancing cancer and impending death.

3. Modern treatment can control cancer pain in almost all patients.

4. If your pain isn't being well controlled, ask your doctor to refer you to a "pain clinic" to see doctors who specialize in pain control.

Nutritional Problems

1. People with cancer often have problems with nutrition.

2. Depression, anxiety, radiation, chemotherapy, surgery, and advancing cancer all can interfere with adequate nutrition.

3. Consultation with a dietitian often may help.

4. The American Cancer Society has a booklet with helpful suggestions on nutrition for the cancer patient.

Psychological Problems

1. Cancer is an emotional crisis for the patient and his family. Finding out you have cancer, facing frightening treatment, and facing possible or impending death are all extremely difficult problems.

2. The physician should help the patient and his family face their problems together. He should help them communicate and grow closer during this crisis.

3. Often additional emotional support is needed—a social worker, psychologist, hospice, etc.

Financial Problems

1. The treatment of cancer is very expensive.

2. We recommend that people make sure their health insurance is adequate for chronic severe illnesses such as cancer.

3. If you are a breadwinner for your family we also recommend life and disability insurance.

4. If you get cancer and don't have adequate or any health insurance, find out if you are eligible for free care at a Veterans Administration Hospital, etc., or are eligible for Medicare, Medicaid, or public assistance to help pay the bills.

7

Introduction to the Diagnosis and Treatment of Cancer

The treatment of cancer has greatly improved in the past several decades. With modern therapy, one in three who develop cancer is cured. Many others live longer or at least feel better with treatment. Doctors are better able to treat cancer today because of two developments: (1) the development of radiation and chemotherapy (where only three decades ago, surgery was the only treatment for cancer), and (2) doctors in surgery, radiation, and medicine have been trained as cancer specialists. We feel it is important for someone with cancer to receive the benefits of improved therapy and the knowledge of cancer specialists. We also believe that the more you understand about cancer, how it should be treated, and how to pick qualified doctors to treat you, the more assured you will be of receiving good care.

In this chapter we introduce general concepts of cancer evaluation and treatment so that you will be better able to understand the chapters on surgery, radiation, and chemotherapy. Several phases of cancer treatment are introduced here that are amplified in subsequent chapters.

—The diagnosis: how is it made? what is a biopsy?
—How is cancer "staged"?
—What are the proven treatments for cancer? (an introduction to surgery, radiation, and chemotherapy)
—How will your doctor decide what treatment you need?
—Who are cancer specialists? What is their importance?
—Why is a team of specialists rather than only one doctor better for many cancers?
—What psychological support is helpful for people with cancer?

The Biopsy

Although your doctor may suspect that you have cancer, he cannot make that diagnosis without a biopsy. Tissue must be obtained and examined under a microscope. The biopsy will show whether a mass or lump is cancer and from what tissue it arose. For example, cancer that originates in the breast is breast cancer whether it is in the breast or has spread to other parts of the body. For more details on how biopsies are done, read the chapter on surgery and the chapter on your particular cancer.

Staging: How Extensive Is the Cancer?

After the diagnosis of cancer is made, your doctor needs to know if the disease has spread. This is called "staging the cancer," and it is important because treatment depends upon the stage of the cancer. Surgery, radiation, or both together are used to treat localized and possibly curable cancers. Cancers that are widespread cannot be cured this way. Chemotherapy is the mainstay of treatment for widespread cancers. The more accurate the staging, the more likely a person is to benefit from therapy. For example, if tests show metastases, a cancer victim can be saved from the side effects of extensive surgery or of high-dose radiation that will not help.

During staging, the doctor attempts to find out: (a) What is the local extent of the cancer? How large is it? How extensively does it invade nearby normal tissues? (b) Whether the cancer has spread to the nearby lymph glands? (c) Whether the cancer has spread to other parts of the body? Different cancers are staged differently. For example, a bone scan is done if the cancer tends to spread to bone; a chest x-ray is needed if it tends to spread to the lungs. More information about how cancers are staged is given in the specific disease chapters.

The Choice of Treatment for Cancer

After careful staging, your doctor must decide what treatment is best for you. Surgery, radiation, and chemotherapy are the three proven treatments for cancer. (Despite all the publicity it has received in magazines and newspapers, immunotherapy is still experimental and unproven.) The choice of treatment depends upon the type and stage of the cancer.

Treatment for Localized,
and Thus Potentially Curable, Cancers

Cancers that are still limited to the area in which they arose are potentially curable. Surgery, radiation, or both together are used to treat localized cancers. For some cancers, such as malignant melanoma, surgery is the treatment of choice because radiation cannot cure the cancer. We call these cancers radioresistant. Other cancers, such as Hodgkin's disease, can be treated so effectively by radiation that surgery is never used.

Many cancers can be cured by either surgery or radiation. The choice of therapy then depends upon which treatment is less toxic and which the patient prefers. For example, early cancer of the larynx (voicebox) can be cured by surgery or radiation. With surgery, speech is lost; with radiation it is not. The choice is clear. Radiation is the standard treatment for early cancer of the larynx. Likewise, early cancer of the lip can be cured with surgery or radiation. Surgery takes a few hours; radiation takes four weeks. Most people prefer surgery.

Surgery and radiation are also used together to treat localized cancers. The former is often more effective against the area where the cancer originates, while the latter can treat the cancer in the surrounding tissues and nearby lymph glands with less disfigurement.

You should read about the treatment of specific cancers in this book. We recommend asking your doctor about the place of surgery, radiation, or both for your cancer before treatment is begun.

Adjuvant Chemotherapy: Chemotherapy for "Localized" Cancers   Adjuvant chemotherapy is the use of chemotherapy in combination with surgery or radiation to treat "apparently" localized cancer. It is used when microscopic nests of cancer cells are likely to be present in distant organs. Radiation or surgery is then used to treat the visible cancer and chemotherapy is used to treat the presumptive microscopic nests of cancer cells in other parts of the body.

We know from past experience that microscopic spread to distant organs has occurred with some cancers even if all tests are normal. With these cancers, although radiation or surgery can treat the visible cancer, most people die from distant recurrences. For example, even in apparently early, localized cases of osteogenic sarcoma, only 15 percent of children are cured by surgery alone because it has already spread to the lungs.

With several childhood cancers, including Ewing's and osteogenic sarcoma, rhabdomyosarcoma, and Wilms' tumor, adjuvant chemotherapy has proven beneficial. In adult cancers it seems to be beneficial for menstruating women with breast cancer that has spread to the lymph glands. For other adult cancers, adjuvant chemotherapy is still unproven as of 1979.

Treatment for Widespread, Incurable Cancer

Chemotherapy is the mainstay of treatment for widespread cancers because it reaches all the tissues in the body. How long someone will live with widespread cancer and how well he or she will feel depend upon how fast the cancer grows and whether chemotherapy will work. Surgery and radiation also have a role in treating widespread disease—they are used to treat symptoms. For example, bone pain from cancer is treated very effectively with radiation.

The choice of chemotherapy for metastatic disease varies for each different cancer. If it can cure a person with widespread disease, high-dose toxic chemotherapy is used. For most cancers, however, chemotherapy is not curative. When chemotherapy prolongs life or merely helps control symptoms, it becomes very important to balance the benefits and the side effects. The less chemotherapy has to offer, the more the doctor and patient need to consider these side effects and the "quality of life." For more information about chemotherapy in general, read the chapter on chemotherapy. For information about the effectiveness of chemotherapy for a specific cancer, read the chapter on that cancer and ask your doctor for more information.

Who Should Be Your Doctor?

Most Americans have a family physician. This is usually a general practitioner or internist, though for some women it may be a gynecologist. Although he can help you through this trying period, he rarely has the formal training, knowledge, or experience to offer you the best cancer care. For the staging evaluation and the planning and administration of treatment, you will need cancer specialists.

The cancer specialists you need to give you good care are determined by the type of cancer you have and its stage. We make recommendations about the particular specialists you need for each cancer in the chapters on specific cancers in this book.

The doctors who specialize in cancer treatment are:

—The board-certified radiation oncologist. He or she has received formal training and is experienced in evaluating people for and giving radiation to treat cancer.

—The board-certified medical oncologist. This physician has received formal training and is experienced in evaluating people for and giving drugs to treat cancer.

—The board-certified gynecologic oncologist. The gynecologic oncologist is an expert in the treatment of cancers of the cervix, uterus, ovaries, and vagina. He or she has received formal training and is experienced in the evaluation and the surgical treatment of these cancers.

—The board-certified surgeon. The board-certified surgeon or surgical subspecialist is a well-trained general surgeon. He or she has received formal training and is experienced in surgery. However, there are not yet any formal training programs and therefore no board certification in cancer surgery. The chapter on surgery in this book helps you to evaluate your surgeon as a cancer surgeon.

More information about finding the cancer specialists you need is available in chapter 4, "Who Should Treat You? Where Should You Be Treated?," and in the specific cancer chapters.

The Team Approach

With most cancers, more than one treatment approach is feasible. For localized cancers, surgery, radiation, both together, and even chemotherapy must be considered. For widespread cancers, while chemotherapy is the accepted treatment, decisions must be made concerning the types and dosages of drugs to use. In addition, surgery and radiation play a role in the control of widespread disease.

The person with cancer is most assured of receiving the best treatment if he is seen by a team of experts. For example, a person with potentially curable cancer of the uterus or of the mouth that can be treated by surgery and/or radiation should be seen by a surgeon and a radiation oncologist. The patient can hear the benefits and side effects of each treatment. Then the doctors and the patient together can decide upon the best treatment. If a particular cancer is treated by surgery, radiation, and/or chemotherapy, all three specialists should see the patient.

Even if there is only one treatment used for your cancer, it pays to have more than one doctor hear about your case. For example, if you have squamous cell cancer of the lung, it can be cured only by surgery. Nevertheless, it is reassuring if your surgeon presents your case at a tumor board. Having your case reviewed by several specialists, even if there is only one accepted treatment, minimizes error. Most cancer specialists realize the advantages of not going it alone and will at least present your case to other specialists at a tumor board conference. A discussion about the benefits of a team approach to your cancer can be found in the specific disease chapters.

How to Choose a Doctor

Two chapters are included on this subject: the first (chapter 4, "Who Should Treat You? Where Should You Be Treated?") discusses the professional qualifications of physicians and the second (chapter 5, "The Doctor-Patient Relationship") deals with what type of interpersonal relationship you should expect. These chapters will allow you to assess not only your doctor's experience but whether he or she is "right" for you. Each of the disease chapters also discusses what specialists you need for a specific cancer.

SUMMARY

1. Cancer must be diagnosed by a biopsy.
2. After diagnosis, cancer must be "staged" to determine its extent.
3. Treatment is based upon the type and extent of the cancer. Accepted treatments for cancer include surgery, radiation, and chemotherapy.
4. Surgery, radiation, or both are used to eradicate and possibly cure localized cancer. Chemotherapy is used to treat widespread cancer.
5. The evaluation, planning, and administering of treatment for cancer is complex. Trained and experienced cancer specialists are needed. Your family doctor does not have the background, knowledge, or experience to offer you the best treatment. A team of specialists best assures you of receiving good care.

8

The Surgical Treatment
of Cancer

Surgery was the first effective form of treatment for cancer. About one hundred years ago, long before radiation or chemotherapy was developed, surgeons were operating upon and curing people with cancer. Since then surgical techniques, anesthesia, and postoperative care have improved, making surgery safer and easier. Very complicated operations not previously possible have become routine.

Despite the development of radiation and chemotherapy, surgery is still prominent in the treatment of cancer. It still cures more people than radiation and chemotherapy combined. In this chapter we will explain how surgery is used and we will try to give enough information to help you choose a well-trained and experienced cancer surgeon.

Surgery and the Patient with Cancer

Surgery plays several important roles in the management of cancer.

—Diagnosis: the biopsy. A biopsy is the surgical removal of a sample of tissue so that it can be examined under a microscope to determine whether a suspicious lump is malignant or benign. Whenever a physician suspects cancer, a tissue sample must be obtained. Benign lumps are usually soft and grow slowly; cancerous growths are usually hard and grow faster. However, it is impossible to be sure that a suspicious lump is benign or malignant without a biopsy. Most biopsies are performed by a surgeon. Many can be done in a doctor's office with just a local anesthesia similar to that used by dentists.

—Staging the cancer: determining the extent of the disease. The surgeon is often important in finding out how far a cancer has spread. For example, in Hodgkin's disease, an operation called an exploratory laparotomy may be done to see if Hodgkin's disease has spread to the abdomen and, if so, to which organs. Also, when a surgeon operates to remove a cancer he or she will carefully examine the nearby areas to see if it has spread. The surgeon's evaluation is often much more accurate than tests and x-rays done beforehand. For example, in half the patients with lung cancer, the surgeon will find that the cancer cannot be removed even though all tests were negative. Likewise, for many cancers in the abdomen, such as cancer of the ovary, stomach, colon, and pancreas, the surgeon can most accurately assess the extent of the disease.

—Curative surgery. Surgery still cures more people than the other two forms of treatment. It can cure cancers that are localized and have not spread to other parts of the body. The types of operation needed to cure specific cancers are discussed in the chapters on those diseases.

—Palliative surgery. Palliation means controlling symptoms, such as pain, to make a person feel better. Surgery is sometimes used to make a patient who cannot be cured feel better. For example, a tumor may be pressing upon and obstructing the bile duct (the tube that drains the bile from the liver into the small intestine), causing jaundice. Even though the cancer is incurable, the patient will feel better and live longer if the obstruction is relieved. Infection will be prevented and the jaundice will disappear.

—Preventive surgery. Surgery plays a role in the prevention of cancer. The surgeon may remove precancerous lesions, such as polyps of the colon or even an entire colon, if they are likely to become cancerous. For example, for people with severe, long-standing ulcerative colitis or familial polyposis of the colon (a hereditary disorder), the risk of developing multiple cancers of the colon is very high. Surgical removal of the colon prevents cancer and saves lives.

How to Choose a Surgeon to Treat Your Cancer

Surgery is crucial in many aspects of cancer management. It is very important that your surgeon be well trained and experienced in performing the surgical tasks outlined in the previous section. Unfortunately, it is difficult to be sure a surgeon is adequately qualified in cancer surgery. It is much easier to choose a doctor for radiation or chemotherapy. In these specialties, physicians who have had formal training and passed an examination in their respective areas can easily be identified. At the present time there are no formal cancer training programs for surgeons, no tests to assess their skills, and no board certification in surgical oncology. You can look in the directory of medical specialists to find board-certified radiation and medical oncologists but not surgical oncologists. However, you can find out if your surgeon is qualified to treat you for cancer.

The board-certified surgeon. The first step toward obtaining good surgical care is to insure that your surgeon is board certified. This means that he or she has had several years of formal training in surgery and has passed an examination that tests skills. Any physician can call himself a surgeon or any other type of specialist. The law only requires that the physician limit himself to surgery or another specialty. This is misleading but legal. Many physicians have their board certificate on the wall of their office. If your doctor does not, ask him if he is board certified. You can also find out by looking in the AMA *Directory of Physicians* or the *Directory of Medical Specialists.* These books should be in your public library or at the state or county medical society office.

The different types of surgeon. There are several different kinds of surgeon. They have been trained to treat and operate upon different areas of the body. Each surgical specialty has its own formal training program, test, and board certification. The type of surgeon you need depends upon what kind of cancer you have. The different types of surgeon are:

—The board-certified general surgeon. The general surgeon has been trained to operate on many areas of the body. He or she is qualified to do surgery for cancers of the breast, esophagus, and many of the organs of the abdomen, including the stomach, colon, rectum, and pancreas, and for malignant melanoma.

—The board-certified thoracic surgeon. A thoracic surgeon is a general surgeon with two additional years of formal training in surgery of the lungs and heart. He or she operates on cancer of the lung and the esophagus.

—The board-certified colon and rectal surgeon. This is a board-certified general surgeon with one or more years of additional training in surgery of the colon and rectum. He or she is very skilled in operating for colon and rectal cancer.

—The board-certified urologist. This specialist has had four or more years of training in diseases of the urinary tract and male sex organs. Only a urologist should operate for cancer of the kidney, bladder, prostate, and testes.

—The board-certified neurosurgeon. He or she has had five or more years of training in diseases of the brain and spinal cord. Cancers of the brain and spinal cord are treated by neurosurgeons.

—The board-certified otolaryngologist. An otolaryngologist has had four or more years of training in diseases of the mouth and throat. He or she does surgery for cancer of the mouth and throat, i.e., cancer of the lip, tongue, and larynx (voicebox). Some general surgeons may specialize in head and neck cancer surgery. (See chapter 19, "Head and Neck Cancers.")

—The board-certified orthopedic surgeon. The orthopedic surgeon has had several years of training in diseases of the bones and joints. He or she should operate for cancer arising from these two areas.

—The board-certified obstetrician-gynecologist. This specialist has had three or more years of training in obstetrics and gynecology. He or she has been trained to deliver babies and care for diseases of the female reproductive organs (the ovaries, the uterus, and the vagina). Gynecologists operate on cancers of the ovary, uterus, and vagina.

—The board-certified gynecologic oncologist. There is a formal training program and board certification for gynecologists who specialize in the treatment of cancer. This is the only formal training program of the many subspecialists in cancer surgery. The gynecologic oncologist has much more training and experience in the treatment of cancer than the obstetrician-gynecologist. (Please refer to chapter 14, "Cancers of the Female Reproductive Organs," for more information about gynecologic oncologists.)

Board certification is not enough.   The board-certified surgeon is well trained and experienced. However, the amount of training and experience in cancer surgery varies considerably. Therefore, finding a board-certified surgeon or surgical subspecialist is only the first step in finding a surgeon who is qualified to treat you for cancer. You need to find out whether he has received any training in cancer surgery, whether he has a special interest in cancer, and whether he is experienced in operating for your cancer. We recommend that you ask your surgeon the following questions:

—Is he a member of one of several societies for surgeons who have trained at cancer hospitals or who have shown ability and interest in the field of cancer? These societies are the Society of Surgical Oncology (James Ewing Society), for general surgeons; the Society of Head and Neck Surgeons, and the American Society for Head and Neck Surgeons, for otolaryngologists, plastic surgeons, and general surgeons; and the Society of Gynecologic Oncologists, for gynecologists. If your surgeon is a member of one of these societies, you can be assured that he is an experienced and respected cancer surgeon. If he isn't, ask if there are surgeons in your community who are. A minority of board-certified surgeons are members of these societies, but many medium-sized and most large cities have at least one such surgeon.

—Has he received any training at a cancer center, such as M. D. Anderson, Roswell Park, or Memorial Hospital? If he has received one or more years of training in cancer surgery at one of these hospitals, he is qualified to treat you for your cancer. Most surgeons have not taken specialized cancer training at these or other hospitals.

—How often does he operate on your type of cancer? For example, if you have breast cancer you want a surgeon who operates for breast cancer more than once every two years. In general, the more frequently your doctor does an operation, the better he will be. If your surgeon has rarely operated on your type of cancer, we recommend that you find someone else. Ask your doctor if there are other, more experienced surgeons in your community. If not, travel to a larger medical center.

—Does he present his cancer cases to a tumor board? Most larger hospitals have regular meetings (called tumor boards) where patients with cancer are discussed. Specialists in the treatment of cancer, including radiation and medical oncologists, attend these meetings. If your surgeon goes to such boards regularly and presents his cases, it should reassure you that he is truly interested in the treatment of cancer. It also shows that your surgeon feels confident enough to discuss his patients with other doctors. The more confident and competent the physician, the more open he can be with other physicians.

If your case is to be reviewed by other doctors, you will get the benefit of other specialists' training and experience. If there is a tumor board in your community and your surgeon does not attend the meetings or present his cases, we would recommend your finding a surgeon who does.

—Would he mind a second surgical opinion? In general, well-trained and confident doctors welcome a second opinion. They realize that their patients' peace of mind is very important.

—Is he referred patients from board-certified radiation and medical oncologists? If your surgeon is sent cancer patients from well-qualified cancer specialists, this is very reassuring. It means that these specialists think highly of him.

—Is the cancer you have ever treated by radiation instead of surgery, or by a combination of surgery and radiation? If so, you should ask your surgeon whether he has discussed your case with a radiation oncologist or whether he thinks you should see a radiation oncologist. If your cancer can be treated by either radiation or surgery, you should see both a surgeon and a radiation oncologist to find out the advantages and disadvantages of each treatment. Experienced cancer surgeons realize the advantage of a team approach. They will not go it alone if the treatment for your cancer isn't only surgery. They also know the importance of involving their patients in treatment decisions.

These questions should be used to guide you in assessing your surgeon's qualifications, to help you decide intelligently whether your surgeon's training, experience, and interest are adequate. We want you to get the best surgeon available to treat you for your cancer.

It is also important that you trust and like your surgeon on a "gut" level. He will be operating upon you and taking care of you after surgery. Your life will be in his hands. No matter how well trained he is, he should not operate upon you unless you feel he is right for you; you must trust him. You should not feel badly about asking for a second opinion or going to see another surgeon for treatment if you don't feel comfortable with your present physician.

Only you can decide if a doctor is right for you. If you are reading this book, you are probably the kind of person who wants to know what's happening to you. Therefore, you want a surgeon who will answer your questions and involve you to some extent in decisions about treatment. You probably do not want a surgeon who asks for blind trust. If you want to be involved in decisions about your care and your surgeon doesn't agree, you probably should find someone who is more responsive to your emotional needs.

In summary, it is important that your surgeon be well trained and experienced in the treatment of cancer. He should also fulfill some of your personal needs. (These are discussed in greater depth in chapter 5, "The Doctor-Patient Relationship.")

Cancer Diagnosis: The Biopsy

The surgeon usually first enters the picture when a family physician, gynecologist, or internist suspects cancer and the patient is referred to a surgeon for a biopsy. The tissue obtained is examined under a microscope by a pathologist, who decides whether the suspicious lesion is malignant or benign. Without a tissue sample, your doctor cannot diagnose cancer.

There are several ways to obtain a sample of tissue. The method used depends both on the size and the location of the suspected cancer. The following are the common biopsy methods:

—Excision biopsy. A suspicious lump is completely removed. This is commonly done for skin cancers and for small breast lumps.

—Incisional biopsy. A lump is only partially removed. This is done when the lump is too large to remove completely.

—Needle aspiration biopsy. A needle is inserted into a lump or cyst to obtain cells or fluid for examination under a microscope.

—Endoscopic biopsy. Endoscopy is used to obtain samples of tissues from areas that would be otherwise inaccessible without surgery. The endoscope is a light-transmitting tube that allows the physician to look at and biopsy lesions in such areas as the back of the throat, the voicebox, the esophagus, the bronchi, the stomach, the bladder, or the colon. Some of the different types of endoscopy are described briefly below. More detailed descriptions are given in the specific cancer chapters.

(a) Laryngoscopy. A laryngoscope is used to look at and biopsy the inside of the mouth and the voicebox.

(b) Bronchoscopy. A bronchoscope is passed through the mouth to look at and biopsy the bronchi, or air passages in the lungs.

(c) Esophagoscopy and gastroscopy. The esophagoscope and gastroscope are swallowed and then used to examine and biopsy the esophagus, stomach, and duodenum.

(d) Cystoscopy. A cystoscope is passed through the urethra to look at and biopsy the bladder.

(e) Sigmoidoscopy. A sigmoidoscope is used to look at and biopsy the lower colon and rectum.

(f) Colonoscopy. A colonoscope is used to check, biopsy, and even remove polyps from anywhere in the colon.

Few of these scopes are managed only by surgeons. Urologists do cystoscopies and otolaryngologists perform laryngoscopies. Most of the other tests are done by internists who specialize in doing these examinations as well as by surgeons.

Some cancers, such as cervical cancer, shed cells that can be collected and looked at under a microscope. For these cancers a surgical biopsy may not be necessary. For cancer of the cervix or lung cancer, cancer cells can be collected by a Pap smear or sputum cytology. If these samples show definite cancer, the diagnosis is established without a biopsy.

Staging: How Far Has the Cancer Spread?

After a tissue diagnosis of cancer is made, your doctor needs to find out how far the disease has spread, or, in medical jargon, "stage" the cancer. It is very important to determine whether the cancer is still localized to its original site, if it has spread to nearby lymph nodes, or if it has spread to distant parts of the body. The treatment needed depends on the stage.

There is no single treatment for a cancer. Cancers that are still localized to the original site or that have spread only to nearby lymph nodes are potentially curable. They are treated by surgery and/or radiation. The goal of treatment is to eradicate completely all cancerous cells. If this can be done, the person will be cured. Extensive surgery, high-dosage radiation, or a combination of both are used. If the cancer has spread to other parts of the body, surgery or radiation cannot cure the person, and would do more harm than good. Careful staging of the cancer, therefore, must come before any decisions about treatment. You should not have a cancer operation until nonoperative tests are done to evaluate the extent of your cancer.

The evaluation can be done by a surgeon, radiation oncologist or medical oncologist. Your doctor must be experienced enough to know what tests to do and how to assess the results. He must know how a cancer spreads to know what tests to order. For example, breast cancer may spread to the lungs or the bones. Therefore, a chest x-ray and often a bone scan are needed before surgery. Oat cell cancer of the lung spreads widely very early, so a liver scan, a bone scan, and a bone marrow biopsy are needed to assess the extent of the disease. Your physician must know how cancer behaves to know how to direct a staging evaluation.

A surgeon has a special role to play in the staging of many cancers. Often the extent of the local cancer can only be accurately assessed by the surgeon at the time of surgery. For example, when the surgeon operates to remove lung cancer, he must look very carefully to see whether in fact it is curable. Half of the time it is not, and there is no value in removing the cancer and most of the lung. Surgery is dangerous and if it cannot cure, it will only do harm. Another example is with cancer of the ovary. When a gynecologist operates for ovarian cancer, he will carefully examine the abdomen for signs of spread. What he finds at surgery determines whether radiation or chemotherapy should be given afterward.

In summary, all people with cancer need to be staged before treatment. This should be done by a well-trained and experienced surgeon, radiation oncologist, or medical oncologist. You need a doctor who knows a lot about cancer to stage you correctly. The surgeon plays a special role in the staging of cancer. Often only he can determine during surgery how far the cancer has spread. He is more accurate than tests or x-rays in assessing the extent of the cancer.

Treatment for Localized, and Thus Potentially Curable, Cancer

If a cancer has not spread to distant areas of the body, it is potentially curable. Treatment options consist of surgery, radiation, or a combination of both. The decision depends upon the size and location of the cancer. The question quite simply is, how can the cancer be completely destroyed with the fewest side effects? In some cases the answer is by surgery, in others it is by radiation, and for still others it is by combination of radiation and surgery. You can refer to the chapters on specific cancers for more detail about what kind of treatment is used to cure a particular cancer.

Since there are several treatments for localized and potentially curable cancer, it is important that you receive the best one for you. Before your surgeon operates, you should ask whether radiation or a combination of radiation and surgery are also used to treat your type of cancer. If so, ask him if he has discussed your case with a radiation oncologist. In fact, when there is more than one treatment used for a cancer, it pays to see the other specialists yourself to get their opinions. For example, if you have a cancer that is sometimes treated by surgery and sometimes by radiation, you should see both a surgeon and a radiation oncologist to hear about the benefits and side effects of each treatment.

Some cancers, such as malignant melanoma, are treated only with surgery. Others, such as Hodgkin's disease or malignant lymphoma, are always treated with radiation. However, many cancers (advanced cancer of the bladder or cancer of the prostate, the lip, the front of the tongue, and the cervix) can be treated with either surgery or radiation, and the choice to some extent should be yours. It partially depends on the size and location of the tumor, but also upon your preference. You need to decide before treatment is started. Afterward, it will be too late.

You need to ask your physician questions about treatment options. You can read about the treatment of a particular cancer in the chapter on that cancer in this book. Even if you find out that we agree with your doctor's recommendations, you will feel better if you fully understand the need and reasons for your treatment. We have seen too many patients bitter about treatment even if they have been cured. For example, we have seen several women with cancer of the breast who have had their breasts removed. Although they are probably cured, they are still bitter about the removal of their breasts. If they were able to go back in time, they would have chosen to have a lumpectomy and radiation instead of a mastectomy. They did not question their surgeons or ask to see a radiation oncologist.

Curative Surgery   Surgery for localized cancers must completely remove all cancerous cells to cure the patient. There are three important principles of curative surgery for cancer.

First, the visible cancer and a generous portion of normal tissue should be removed. Cancer often spreads microscopically beyond the area of visible cancer. If all the cancer cells are not removed, the disease will recur and the chance for cure is lost. This means that good cancer surgery involves removing normal tissue, which may be disfiguring, as in the case of head and neck or breast surgery. Cancer surgery must be extensive. As a patient, you face a choice between losing your life to cancer and accepting disfigurement from the removal of normal tissue.

Second, the cancer surgeon will attempt to remove the visible cancer, the nearby normal tissue, and the nearby lymph glands all in one piece. This is called an "en bloc" resection. The reason for it is to minimize the chance of cancer cells shedding into the wound.

Finally, nearby lymph glands are usually removed even if they are not enlarged. There is controversy about whether this is necessary. The lymph nodes are removed because although they may appear normal they can still contain nests of cancer cells. Ask your surgeon whether he intends to remove the lymph nodes draining the cancer. You can also refer to the chapters on specific cancers to find out whether lymph nodes are routinely removed with your kind of cancer.

Find out about your surgery beforehand.   Your surgeon wants to cure you. Therefore, he will probably plan a fairly extensive operation. However, you are the one who must undergo and live with the results of the surgery. You should ask your surgeon about his plans and what they mean for you. Cancer surgery is not emergency surgery; it does not have to be done in a matter of hours or even days. You have time to see another surgeon for a second opinion. If it does nothing else, a second opinion will give you more confidence in your surgeon. We find that people accept and adjust better if they understand and agree with the surgeon's plans before the operation. It does not pay to be dissatisfied and angry afterward. It is too late to change things then.

The biopsy and surgical treatment need not be done on the same day. Many surgeons have the person with possible cancer sign a dual consent form for a biopsy and surgery to remove the cancer if needed. Tissue samples obtained during surgery can be looked at very quickly by a method involving what are called frozen sections. This method allows the surgeon to do both a biopsy and definitive surgery during the same operation if the biopsy shows cancer. For example, instead of just a breast biopsy, a radical mastectomy is done if the biopsy is positive. A woman with suspected breast cancer can have a biopsy and wake up without a breast. We think people adjust better if they have had some time to think about things, to get a second opinion, and to come to terms with their cancer and the treatment needed for it. There is no proven medical benefit gained from dual consent operations unless extensive surgery is necessary to obtain a biopsy.

For some cancers, such as cancers of the mouth, throat, breast, uterus, and cervix, the decision to sign a consent for a biopsy and removal of the cancer at the same time is up to you. You do not lose your chance for cure by waiting a few days to think about things and get a second opinion. For some cancers, however, the biopsy and the treatment must be done at the same time. For example, if you have cancer in the abdomen, the surgeon may have to operate to get a biopsy, make the diagnosis, and perform definitive treatment all at the same time. You do not want to undergo two major operations to treat your cancer when one will do.

Cancer recurrence: the need to be followed closely after surgery. After surgery or radiation for cancer, you should be followed closely by your doctor. It is important to detect a recurrence of the cancer as soon as possible. Early detection and treatment of recurrent cancers offer a better chance for control or even cure.

If a cancer comes back near where it first started, the physician must decide whether it has spread. If there is no evidence for spread, every effort should be made to try again for a cure. Although cure is improbable, it is not impossible. If the cancer has spread to other areas, radical treatment for the local recurrence is not indicated. Palliative rather than curative therapy is needed.

Palliative Surgery Surgery can be used for palliation, that is, to treat symptoms and make people feel better if a cure is impossible. The aim of palliative surgery is to treat symptoms with as little discomfort as possible. No attempt is made to remove the cancer completely; the goal is to control it so that a specific problem is solved. For example, if a cancer presses on the bowel and obstructs it, the surgeon can divert the colon around the obstruction. The cancer is not removed, but the pain from the obstruction is relieved. The surgeon must always weigh the nonmonetary cost of treatment, which includes hospitalization and the time to recover from surgery, with the benefits.

It is important to have an experienced surgeon for palliative surgery. If a cancer patient is sick and has only weeks or months to live, it is difficult to decide whether surgery, radiation, chemotherapy, or no treatment is best. There are no rules about palliative surgery. A good surgeon can judiciously use surgery to help make the remaining days, weeks, or months more tolerable for the incurable cancer victim. Sometimes palliative surgery can even prolong life.

Preventive Surgery   Surgery is important in the prevention of cancer. The removal of precancerous growth saves some people from developing and possibly dying of cancer. For example, the removal of precancerous moles on the skin, areas of leukoplakia in the mouth, or polyps of the colon prevents cancer. There also are diseases that are associated with a very high risk of cancer. For example, most people with severe, late, ulcerative colitis (an inflammatory disease of the large bowel) or with familial polyposis (a genetic disease of the large bowel) develop cancer. Surgical removal of the entire colon with a colostomy is traumatic but is indicated. It saves the lives of many with these diseases of the bowel.

SUMMARY

1. Surgery has an important place in the management of cancer.

2. Surgery is usually needed to diagnose cancer and is important in seeing how far it has spread. It is used to cure cancer and to palliate those who are incurable. It even has a role in cancer prevention.

3. It is important to have a surgeon who is well trained and experienced in the management of cancer. There are no formal training programs, and thus no board certification, in cancer surgery. In order to be sure your surgeon is qualified, you must ask many questions. You must find out about his or her background and experience.

4. Before you accept any treatment, check out the alternatives. Many cancers can be treated with either surgery or radiation. It pays to find out the advantages and disadvantages of each approach for your cancer. You should play an active role in deciding what treatment you should get.

9

Radiation Treatment for Cancer

Radiation was discovered late in the nineteenth century. Scientists soon found that it could damage normal tissues. Early in this century, it was discovered that radiation could also damage and even completely destroy cancer. Radiation will affect cancer and normal tissue in varying degrees. However, damage to the cancer can be maximized and damage to normal tissues minimized by confining the radiation as much as possible to the area of the cancer.

There has been tremendous progress in radiation treatment of cancer in the past decade. This is due to several factors: (a) doctors have learned from experience how much radiation normal tissues can tolerate; (b) new machines have been developed to deliver more radiation to the tumor and less to the normal surrounding tissues, so the cancer is damaged much more than the normal tissues; and (c) doctors have learned which tumors respond well to radiation.

The old radiation machines delivered more radiation to the skin and surrounding tissues than to the tumor. People receiving radiation repeatedly got severe skin burns. This has given radiation a bad name. People who must receive radiation now remember stories about the horrors of radiation therapy. But new machines deliver much more radiation to the tumor than to the skin and other normal tissues, making the horrible burns a thing of the past. In short, with years of experience and with new radiation machines, the benefits of radiation have increased tremendously. Tumors are now treated more effectively with fewer side effects to the patient.

More than half of all cancer patients will receive radiation treatment at some time for their cancer. Some will receive radiation in an attempt to eradicate the cancer and cure them, while others will receive it for palliation or to make them feel better. Radiation alone is currently used in about one-third of patients who have localized and potentially curable cancer. The other two-thirds are treated with surgery or a combination of surgery and radiation. Radiation also plays an important role in palliation, or making the patient feel better. When the cancer is incurable, radiation can effectively control pain due to bone metastases and brain damage from brain metastases.

Radiation and surgery are both local forms of therapy used to cure localized cancers. They cannot be used to eradicate cancers that have spread to distant parts of the body. The decision to use either surgery or radiation to treat a localized, potentially curable cancer depends upon which can do the job better. This is determined by the type and size of the cancer. If both can do the job equally well, the treatment that can do the job with the fewest side effects to the patient is chosen. For other cancers the choice is clear. More and more, surgery and radiation are used together. Often, surgery is more effective in treating the site of the largest mass of cancer, while radiation can more effectively destroy nests of cancer cells that have spread to nearby tissues and lymph glands. For more information about the place of radiation and/or surgery in the treatment of a specific cancer, read the chapters on specific cancers and ask your doctor.

Principles of Radiation Therapy

We will briefly outline principles that guide the radiation oncologist in treating a cancer patient. We feel that you will more easily understand why radiation is being administered in a particular fashion if you understand these important principles.

—The higher the dosage of radiation, the greater the damage to the cancer cells and the normal cells in the surrounding tissue. Radiation dosage is usually measured in rads. High doses are usually used when the aim is to cure the person with cancer. Lower doses are used in the patient with widespread cancer, where the aim is palliation or control of symptoms such as pain.

—Radiosensitivity. The term *radiosensitivity* can be applied to a cancer in two ways. It can be used to define how much radiation is needed to kill a specific cancer. For example, if cancer A can be completely eradicated with 3,500 rads while cancer B requires 6,000 rads, we can say that cancer A is more radiosensitive than cancer B. The radiosensitivity of a cancer depends upon several factors, of which the tissue from which it arose and size are probably the most important. The larger the cancer, the more radiation is needed to eradicate or completely destroy it.

Radiosensitivity can also be defined in another, more practical way— as the relative sensitivity of a cancer and the normal surrounding tissue to radiation. A radiosensitive tumor will be destroyed by radiation that the normal surrounding tissue can tolerate, while a radioresistant tumor cannot be destroyed by the dosage of radiation that the normal surrounding tissues can tolerate. This definition is practical, since it tells the radiation oncologist whether a cancer can be effectively treated or eradicated by radiation. For example, tumors A and B can both be eradicated by 4,000 rads. Cancer A is located in an area where the normal tissues can tolerate 6,000 rads. This is a radiosensitive tumor, since it can be eradicated. We can deliver 4,000 rads, kill the cancer, and not destroy the normal tissue. Cancer B can also be eradicated with 4,000 rads, but it arose in an organ (such as the liver or the kidney) that can only tolerate 3,000 rads. Radiation cannot eradicate this cancer because the normal tissues cannot tolerate the dosage needed. Obviously, this latter definition is much more important than the former in guiding the radiation oncologist.

Physicians, including radiation oncologists, often speak of the therapeutic ratio of a treatment. This refers to the benefit versus toxicity of a treatment. The therapeutic ratio in radiation therapy is defined as the tolerance of normal tissues around the cancer compared to the quantity of radiation needed to kill the cancer. If the ratio is greater than one, then the cancer can be eradicated; if it is less than one, it cannot be. For example, if a cancer requires 5,000 rads to be destroyed completely and the normal tissues can tolerate 6,000 rads, radiation can eradicate the cancer. However, if the numbers are turned around—if the cancer needs 6,000 rads to be completely destroyed and the normal tissues can only tolerate 5,000 rads—radiation cannot eradicate the cancer and cure the patient.

—Radiocurability. The term *radiocurability* refers to the possibility or probability of curing a cancer with radiation. Radiocurable cancers are radiosensitive and are still localized to their site of origin and neighboring tissues. Some radiosensitive cancers, such as Hodgkin's disease or a small cancer of the lip or tongue, are usually radiocurable. These can be completely eradicated and usually have not spread to other parts of the body. Other radiosensitive cancers, such as Ewing's sarcoma or rhabdomyosarcoma, are rarely radiocurable. Even when these cancers appear to be localized, there are usually microscopic nests of cancer cells present in distant sites.

—Toxicity from radiation therapy. The toxicity from radiation depends upon the dosage of radiation administered, the area receiving the radiation, the size of the area being radiated, and how the person responds to the radiation (which varies considerably from person to person). Radiation oncologists know from experience what side effects to expect from a specific course of radiation. The greater the possible benefit of radiation, the more toxicity the radiation oncologist and the patient will accept. If cure is possible, many side effects are accepted. If radiation is used to control a problem in a patient who is dying of cancer, many fewer side effects are accepted. Toxicity will be discussed further later in this chapter.

—Curative radiation. When radiation is used in an attempt to cure a person with a localized cancer, high doses are administered to a fairly large area. The higher the dose administered to the visible cancer, the greater the chance of killing all the cancer cells; the larger the area radiated, the greater the chance of eradicating small nests of cancer that have spread to neighboring tissues. Therefore, if you receive radiation for a localized cancer with the aim of curing you, the radiation will be administered to a much larger area than the visible cancer.

—Palliative radiation. When radiation is used to control symptoms in a patient who has widespread disease and who is therefore incurable, low doses of radiation are used to fairly small areas. The object is to use as little radiation as possible to control the problem. It is not important to eradicate all the cancer cells in the area. For example, if the person has pain because of metastases to bone, all that is required is to control the cancer enough that the pain goes away. It is not important to kill all the cancer cells.

The Board-Certified Radiation Oncologist

Radiation plays an important role in the treatment of cancer. Decisions concerning radiation are complex. Someone must decide whether radiation should be used or not, and if so how. The planning and administration of radiation are complicated. Decisions concerning the type of machine to use, the dosage to administer, and the area to be radiated are complex. It is important that the right decisions be made. A board-certified radiation oncologist is a physician who has received three or more years of formal training in the use of radiation to treat cancer and has passed an examination in this area. Like the medical oncologist, he has been trained and is experienced in evaluating the extent of, or staging, cancers as well as in using radiation to treat them. He has also been trained to use radiation in combination with surgery and chemotherapy to best treat each patient. A board-certified radiation oncologist is the physician most qualified to evaluate you for, plan, and administer radiation for cancer.

Most physicians treating cancer patients with radiation are board-certified radiation oncologists. Still, it is important for you to be sure. Many doctors will display their board certificate on the wall of their office. If you physician does not, you should ask him if he is a board-certified radiation oncologist, or if you feel too inhibited to ask him directly, you can find out by looking in the AMA *Directory of Physicians* or in the *Directory of Medical Specialists*, copies of which are available either in your public library or in the library of the state or county medical society.

The Board-Certified Radiologist

A board-certified radiologist is a physician who has received three or more years of formal training mainly or exclusively in the use of x-rays for diagnosis: he has been trained to interpret x-rays. If he is older and was trained years ago, he may also have had some formal training in the use of radiation to treat cancer. Radiation is a new field. In the past, radiologists administered radiation for cancer. On the average, however, they had only about nine months of training in the use of radiation to treat cancer.

Some board-certified radiologists do diagnostic radiology and also administer radiation to treat cancer. These physicians have had less training than board-certified radiation oncologists, and are only doing radiation treatment for cancer part time. We do not advise your being evaluated for and given radiation by such radiologists. Chances are, they are not as expert in the use of radiation to treat cancer as board-certified radiation oncologists. There are, however, some board-certified radiologists who devote themselves exclusively to the treatment of cancer. Radiologists who belong to the American Society of Therapeutic Radiologists do radiation therapy for cancer full time. Although they have had less formal training than board-certified radiation oncologists, they have had years of experience. Many are excellent and give as good treatment as radiation oncologists. Others, however, have not kept up to date and do not offer adequate treatment for cancer. Therefore, we recommend that people be evaluated for and treated by board-certified radiation oncologists if possible. If you are being seen by a radiologist, at least be sure that he does radiation treatment for cancer full time.

The Different Types of Radiation

In this section we will describe the various machines or types of radiation that are being used to treat cancer patients.

Orthovoltage Radiation

Orthovoltage radiation was the first method used to treat cancer patients. Its main disadvantage is that because orthovoltage x-rays do not penetrate well, the skin and surrounding normal tissues receive more radiation than the tumor in the body. It is this method that, in the past, caused the severe skin burns that gave radiation a bad name. Orthovoltage radiation machines are still occasionally used for symptom relief; for example low doses of orthovoltage radiation can relieve bone pain without causing severe skin burns.

Cobalt and Linear Accelerators

These two machines deliver much more radiation to the cancer and less to the skin and normal surrounding tissues than the older orthovoltage x-ray machines. Most people with cancer are now being treated with cobalt or linear accelerator radiation.

Neutron Radiation

This is a new and still experimental form of radiation that is currently being evaluated. Neutron radiation delivers a high dose of radiation to the cancer, much like the cobalt and linear accelerator machines, but may be more effective against cancers that do not respond well to these other two machines.

Implantation of Radiation

Radiation can be administered by directly implanting radioactive material into the cancer. Seeds, capsules, wires, needles, or pins are made radioactive and then inserted into the cancer. Implants deliver a very high dose of radiation to the cancer and very little to surrounding tissues. The implants are removed after the dose of radiation is delivered. Cancers of the mouth, cervix, and uterus are often treated by implantation of radiation. Some cancers are treated with both external radiation and implants.

How Is Radiation Given?

External Radiation

The radiation oncologist will first spend time with the patient, planning the dosage and area to be radiated. The patient lies under the machine, x-rays are taken, and marks are put on the patient to outline the area to be radiated. This may take several hours. Then the person comes in (usually on weekdays) and receives radiation for a matter of minutes. Radiation is usually administered for two to six weeks, depending on the dosage given. The patient is not hospitalized unless he or she is very sick from the cancer.

Radiation by Implantation

A person must be hospitalized to receive radiation by implantation. The implants must be carefully inserted by the radiation oncologist, and the patient must be isolated from other people because he is a source of radiation and is therefore dangerous to others. That is the main reason for hospitalization. The implants are kept in for several days and then removed when the needed dosage has been administered. Depending on the area implanted, there may be pain involved. For example, if implants are made into the pelvis for advanced cancer of the cervix or uterus, the patient will feel some pain when they are put in and removed. However, for treatment of earlier stage cervical or uterine cancer or for cancer of the tongue, there is minimal discomfort from the implants.

What Can Radiation Do for You?

Radiation is used to cure people with localized cancers and to make people with widespread or incurable cancer feel better by controlling symptoms. Whether radiation is used for cure or for palliation, it should be used because it can do the job better than other methods such as surgery or chemotherapy. In each situation it is important that the patient be treated with the best method. This often involves the patient's being seen by several specialists and a decision from a team of doctors.

Curative Radiation

Radiation and surgery or both are used to cure localized cancers. The choice simply depends upon which can do the job better. The treatment that can eradicate the cancer with the least side effects should be used. Doctors know from past experience the advantages and disadvantages of using radiation, surgery, or both for various tumors. However, for many cancers doctors don't know which is better, and therefore clinical trials are in progress to evaluate different forms of treatment. (For information about the usual treatments for specific cancers, you should read the chapters on specific cancers in this book and also ask your doctor.)

Some tumors, such as malignant melanoma, are very radioresistant and so cannot be eradicated by radiation. These cancers are treated by surgery. Many cancers are radiosensitive and can be treated with either radiation or surgery. For example, early cancer of the prostate, early cancer of the breast, and small cancers of the lip or the front of the tongue can be treated by surgery or radiation. We advise seeing both a surgeon and a radiation oncologist to hear the advantages and disadvantages of each approach. The patient, with his physicians' information and advice, should decide which treatment suits him best.

In other cases, the choice is obvious. Early cancer of the larynx (voicebox) can be eradicated by surgery or radiation. With surgery, the patient must learn to speak again and has a permanent hole, or stoma, in his throat. Radiation can eradicate the cancer while preserving the person's voice and without a stoma. Obviously, radiation is the treatment of choice for early cancer of the larynx.

More and more, surgery and radiation are used together. Surgery is more effective than radiation for large areas of cancer, while radiation is often more effective to treat microscopic nests of cancer cells in the surrounding tissues or lymph glands. Combining surgery and radiation is accepted treatment for advanced cancers of the uterus, the tongue, and other areas of the mouth and throat. There are clinical trials evaluating the use of radiation and chemotherapy for other cancers, such as advanced cancer of the rectum and colon.

Consider Treatment Options Carefully before Treatment Is Started   Before you receive radiation, surgery, or both for potentially curable cancer, you should make sure you have heard the whole story. Your physician will either be a surgeon or a radiation oncologist. Ask before treatment is started whether there are other ways of treating your cancer, and if so what they are. For example, if you have a cancer of the tongue and have seen a radiation oncologist, it pays to see a surgeon. You can hear from both these specialists the advantages of their treatment and then decide with them how to be treated. Many radiation oncologists prefer to work with teams. They will have you see a surgeon and even a chemotherapist and plan therapy together. Usually the well-trained and confident specialist realizes the advantage of a team approach in the treatment of cancer. If, for example, your radiation oncologist is seeing you alone, you should ask him whether he has discussed your case with a surgeon or a group of surgeons at a tumor board. You must find this out before treatment is started.

Palliative Radiation

People with widespread and therefore incurable cancer develop many complications. Some of these problems are best treated by radiation. The aim with palliative radiation is to treat the patient with as little radiation as possible that is still effective. Just as with curative radiation, it is important to use radiation for palliation only if it can do the job better than surgery or chemotherapy. We cannot describe all the situations where radiation is used, but radiation is commonly used to control bone pain from metastases and bone metastases. For these two problems radiation often is more effective than other forms of treatment.

The Toxicity from Radiation

Early and Late Radiation Toxicity

Radiation causes damage to normal tissues. The side effects appear while radiation is being administered or soon afterward and usually are only temporary. These are referred to as the early side effects of radiation.

Radiation can also damage blood vessels. Slowly, over a period of months to years, they close off and stop giving nourishment to the tissues they supply. The organ or organs involved become damaged, and this damage is usually permanent. These are referred to as the late side effects of radiation. They occur months to several years after radiation has been completed.

Both early and late damage to normal tissues occur only in the area that receives radiation. For example, the tissues of the mouth can only be damaged if a tumor in the area of the mouth is being treated. Likewise, the kidney should only be damaged if a tumor in that area is being treated. The radiation side effects that a cancer patient worries about and experiences are therefore closely related to the area radiated, and therefore vary greatly from patient to patient. In addition, all people who receive radiation may have so-called general side effects, such as loss of appetite, fatigue, nausea, and vomiting, although these also vary somewhat, depending on the dosage and the area radiated.

Early, or Acute, Radiation Toxicity We cannot describe every side effect of radiation, but we will list the major ones that occur during or soon after radiation. The list is quite extensive and may scare you. Please remember that normal tissues can be damaged only if they are in the area near the cancer being radiated. For example, if you are receiving radiation to your leg for bone metastases, you will not suffer side effects in the lungs, stomach, or mouth. Also, there is a great variation in the degree of toxicity that patients suffer. This depends partly on the dose of radiation and how the person responds to it. Two people may receive the same radiation to the same area, and one can have serious side effects but the other not. Most patients receiving radiation feel neither completely well nor very sick.

The early side effects of radiation will be described according to the areas radiated. These are:

—Radiation to the head. People lose their hair temporarily and can develop inflammation and sores in their mouth.

—Radiation to the neck. Radiation to the neck may cause temporary irritation to the back of the throat and esophagus, making it difficult to eat.

—Radiation to the lungs. Radiation to the lungs often causes temporary irritation to them. People develop a dry cough and even some shortness of breath. This usually occurs soon after radiation is finished and usually is temporary.

—Radiation to the upper abdomen. Radiation to the upper abdomen may cause loss of appetite, nausea, and vomiting while radiation is being administered. Drugs to prevent or decrease the nausea and vomiting are often given to minimize this side effect.

—Radiation to the lower abdomen. Radiation to the lower abdomen may irritate the bowel and cause watery diarrhea and/or abdominal cramps. The bladder may also become irritated. The person may have pain on urination, frequent urination, or even some blood in the urine.

(a) The ovaries. The ovaries, situated in the lower abdomen, are sensitive to radiation. Therefore, radiation in this area to any degree will cause sterility (the inability to have a baby) and induce early menopause by interfering with the production of hormones. Women receiving radiation to the lower abdomen will commonly stop menstruating and go through the change of life no matter what their age. Ask the radiation oncologist about this before radiation is begun.

(b) The testicles. The testicles are also sensitive to radiation but are shielded since they are outside of the abdomen. However, if the testicles are radiated, the man will become sterile (unable to father children). But production of male hormone usually continues, and therefore there is no problem with impotency or sexual function.

—Radiation to the extremity. Radiation to an arm or leg usually has very few side effects. The main side effect is irritation to the skin, which occurs no matter where radiation is administered since the skin covers the whole body. Radiation to any bone or cartilage in children can interfere with growth.

—Skin toxicity. The skin overlies the whole body, so some area always receives radiation. With the new machines, much more radiation is delivered to the cancer and less to the skin. Therefore, skin damage is usually limited and not very serious. Skin exposed to radiation will become tanned or sunburnt, but usually is not damaged beyond this.

—Damage to the bone marrow. The bone marrow is where blood is made. Radiation damages bone marrow in the area being radiated; the degree of damage parallels the width of the area being treated. In an adult, blood is made mainly in the bones of the pelvis, spine, ribs, and skull. The radiation oncologist will check your blood count regularly to be sure it is not too low from the radiation. You may need a red cell transfusion if you become anemic. Infrequently, the platelets, which are vital to prevent and control bleeding, may become too low and you will require one or several platelet transfusions. Likewise, your granulocytes, which fight infection, may become very low. You may even develop an infection and have to be hospitalized. Usually this does not happen, because the radiation oncologist knows from experience how much radiation a person can tolerate. He or she checks your blood counts and stops radiation if the marrow is being damaged too much.

Generalized Toxicity, or Side Effects, from Radiation   There are some side effects from radiation that are not as closely related to the area radiated as those just described. People receiving radiation may feel tired, lose their appetite, or become nauseated and vomit. These side effects do depend somewhat upon the area and dosage used, but they can occur after radiation to almost any area. Usually radiation to the abdomen causes more of these side effects than radiation to the neck, for example, but they can occur after radiation to any part of the body.

The Late Side Effects of Radiation   Some side effects occur months or years after radiation is completed. Permanent damage to organs is not very frequent because doctors know from experience how much radiation normal tissues can tolerate and use a lower dosage. However, people's normal tissues vary in their tolerance. Therefore, the doses that are safe for most patients can cause permanent damage in some. We will not list all the problems with permanent damage except to remind you that damage occurs only to organs that have received radiation and that this permanent damage is not frequent. This permanent damage is due to the destruction of blood vessels; the organ becomes scarred and doesn't function. For example, if an area of the esophagus becomes permanently damaged, it will become narrowed and the person will have trouble swallowing food. Another example would be permanent damage to the salivary glands after radiation to the mouth, so that the patient will have to live with a dry mouth and have problems with his or her teeth, as saliva is very important in maintaining the teeth and preventing cavities. If a kidney receives too much radiation and is permanently damaged, the patient develops high blood pressure; if both kidneys are damaged, he or she can go into renal failure.

Radiation is a carcinogen. All people who receive radiation are more prone to develop cancer. No matter which area is radiated, there is a slight increase in the incidence of acute leukemia. In addition, in the area that has been radiated a tumor of the bone or soft tissues may develop.

Radiation to Bones in Children

Radiation to bones or cartilage in children will interfere with growth. This is avoided as much as possible, of course, but bones may have to be radiated to cure children of very malignant cancers. Radiation to the spine will result in a decrease in growth, so that the child will not grow to his normal height. In addition, this can cause deformities such as curvatures. Radiation to the skull may interfere with the skull development, and radiation to the mouth may interfere with the development of teeth. This is very disturbing, but most parents and older children will accept these problems if radiation can save the child's life.

SUMMARY

1. Radiation therapy, like surgery, is a local form of treatment directed to a specific area of cancer. More than half the people with cancer will receive radiation treatment.

2. Radiation, surgery, or both are used in an attempt to cure localized cancers. The treatment that does the job best should be used. At present, about one in three localized cancers is treated with radiation.

3. Radiation is also used to relieve symptoms in people with widespread, incurable cancer.

4. The board-certified radiation oncologist is a physician who has had

formal training and passed an examination assessing his competence in using radiation to treat cancer. He is the physician best qualified to evaluate you for, plan, and administer radiation therapy.

5. The toxicity with radiation varies considerably. Radiation will damage only normal tissues that receive radiation, not all tissues in the body, so most side effects occur only in the area radiated. People receiving radiation do not feel completely well; neither do most feel very ill. Usually within a month or two of the radiation, people feel completely normal again.

6. Radiation side effects are much less severe today than ten or fifteen years ago. Radiation oncologists have more experience using radiation, and new machines deliver more radiation to the cancer and less to normal tissues.

7. The benefits of modern radiation treatment far outweigh the toxicity, or side effects. Radiation cures many people and makes many others feel better.

10

Chemotherapy

THE USE OF DRUGS AGAINST CANCER

Chemotherapy, a word shortened from "chemical therapy" means the use of hormones or drugs to treat disease. Nontoxic hormones, which are natural chemicals produced by endocrine glands, selectively damage some cancers, such as breast and prostate cancer. Hormones and drugs used for chemotherapy reach all tissues of the body and are used to treat widespread cancers. In contrast, surgery and radiation are only effective as local treatments. Combinations of surgery, radiation, and chemotherapy are increasingly being used to control cancer.

Chemotherapy is a relatively new field. Only thirty years ago there were no drugs to treat cancer, and not surprisingly there were no medical oncologists (doctors who specialize in treating cancer with drugs). In 1941 Dr. Charles Huggins discovered that the female sex hormone, estrogen, could shrink prostate cancer. Pain often disappeared overnight —a minor miracle. He received the Nobel Prize for his work.

In World War II, nitrogen mustard was discovered as a by-product of the U.S. effort to develop chemical warfare agents. It was active against Hodgkin's disease. Next methotrexate, an antivitamin, was found to be effective against acute leukemia in children.

In the past twenty years there have been dramatic developments in cancer chemotherapy. Many drugs have been developed that are effective against cancer, and doctors have learned how to use them to help people with cancer. The new specialty called medical oncology was developed because, with the many new anticancer drugs, the need arose for physicians with specific training in their use.

The Board-Certified Medical Oncologist

The board-certified medical oncologist is a doctor who has been trained to direct all aspects of cancer care. He or she specializes in using chemotherapy to treat cancer. Medical oncologists receive training in internal medicine for two or three years before they take an additional two years of training in adult cancer medicine. You should be evaluated by a board-certified medical oncologist if you have widespread cancer or one of the localized cancers that are treated with chemotherapy. If you have a cancer arising from the bone marrow or lymph nodes, such as leukemia or Hodgkin's disease, you may be sent to either a board-certified hematologist or a medical oncologist. The board-certified hematologist has been trained to treat cancers that arise from the bone marrow and lymph nodes but has not received formal training in the treatment of other cancers.

Children with cancer should be evaluated and treated by a pediatric oncologist. A pediatric oncologist has received training both in pediatrics and in cancer chemotherapy for children. He or she is the pediatric equivalent of a medical oncologist.

The board-certified medical oncologist and pediatric oncologist are more than just experts in the use of anticancer drugs; they are trained in all aspects of the care of the person with cancer. They are familiar with how to test for spread of cancers and how to deal with problems such as pain, lack of appetite, depression, and the other emotional responses to cancer. They also know the local community resources that can help people with cancer, such as what the American Cancer Society offers and what home nursing, financial, transportation, and psychological services are available.

A board-certified medical or pediatric oncologist should evaluate people with cancer who need chemotherapy. If chemotherapy is toxic or complicated, it should be given by the oncologist. If it is simple it can be given by a family physician, internist, or pediatrician.

If the oncologist gives the chemotherapy himself, he, in fact, becomes your primary doctor. You will need not only a doctor who is an expert chemotherapist but also one who can help you through an emotionally difficult time. No doctor can fit the psychological needs of all people. Therefore, neither you nor your oncologist should feel badly if he is not the right doctor for you. You need a doctor whom you trust and can talk with easily. If you are reading this book, you probably want a medical oncologist who will be open with you—one who will give you the facts and allow you to help make decisions about your treatment. Ask to be referred to another oncologist if your doctor does not fit your personal needs.

The Medical Oncologist, a Cancer Treatment Team Member

More and more cancers are treated with a combination of surgery, radiation, and chemotherapy. Surgery and/or radiation treat local areas of cancer, and chemotherapy is used to kill cancer cells that have spread to other parts of the body. When surgery was the only treatment for cancer, surgeons alone evaluated and treated people with cancer. Now, however, with three forms of treatment to choose among or use together, decisions are more complex. There is an increasing need for people with cancer to be evaluated and treated by a team of specialists.

Each of the specialists on the team knows one area best. The team approach offers the benefit of opinions from several experts. There is less chance for error, since different treatment approaches are carefully considered. Finally, as explained in the chapter on surgery, it is difficult to be sure that your surgeon is qualified to treat you for cancer. However, if a surgeon is part of a team with board-certified radiation and medical oncologists, you can be more assured that he or she is qualified. These cancer specialists would not work with a surgeon who was ill trained or inexperienced in cancer surgery.

A person with cancer does need a single primary physician. A person will be sent to a surgeon, a medical oncologist, or a radiation oncologist who will be the primary doctor, but he or she may still be evaluated by a team of specialists. The chapters on specific cancers in this book indicate whether a team approach is important for a particular cancer. If your doctor seems to be going it alone but you would prefer a team approach, ask him to refer you to one of the other specialists for an opinion. This is very important if your cancer is usually treated by a team of experts. Make sure you are fully evaluated before your treatment starts.

Principles of Cancer Chemotherapy

Chemotherapy is usually given in a doctor's office. It is given by mouth, intravenously, or into a muscle; the method depends upon the drug. Chemotherapy is never painful. Only a few patients (such as those with acute leukemia or testicular cancer) need to be hospitalized to receive chemotherapy.

The length of treatment varies tremendously, depending upon the type of cancer, how well you respond, and other factors. If the drugs work well, chemotherapy is usually given for long periods of time. If you are taking chemotherapy and the cancer is growing, or "progressing," the therapy is ineffective and should be stopped or changed. People on chemotherapy whose cancer is stable (neither getting larger nor getting smaller) may be responding to treatment. However, cancers can also stop growing in the absence of therapy.

Cure is a word used cautiously by the medical oncologist. A patient with widespread cancer who receives chemotherapy is considered cured if he or she obtains a complete remission and if the cancer does not return for several years after the chemotherapy has been stopped. Different cancers return either quickly or slowly after therapy is stopped. For example, a person free of Hodgkin's disease five years after chemotherapy is probably cured. An adult in remission from acute leukemia five years after treatment may or may not be cured. A man with testicular cancer who is free of disease two years after finishing therapy is probably cured. Each cancer is different. Remember that a complete remission does not mean a cure.

There are six principles or concepts that guide the medical oncologist in planning chemotherapy. If you understand these principles, it will help you to understand how and why you are treated in a particular way.

(a) Anticancer drugs harm both normal and cancerous cells. Efforts to develop drugs that selectively attack cancer cells and leave normal cells unharmed have failed. This is not too surprising. Cancer cells have few differences from normal cells on a biochemical level.

(b) The higher the dosage, the more damage is done to both cancerous and normal cells. The medical oncologist knows from experience how much of a drug your body will tolerate. He or she also knows whether it is to your benefit to use high-dose toxic chemotherapy. If chemotherapy can either cure you or greatly prolong your life, high-dose treatment should be used, and most people accept it. For the many cancers that do not respond well to chemotherapy, high-dose toxic chemotherapy is not effective and usually does more harm than good.

(c) Anticancer drugs harm or kill more dividing cells than resting cells. Cell division is the creation of two cells from one. For a cell to divide, the chromosomes must be duplicated and many enzymes must be made. Cells undergoing division are prone to damage by anticancer drugs. In the adult, the only rapidly dividing normal cells are in the bone marrow (where blood is formed), in the lining of the gastrointestinal tract, in the hair follicles, in the testes, and in the skin. The most common side effects from chemotherapy occur in these organs and are described later.

You might guess that most cancer cells are dividing rapidly, since untreated cancer continues to grow until it kills. However, we have found that with most cancers, many cells are not dividing. Cancers that do not respond to drugs often have only a few dividing cells. The resting cancer cell is not usually harmed by anticancer drugs. In some fast-growing cancers, such as acute leukemia, Hodgkin's disease, and testicular cancer, most of the cells are dividing. Therefore, drugs work well, and can cure many people with these cancers. Unfortunately, in most of the common adult cancers only a few cells are dividing at any one time, so chemotherapy does not usually work well.

A major thrust of research in cancer chemotherapy is to develop drugs that attack nondividing cancer cells. Unfortunately, at this time there has been no major breakthrough.

(d) Larger cancers have fewer dividing cells. The larger the cancer, the fewer cancer cells are dividing. Likewise, the smaller the cancer, the more cancer cells are dividing. Since chemotherapy is more effective against dividing cells, we would expect it to work better against smaller tumors. This has been shown in mice with cancer. For example, in mice chemotherapy may be ineffective against tumors large enough to be seen or felt. But if the visible tumor is removed by surgery or treated with radiation, chemotherapy is then effective against the small nests of residual cancer cells. These animal experiments have shown the benefits of using chemotherapy after surgery or radiation and provide the experimental basis for trying similar studies in people.

(e) Chemotherapy can be used to treat residual nests of cancer cells after surgery or radiation (adjuvant chemotherapy). The surgery or radiation treats the bulk of the cancer and the chemotherapy treats any residual microscopic clusters of cancer cells. These microscopic nests of cancer cells are hoped to be dividing rapidly, and thus to be very susceptible to the drugs.

Adjuvant chemotherapy has been tested in people for about ten years. It is of proven value and is standard treatment for several childhood cancers, including Wilms' tumor, rhabdomyosarcoma, Ewing's sarcoma, and osteogenic sarcoma (see chapter 23, "Cancer in Children"). The place of adjuvant chemotherapy in the treatment of adult cancers awaits further clinical trials. Only in advanced breast cancer involving the lymph nodes have clinical trials shown the probable benefit of adjuvant chemotherapy. For cancers for which there is no effective chemotherapy, adjuvant chemotherapy will probably not work. For example, adjuvant chemotherapy will probably not be of benefit for non–oat cell lung cancer or colon cancer.

More and more people are receiving adjuvant chemotherapy after surgery or radiation in the often vain hope that it will be of help. We advise that you carefully consider not taking such therapy if you do not have a cancer that is responsive to chemotherapy. Ask your medical oncologist why he recommends therapy. Just because you have a malignant cancer is no reason to take adjuvant chemotherapy. If the drugs do not combat the cancer effectively, all they can do is cost you money and time and give you unpleasant side effects. The use of adjuvant chemotherapy for specific cancers is discussed in the specific disease chapters in this book.

(f) Chemotherapy can be given as a combination of several anticancer drugs to control a cancer more effectively. This way, damage to the cancer can be increased without increasing toxicity to normal tissues. The dosage of any one anticancer drug is limited to how much the body can tolerate. If there are two or more drugs that are effective against a cancer with different side effects, they can often be more effective together than alone. We can use the maximal dosage of each drug if the side effects are different. For example, Cytoxan, vincristine, and prednisone have different toxicities, but they are each effective against malignant lymphomas. By using the three drugs together, combination chemotherapy can attack the lymphoma more effectively, so the patient will probably live much longer.

There are only a few cancers for which combination chemotherapy has been shown to be definitely better than less toxic single drugs: acute leukemia in children and adults; malignant lymphoma, including Hodgkin's disease and non-Hodgkin's lymphomas; testicular cancer; breast cancer; oat cell lung cancer; soft tissue sarcomas; and most of the childhood cancers, including Wilms' tumor, neuroblastoma, Ewing's sarcoma, and osteogenic sarcoma.

Many oncologists recommend combination chemotherapy for cancers in which its value is very dubious. You should question your oncologist carefully about the benefits of combination chemotherapy for your particular cancer. You should also refer to the chapters on specific diseases for more information about the use of combination chemotherapy for specific cancers.

What Can Chemotherapy Do for You?

When people with cancer are faced with chemotherapy they want to know what it will do for them. How can it help and at what price? The following information summarizes chemotherapy—its triumphs, its failures, and its price. For more details about the chemotherapy of particular cancers, we refer you to the chapters on the different cancers, and we suggest you get more information from your medical oncologist. The effectiveness of chemotherapy for a particular cancer can change at any time as new drugs appear. Therefore, although most of the information in this chapter will be valid when you read it, please remember that there may be new developments. Use this information as a guide and then find out from your medical oncologist whether the treatment for your particular cancer has changed since this book was written.

Cancers That Can Be Cured with Chemotherapy

There are a small but increasing number of cancers that can be cured by chemotherapy. Most require high-dose combination chemotherapy that is toxic and difficult to give. If you have a cancer that can be cured with chemotherapy, you need the best possible treatment and should be treated by a board-certified medical oncologist. If your child has a curable cancer, he or she should see a pediatric oncologist. A board-certified hematologist can treat you if you have a leukemia or lymphoma. It pays to be treated by a well-trained and experienced specialist; otherwise, you will decrease or lose your chance for cure. If you have a curable cancer and need chemotherapy, you should at least travel to a community that has a board-certified specialist in cancer chemotherapy.

At this time, the following cancers, even though widespread, may be cured by chemotherapy: malignant lymphomas, including Hodgkin's disease and non-Hodgkin's lymphoma; acute lymphatic leukemia in children; testicular cancer; choriocarcinoma in women; and several childhood tumors. In addition, a few women with ovarian cancer and adults with acute nonlymphocytic leukemia are cured by chemotherapy. By the time you read this book, we hope that more cancers will be added to this list.

Doctors approach cancers that can be cured aggressively and try to give as much chemotherapy as a person can tolerate. This means the person will get sick from the therapy. He or she may even need hospitalization to treat complications such as infection or bleeding. Most people accept these side effects when drugs can offer a chance for cure. It's quite simple. If chemotherapy can save your life, you will probably be willing to face many unpleasant side effects. Aggressive chemotherapy is usually given for not more than one year. For a young person, one year of misery from therapy is a small price to pay for a normal life afterward.

Cancers for Which Chemotherapy Can Prolong Life and Make You Feel Better

For some cancers that chemotherapy cannot cure, it can prolong life and help people to feel better. Since cure is impossible, you and your oncologist should carefully weigh the benefits and side effects of chemotherapy. For example, it may not pay to take toxic chemotherapy for a chance to live six months longer if you will be sick much of the time from the therapy with nausea and vomiting and a sore mouth. Because the benefits of chemotherapy are less with these cancers, the side effects must be carefully considered and weighed against the benefits. The least toxic therapy that will prolong survival is given so people can enjoy their additional time. Many people fear chemotherapy. They are afraid of the severe nausea and debility. Often these problems are more related to advanced cancer than to drugs. The side effects of drugs are related to the doses and the types of drugs used. You can take chemotherapy with few or no side effects.

At the present time, chemotherapy may prolong life and help you feel better if you have one of the following cancers: cancer of the breast, prostate, thyroid, kidney, or uterus, acute leukemia in adults, multiple myeloma, oat cell cancer of the lung, cancer of the ovary, and some sarcomas. Almost all children with cancer live longer with chemotherapy. You should refer to the chapters on each of these cancers for more details and ask your doctor about what chemotherapy can offer you.

If you have one of these cancers, your chemotherapy should be planned by a medical oncologist. Then, depending on the complexity of the treatment, sometimes can be given by your family physician. For example, in acute leukemia in adults, the chemotherapy must be given by experienced specialists. In contrast, prostate and thyroid cancer can be treated with hormones that can be given by your family doctor. He or she can treat you and consult with the oncologist if problems arise.

Cancers for Which Chemotherapy Is Not Very Effective

For many of the common adult cancers, chemotherapy is not very effective—it offers only a small chance for a temporary response. For some it offers almost nothing. When the benefits of chemotherapy are so minimal, the side effects must be very carefully considered. If you have a cancer that is not known to respond well, we recommend low-dose, relatively nontoxic chemotherapy or no chemotherapy at all unless you want to try experimental therapy.

The following cancers usually do not respond well to chemotherapy: cancers of the mouth, esophagus, stomach, colon, rectum, pancreas, bladder, cervix, liver, skin, or brain, non–oat cell cancers of the lung, or malignant melanoma. Though most people with these cancers do not benefit from chemotherapy, occasional patients live longer and/or feel better. There is always the hope that you will be one of these lucky people.

What Should You Ask the Medical Oncologist about Chemotherapy for Your Cancer?

When you are being evaluated for chemotherapy by a medical on-cologist, you should find out what kind of therapy he or she is planning to give you and why. If you are reading this book, you probably want to know the facts about your cancer and the treatment you are receiving. You probably want to understand what's happening and have some con-trol over your therapy.

You should find out from the medical oncologist what chemotherapy can be expected to do for you. Can it cure you? Can it prolong your life? Can it make you feel better? For example, almost half the people with advanced Hodgkin's disease are cured with chemotherapy. But by con-trast, only rarely is a woman with ovarian cancer cured.

You should also ask about what side effects your doctor expects. This becomes very important when the aim of therapy is to make you feel better. For example, the chances of temporarily helping a person with colon cancer are only about 20 percent. You may decide to take chemo-therapy if the side effects are not severe. Answers to these questions may help you decide whether to take chemotherapy and, if so, what kind.

If you have a cancer for which chemotherapy can only temporarily make you feel better, the question concerning when you should be treated arises. If you have widespread cancer but are feeling well, should you start chemotherapy? Should you wait until you start to get sick? In the past doctors have not used chemotherapy for palliation until problems such as pain occurred. However, more and more oncologists are giving chemotherapy for progressive widespread disease in the absence of symptoms in the hope that it will help patients. However, there is no proof that this works. The disadvantage is that when people who feel well take chemotherapy, they have to go to the doctor's office and take drugs that usually have some unpleasant side effects. We think you should question the advisability of taking chemotherapy if you feel well and the aim of treatment is palliation. For cancers that respond better to chemotherapy, giving it early when the cancer is smaller and the person is in better condition is quite reasonable.

Although board-certified medical oncologists have received several years of formal training and have experience in chemotherapy, they don't all treat patients the same way. They have been trained at different centers and their personalities are different. Some medical oncologists can accept impending death better than others. In general, they will treat you the way they would want to be treated themselves. If you feel uncomfortable with your medical oncologist's approach to your cancer or with his personality, ask to see another doctor. You must trust, agree with, and be able to talk with your medical oncologist. Ask for a second opinion whenever you doubt his recommendations. Most confident, well-trained doctors welcome a second opinion. They realize that the patient's peace of mind is extremely important.

Toxicity from Chemotherapy

It is a common misconception that all patients receiving chemotherapy get very sick. Side effects of chemotherapy vary tremendously, depending upon the type and doses of drugs used, your condition, and how you respond to these drugs. For example, if you are nauseated from widespread cancer, you will probably get sicker than if you are feeling well. Also, two people in the same condition and with the same cancer can react very differently; one can get very sick and the other suffer no toxicity at all from the same treatment.

Your medical oncologist knows from experience what side effects to expect from treatment. In our experience it has been necessary to warn our patients about the expected side effects from chemotherapy, because most people fantasize worse side effects than those that actually occur. Many patients receive chemotherapy and have either no or few side effects. They are able to work and perform most or all of their normal activities while receiving chemotherapy.

Some of the more common side effects of cancer chemotherapy are described below. Remember that no one gets all these side effects. We urge you to ask your physician about what side effects you can expect. If you are to receive a single drug in low doses, he will probably tell you he expects few if any side effects. If you are to receive high-dose combination chemotherapy, as for testicular cancer, he will tell you that you will get very sick. In fact, you will be so sick that you will want to stop treatment even though the treatment may be curative.

Remember that this list is general. It does not tell you what side effects you can expect from your specific therapy.

—Decreased appetite, nausea, and vomiting. Many anticancer drugs cause loss of appetite and nausea. Your physician may give you a drug to help control the nausea and vomiting. Your appetite may be diminished for several days. The nausea and vomiting usually last for less than a day but can also persist for several days. Your doctor should warn you about this and may hospitalize you to control vomiting and prevent dehydration.

—Mucositis; sores in the mouth. Several drugs, such as methotrexate, bleomycin, Adriamycin, and Daunomycin, may cause temporary sores in the mouth.

—Diarrhea. Drugs such as 5-Fluorouracil, used for breast and colon cancer, can cause diarrhea, cramps, and bloating. However, most people taking the drugs do not have this problem.

—Hair loss. Several drugs cause temporary hair loss. Your doctor should warn you if he expects your hair to fall out. You may want to order a wig before you lose your hair. Then you will have it when you need it and it can be matched to the color of your own hair. The drugs that commonly cause hair loss are cyclophosphamide, Adriamycin, Daunomycin, and vincristine. With vincristine, hair loss can be reduced by placing a tourniquet around your head during the injections. This decreases the scalp circulation and prevents the drug from killing the hair roots.

—Bone marrow suppression. Most drugs used to treat cancer interfere with bone marrow growth. Red blood cells, platelets, and white cells are made in the marrow. Your doctor will obtain blood counts often during and after chemotherapy to check on the status of your blood. You may need transfusions of either red cells or platelets with high-dose chemotherapy.

Chemotherapy also lowers the white cell count, making a person prone to serious infections. If you are receiving chemotherapy and develop a fever or chills, you should call your doctor immediately. You could have a bacterial infection because your white blood count is low from chemotherapy. This is an emergency. Because your resistance to infection has been lowered by chemotherapy, the infection can spread very rapidly and kill you in a matter of hours. If your doctor suspects an infection, he will give you antibiotics and probably put you in the hospital. You need to be carefully observed and take intensive antibiotic treatment.

—Nerve damage. Two drugs, vincristine and vinblastine, cause nerve damage. Early damage appears as numbness of the toes or fingers. This can progress to weakness and even paralysis. Your doctor should check for this before each dose of these drugs. If you think you are getting weak or have severe constipation with these drugs, tell your doctor. He will adjust the dosage or stop the treatment until you recover.

—Fertility. Many anticancer drugs damage both the ovaries and testes. In men, the production of sperm may be decreased or cease altogether. This may be temporary or permanent. If you are a young man who still wants to father children and are being treated for a potentially curable tumor, you may want to have sperm frozen. You can then father a child after receiving chemotherapy.

Chemotherapy also damages the ovary. Women may stop ovulating and menstruating during chemotherapy. They may experience hot flashes or other signs of menopause. Damage to the ovary may be either temporary or permanent.

—Risk to future children. Anticancer drugs damage DNA, the genetic material of our cells. If the mother or father has received chemotherapy, there is at least some increased risk of having a child with a birth defect. Thus far, children of people who have received chemotherapy have not had an increased incidence of birth defects, so the risk may be small. However, the genetic damage may show up in future generations.

—Chemotherapy in the pregnant woman. Chemotherapy can damage the fetus. A fetus is most sensitive to damage in the first three months of pregnancy. We suggest therapeutic abortions for women who must receive chemotherapy in their first trimester. Chemotherapy later on may also cause damage, but normal children have been born of most mothers who received chemotherapy during the last few months of pregnancy.

—Damage to the skin and soft tissues. Several drugs are given intravenously that are very irritating if they leak out of the vein into the surrounding tissues. These drugs are actinomycin, Adriamycin, Daunomycin, vincristine, vinblastine, and nitrogen mustard. If you are receiving one of these drugs intravenously and have any pain during the injection, tell your doctor. He should stop the injection, check the intravenous site, and probably change the site. Leakage of the drugs into the soft tissues always causes a painful sore, and can often cause a severe ulcer that does not heal for months.

—Increased risk of another cancer. Many of the anticancer drugs are carcinogens—they promote the development of cancer. If you have been treated and cured of one cancer with chemotherapy, you have a slightly higher chance of developing a second cancer. But we feel that this risk is small compared to the benefit from curative chemotherapy.

—Toxic interaction with other drugs. There are many drugs that interact with chemotherapy. For example, aspirin and blood thinners, or anticoagulants, can be very dangerous if you are receiving chemotherapy. Chemotherapy can lower the number of blood platelets, whose function is to prevent and control bleeding. Aspirin and anticoagulants both can cause bleeding. If you are taking anticancer drugs, ask your doctor about the safety of other drugs you use. Do not take any new drug, including those than can be purchased in a drug store without a prescription, without first asking your oncologist.

—Other side effects. There are other side effects with individual drugs. You should ask your medical oncologist or pediatric oncologist what side effects to expect from the drugs prescribed for you or your child.

Experimental Chemotherapy:
What Does It Offer a Person with Cancer?

It is extremely difficult for both the medical oncologist and the patient to accept the grim facts when the patient is dying from cancer and there is no effective treatment. It is tempting for the physician to try high-dose chemotherapy and for the patient to ask for experimental therapy. Unfortunately, experimental treatment hurts more often than it helps unless there is a new, very promising form of therapy. We recommend that you not take experimental therapy unless your oncologist really feels that something promising is available.

Progress in cancer chemotherapy depends solely upon the use of new, unproven drugs. Experimental chemotherapy is often offered to people with cancer in this country, since there is no good treatment for many cancers and doctors are testing many new drugs. Experimental chemotherapy does offer hope. If you have a cancer for which currently available drugs do not work, or if your cancer has not responded to standard treatment, a new drug may be your only chance. However, there are risks with experimental chemotherapy. Since these are new drugs, doctors know less about their side effects and about how useful they may be.

Experimental chemotherapy is discussed in greater detail in chapter 24, "Experimental Treatment for Cancer." We explain there the possible benefits and risks of different types of experimental chemotherapy. We urge caution. Experimental therapy can help only a few people with cancer, and it can harm many.

SUMMARY

1. Chemotherapy is the use of chemicals and hormones to treat disease.

2. Chemotherapy reaches all tissues of the body. It is used to treat cancers that are widespread. In contrast, surgery and radiation are used to treat localized cancers.

3. The board-certified medical oncologist has been trained and has passed a test assessing his knowledge in the use of chemotherapy to treat adults with cancer. The board-certified pediatric oncologist has had similar training in the use of chemotherapy to treat children with cancer. The board-certified hematologist is trained and qualified only to treat cancers arising from the marrow and lymphoid tissues—malignant lymphomas, the leukemias, and multiple myeloma. The appropriate specialist should examine you, plan, and, if the treatment is complicated or toxic, actually give the drugs.

4. Chemotherapy can cure some cancers, prolong life for some cancer patients, and improve the quality of life for others. The greater the potential for benefit, the more side effects are worth tolerating. If chemotherapy can cure a cancer, it pays to try to withstand even very unpleasant side effects. If it can offer only temporary relief of symptoms, the side effects of the treatment should be carefully considered. Too many people are currently being treated with toxic chemotherapy for cancers that usually do not respond.

5. Carefully consider the benefits and risks of experimental chemotherapy if it is offered. Find out if you are to enter a phase I, II, or III trial before you take any experimental treatments. (See chapter 24, "Experimental Treatment for Cancer.")

11

Cancer "Quackery" and Other Unproven Methods of Cancer Treatment

When Caroline's parents were told that their seven-year-old daughter's abdominal lump was cancer and not just a simple infection or benign cyst, they were aghast. She had always been healthy, and still looked like a normal, active child.

Caroline and her parents were sent to a pediatric oncologist, a specialist in the treatment of childhood cancer. The pediatric oncologist examined the child and had her seen by a radiation oncologist and a pediatric surgeon. He made a series of tests to see if the tumor had spread. Then he met with her parents and explained that Caroline had a rhabdomyosarcoma, a rare and very dangerous childhood cancer that grows quickly and spreads early. For Caroline to have her cancer treated and possibly cured, she needed surgery followed by radiation to the area of the cancer. Then she would receive chemotherapy to treat the tumor cells that had spread through the bloodstream and lymphatics to other parts of the body. The doctor explained that the radiation would have short- and long-term side effects that included nausea, weakness, diarrhea, and possibly growth problems. Chemotherapy would make Caroline lose her hair and vomit for two to three days after each course. With therapy cure was possible. Without it, Caroline would die, probably within a year or two.

Caroline's parents were frightened and did not want to believe her doctor. Not only did their daughter have cancer, but the treatment recommended would make her sick and had only one chance in three of curing her. They went home to think about this horrible and terrifying situation.

One of their friends told them about a treatment not given by physicians that was simple and nontoxic and could cure any cancer. He had a relative who was told by physicians that he had terminal cancer, but he was cured by this treatment. Caroline's parents wanted an easy solution. They wanted to believe their friend. Faced with the choice between an imperfect and toxic treatment and a sure, easy cure, they did not return to the pediatric oncologist for standard treatment. Instead, they traveled to a "cancer clinic." They saw the "doctor" who had the miracle "cure." After talking to him, they readily accepted all he said. Caroline was started on a special diet and given high doses of an unknown "vitamin."

For six months Caroline felt well taking the secret medication and following a strict vegetarian diet. However, the lump got larger and Caroline became sick; her appetite became poor, she started losing weight, and she became very tired. Her parents worried and had second thoughts about the treatment they were giving their daughter. They took her back to the pediatric oncologist.

The doctor examined Caroline and then ordered a liver scan, a chest x-ray and a CAT scan. He told them that the tumor had spread to her liver and lungs and that she would die. Chemotherapy could help delay death but could not cure her. The periatric oncologist was angry. He told Caroline's parents that he had tried to contact them when they did not return for treatment and that he had even called the hospital lawyer to see if he could obtain a court order to have the child treated. The lawyer had not been anxious to get involved in such a complex issue, and the doctor had not looked into it further. Now he was sorry.

Caroline received chemotherapy and felt better for a short time, but died five months later from her cancer. Four years after her death, her parents and her doctor still feel guilty. The cancer "quack" who "treated" Caroline and took away her only chance for cure is still treating cancer patients. He is protected from the law by loopholes, by the difficulty of getting people to testify against him, and by powerful friends.

Quack treatment for cancer can be dangerous even if the treatment itself has no side effects. In Caroline's case, her one chance in three for cure was lost because her parents chose the "sure cure." Many quack treatments are without side effects; in fact, that is their appeal. But their major side effect can be an earlier than necessary death if they are used instead of a treatment that has been proven effective.

Why Do People Go to Cancer "Quacks"?

Each year more than half a million Americans discover they have cancer. The shock of having cancer, our most dread illness, provokes different actions and reactions in each of us, but panic and desperation must be an almost universal reaction to the word cancer. Cancer is frightening not only because it makes us face our own death but also because of all the real and imagined suffering associated with it. There is certainly real suffering whether a patient is cured or not. At the very least, he or she has to face a very real emotional crisis. If the patient is not cured, death may come slowly. While doctors can usually control many of the complications, such as pain, cancer deaths often involve a long period of slow decline; the person becomes weaker and more dependent on others. This is a difficult time for most people. It is easier to think of a quick, painless death from a heart attack than to face a slow decline with cancer.

People are afraid of the proven methods of cancer treatment. Cancer surgery is often mutilating. The terms *radiation* and *chemotherapy* conjure up visions of all sorts of disastrous side effects. There is certainly some truth to these fears, although cancer surgery is often not mutilating and radiation and chemotherapy for most cancers are much less toxic than imagined. Still, cancer is terrifying and difficult to face. Everyone who must face it will wish for an "easy" escape. No physician can promise a cure. At present, one of every three cancer patients in the United States is cured. That means that two of three will die from cancer.

Some people still feel that all cancers are incurable and that their doctors are lying to them to make it easier to accept the future. It is certainly simpler for people to believe they can be cured easily with a treatment that has no side effects and always works. The allure of such a promise is reflected by the many thousands of Americans who turn to cancer quackery each year. In this chapter we present our own biased and angry views about cancer "quacks," who make money off the fears of frightened and gullible people.

We define cancer quackery as the deceitful use of unproven methods to treat cancer. The treatments normally used by physicians—surgery, radiation, and chemotherapy—have been evaluated by scientific trials with patients to prove their effectiveness. There is no doubt that offering the false hope of an easy, nontoxic, but expensive "sure" cure can help relieve anxiety in cancer patients. Most people with cancer feel wonderful while taking quack treatments, since they believe they'll be cured and are taking substances without side effects. The escape is usually short-lived, however. The cancer continues to grow, and the victims become sick and return to their original physicians.

The history of false methods of cancer treatment dates back many centuries. Many fads, natural products (such as cobwebs with arsenic powder), herbal teas, special (usually vegetarian) diets, large doses of vitamins, and machines (such as the orgone box) have been sold to cancer victims over the years. While the "treatments" have changed, the sellers of these products have employed the same methods to push their wares, and typically have profited greatly from their dedication to cancer patients.

We have never seen "quackery" or other unproven treatments control a cancer. Between 10 and 20 percent of our patients try these methods. Some do so because they fear both the cancer and the treatment that we recommend. For some, orthodox treatments have not worked. Others need the illusion of a easy, 100 percent effective cure.

The Cancer Quack

Cancer quacks range from uneducated, untrained people to scientists and doctors. Quack treatments are often expensive, and many cancer quacks use their methods to get rich. A special diet and vitamin supplements may cost $1,500, and health insurance does not cover unorthodox treatments.

Although the personalities and sales pitches of cancer quacks vary, they tend to share many characteristics:

—They have unusual degrees after their names.

—They do not publish the results of their treatments in scientific or medical journals, but use testimonials from patients who state that they have been cured.

—They usually have one treatment that works for all cancers. The treatment is often the practitioner's secret, personal medicine.

—They often claim to be persecuted by the government or by doctors.

—They offer sure success with no side effects.

—They are often flamboyant, charismatic people.

—They often claim to have special tests to evaluate your cancer that are different from the tests that doctors normally use.

—They are willing to treat you without a biopsy proving you have cancer. The only way to diagnose cancer is to have some tissue removed and examined under a microscope. Many of the people "cured" by quacks only thought they had cancer. They came for treatment and are still alive and tell others they were cured of a cancer they never had.

We can all learn from the successful cancer quack. He fills a need that physicians should fill. No doubt some doctors are too scientific and don't offer enough emotional support and hope. The quack fills this gap. But even if all physicians were understanding and gave maximum support to people with cancer and to their families, the allure of the magical, easy cure would remain.

Other Unproven Treatments for Cancer

Whether an unorthodox treatment is fraudulent quackery for profit or involves the use of an unproven therapy advocated by someone who sincerely believes in it and wishes to help others, it is dangerous for the patient. The use of unproven methods of cancer treatment is rapidly increasing in the United States, while trust in many institutions, including the medical profession, is declining. The myth of the self-sacrificing and infallible doctor is rapidly fading. Some doctors may be too interested in money, some may be cold and impersonal, and all make mistakes. But we find it impossible to believe, as cancer quacks often say, that organized medicine has refused to acknowledge cancer treatments that work. When doctors get cancer, they take the same treatments they recommend.

The cancer patient hears about unproven treatments from many sources. Often acquaintances, friends, or relatives bring up the subject and talk of people who have been "cured" with these easy forms of therapy. There are many books and magazines on the subject, often in health food stores. People who believe in these unproven methods of treatment are given free publicity on television and radio. The cancer victim is bombarded with misinformation.

There are also associations committed to the use of unproven methods of cancer treatment. One of the largest is the International Association of Cancer Victims and Friends, which was founded in California in the 1960s. This organization aims to convince the public that these unproven methods of treatment are effective and to make these treatments legal. It has been successful at this in a number of states. This organization is mainly interested in Laetrile, one of the most widely used unconventional cancer treatments.

Laetrile

Laetrile is a compound made from apricot pits. It is sold under various names, including Laetrile, vitamin B_{17}, or nitriloside. The purported active ingredient is cyanide, a well-known poison, which is attached to a compound known as amygdalin. The cyanide cannot act unless it is freed from its attachment. This release of cyanide supposedly occurs only in cancer cells. Therefore, the cancer cells are poisoned with cyanide, whereas normal cells are unaffected. There is no scientific evidence that this occurs. Laetrile is certainly not a vitamin, a substance the body does not make but needs in small quantities.

In many research centers, Laetrile has been shown to be ineffective against animal cancers. Therefore, it has not been scientifically tested on humans with cancer. Still, it is dispensed in many clinics and offices in this country and in Mexico. In the experience of the cancer doctors in our clinic, no cancer patient who has taken Laetrile has improved, and no tumor has gotten any smaller. The patients' time and money are lost. In some cases, treatment that might have been effective was not used because the patient turned to Laetrile.

J.H. was sixty-seven, had retired three years earlier, and was enjoying life. Two years previously, he had had a cancer of the colon removed and had done well. He had just been told by his family doctor that his liver was getting larger and that a liver scan showed that his colon cancer had spread to his liver. His doctor sent him to a medical oncologist, who gave him some very depressing news: there was no way of removing the cancer by surgery. Chemotherapy for colon cancer was not very effective. Since J.H. still felt well, the medical oncologist recommended no treatment until he began to have symptoms from the cancer. Then J.H. could start 5-Fluorouracil, a relatively nontoxic and safe drug that might make him feel better and prolong his life. However, it could not cure him. When J.H. asked, the oncologist told him he would probably die within two years.

Although he felt well, J.H. found it impossible to live knowing the cancer was growing without receiving some treatment. He asked to see a second medical oncologist, who gave him the same advice. The second doctor, sensing J.H.'s anguish, told him he could start treatment right then, although there was no proof that this was better. J.H. was told that experimental therapy would probably just make him feel worse. There were no drugs under study that were likely to be effective against his type of cancer.

One of his friends told J.H. that there were safe, effective treatments for cancer that were not licensed in the United States but were available in Mexico and other countries. The friend said he knew of many people who were cured when regular doctors had told them they would soon die of cancer. J.H. could not resist, and he flew to Mexico to receive the miracle drug. It cost him three thousand dollars for a two-week treatment. He went alone, leaving his wife behind, since he was living on a very slim pension and they could not afford two air fares. He felt much better while at the Mexican clinic. This often happens with unconventional treatments because of the very optimistic attitude of the people who give them and because people want to believe that they can be cured.

When he returned home, J.H. still felt well but some pain had started in the right side of his abdomen. His liver was getting larger. He soon went back to his oncologist because he was starting to feel weak. He took the 5-Fluorouracil, which did not control the cancer, and he died two months later.

J.H. had taken Laetrile. It did no harm because there was no effective conventional treatment. However, he spent three thousand dollars and two weeks of his time, both of which were important to him. Health insurance, of course, will not cover unproven methods of treatment.

A.H. was a thirty-one-year-old woman with acute lymphocytic leukemia. Chemotherapy gave her a two-year remission. Then the disease recurred. Even with further treatment, she would die in the next few months. Friends told A.H. of Laetrile, and she went to Mexico with her husband for a two-week treatment. She returned very ill, in a wheelchair, and died several days later. The treatment cost two thousand dollars. Even worse, she missed spending her last two weeks with her family. Her husband, despite A.H.'s poor response to Laetrile, still believed in it because "other people looked so good" in the Mexican clinic.

A.H.'s story typifies the experience of people who have taken Laetrile. Her husband's response to Laetrile's failure shows how testimonials can be obtained. Very often, relatives, close friends, and spouses believe these treatments work even if their loved one died soon afterward. There is a feeling of being saved, much like a religious experience, at these clinics, and very few of the surviving relatives or friends ever harbor any negative feelings. We are impressed by how much good will remains after these treatments fail. Some of the people dispensing Laetrile tell patients that radiation and chemotherapy are responsible for Laetrile's failure.

One of the problems we have when our patients ask about Laetrile is that we cannot say absolutely that it does not work. We say it has not helped our patients who have tried it, but since it has not been put through a large trial in the United States, we cannot state conclusively that it does not ever work. Many people then say, "What do I have to lose? I'll try it." It is usually nontoxic. Except for the expense, if you have tried conventional treatments you really have little to lose. However, if you try Laetrile instead of treatments that can cure you or help you to live longer, you may pay with your life.

Laetrile may have some side effects. If you take it by mouth, large doses can be dangerous. People have obtained B_{17}, or Laetrile, from health food stores, have gobbled too many pills, and have died from an overdose of cyanide. Also, many physicians giving Laetrile prescribe a low-protein, low-calorie diet. Even in a normal person this can cause malnutrition. In a person with cancer, it leads to rapid deterioration.

In general, the practitioners who prescribe Laetrile are careful with the dosages. When given intravenously there is less chance of cyanide poisoning, but some of the Laetrile has been contaminated by bacteria. Therefore, you could get a bad infection from intravenous Laetrile. However, serious side effects are rare.

Why, then, if Laetrile is relatively nontoxic, is it not available in the United States? The Food and Drug Administration is charged with proving drugs to be effective before they can be licensed. Laetrile is used in other countries because they have less protection. The Food and Drug Administration has not allowed Laetrile to be manufactured or sold in the United States because it is not effective. The FDA, however, can control only those drugs that cross state lines, and the many organizations committed to unproven treatments are fighting to get Laetrile approved within states. We can see one major advantage to this: people who would take Laetrile anyhow could then get it without traveling long distances. A possible disadvantage is that more people would try it because it would be cheaper. We will have to wait to see whether legalizing Laetrile would end up being harmful.

Diet Therapy

Laetrile is probably the most popular unproven cancer treatment now, but other approaches are also used, often in conjunction with Laetrile. Special diets play a big role. Often the diet is very restrictive, and may exclude meat and other high-protein foods and include large quantities of carrot or grape juice. While natural foods are good for you, there is no evidence that any diet can make a cancer shrink. In general, these diets will not harm you unless they are so restrictive that you don't get the vitamins, calories, and protein that you need. Some vitamins, such as A and D, build up in your body and can make you sick if you take too much. Large doses of vitamins B, C, and E are probably not harmful but, again, there is no strong evidence that they work on established cancers.

Enemas

As part of the general unproven approach to cancer treatment, enemas are prescribed to clean out the bad products in the bowel. Very often, repeated enemas with strange substances such as coffee are used.

There are many more unproven approaches to cancer, but Laetrile is the current mainstay. Diet, vitamins, and enemas are supplements. Buying and preparing special foods and taking Laetrile and enemas will take up most of the day and will probably take your mind off your cancer.

From our standpoint, cancer quackery and unproven methods of treatment do not work. Therefore we do not recommend them. What you have to lose by trying unorthodox therapy depends on your situation. Cancer usually starts in one area and can be cured with surgery or radiation before it spreads. If you turn to cancer quackery when you have a small, curable cancer and then come back to the doctor after your tumor has spread, you've probably lost your chance for cure. Cancer quackery has cost you your life. If the cancer has already spread, doctors can only rarely cure you. However, chemotherapy cures some widely spread cancers, such as Hodgkin's disease, and the earlier you are treated the better your chances are. If you wait and try unproven methods of treatment and then come back months later, very sick, doctors probably will not be able to help you very much. But if you are dying of cancer and your doctors have little or no treatment to help you, turning to unconventional therapy is not as bad. It may even make you feel better because of the hope that is offered. However, unproven treatments are expensive and aren't covered by insurance.

If you have to try unorthodox treatment because you can't face not trying the "sure cure," make sure that you do not rob yourself of your only chance for cure with conventional treatments. Take the standard therapy first, or take both together. Why not have the surgery for your colon cancer (which cures half of patients) and then take Laetrile or vitamins or go on a special diet? Many doctors, although they are against quackery, will tolerate it as long as you take orthodox treatment as well.

SUMMARY

1. Conventional treatments for cancer—surgery, radiation, and chemotherapy—are imperfect. They don't always work, and they have side

effects. However, one cancer patient in three is currently being cured by these methods of treatment.

2. Cancer "quackery" is the deceitful use of unproven methods to treat cancer.

3. The lure of cancer quackery is the offer of a perfect treatment. A quack says that there is only one treatment, no matter what type of cancer you have, and it always works and is safe.

4. The cancer quack is usually in it for the money, though some really believe in their treatments.

5. If you turn to cancer quackery and have a treatable or curable cancer, it may cost you your life.

6. Laetrile, strict diets, huge doses of vitamins, cleansing enemas, and hypnosis are currently the most popular unproven treatments for cancer.

7. We have never personally seen a cancer respond to unproven treatments.

8. Unconventional therapy is expensive, as it isn't covered by medical insurance.

9. If you wish to try unorthodox treatment, our advice is to try proven treatments first, or both together. Don't lose your chance for cure.

12

Breast Cancer

While taking a shower, B.W., a sixty-one-year-old housewife, felt a lump in her left breast. She was frightened, and rather than do what she knew was necessary, she denied the lump was there. Six months later, she went to her doctor when her husband noticed the growing lump in her breast. Her doctor felt a hard mass and enlarged lymph nodes in her left armpit. He immediately referred her to a surgeon, who was sure B.W. had breast cancer because the lump was very hard.

The next day she was admitted to the hospital. Under local anesthesia the surgeon removed some tissue from the breast mass (a biopsy). As expected, it showed cancer. That evening the surgeon told B.W. and her husband she had breast cancer and he recommended a mastectomy. A series of laboratory tests showed no metastases. Three days later she had a modified radical mastectomy, and her breast and the lymph glands under the arm were removed. The cancer was four inches in diameter, and five lymph glands under the arm (axillae) contained cancer.

B.W. recovered well physically from the surgery. However, the shock of having a life-threatening illness and losing her breast left her extremely depressed and anxious. Despite an understanding and loving husband, she felt no better after she went home although she attempted to be brave and cheerful. She did not share her feelings with her husband; she felt she would get over her problems. She worried about death and what would happen to her husband. She was also ashamed of her altered physical appearance; she could not look at herself in the mirror without her clothes on. She assumed that her husband was also repulsed by her scar and she never let him see it.

B.W. saw her surgeon regularly. He examined her thoroughly, asked her how she was doing, and assured her all was well. She never told him of her anxiety and fears. She felt that he was too busy and that it was not his responsibility to do more. For two years, she was physically well, but her depression and anxiety continued. She was withdrawn, rarely saw old friends, and found little reason to go on living.

B.W. noticed increasing shortness of breath and loss of appetite. The cancer had recurred in her lungs and liver. She was referred to a medical oncologist, who treated her with anticancer drugs. Her breathing and appetite improved, and for eleven months she felt fairly well. Then the cancer began to grow again. She died four months later.

This story is repeated too often. Many women are too paralyzed by the frightening possibility that they have breast cancer to seek help early. Often a breast mass is not cancer. The lump may be benign, and ignoring it is not harmful. However, approximately 100,000 women each year develop breast cancer. "I knew it was cancer and just couldn't bear to find out" is a story doctors hear every day. If you feel a lump in your breast, you should see your doctor immediately. It may be cancer.

When B.W. first felt her lump it was already quite large. The cancer had probably already spread to other organs, and was therefore incurable. A cancerous breast lump large enough to be felt by chance has often already spread and is incurable. You should be examining your own breasts each month to detect breast cancer early, when it is still curable.

Too often, women like B.W. suffer in silence. Fear of recurrence and death are universal. The loss of a breast, an organ so emphasized in our culture, is very difficult to adjust to. After a mastectomy, many women are ashamed of their bodies, and fears of loss of sexual appeal are very common. B.W. did not seek help, nor was any really offered. Consequently, during her two years of good health, she was miserable. She was preoccupied with her fears rather than coming to terms with them. Her story is not unusual. We have seen many people who had cancer years ago and who are almost certainly cured, but who remain preoccupied with fears—of recurrence, of suffering, of death, or of loss of love because of a mastectomy.

If you are one of the millions of American women who will develop breast cancer, your story can be different. With regular examinations, breast cancer can often be diagnosed early, when the chance for cure is good. You also need not face your fears alone; there are people to help you. You must, however, take the responsibility and initiative to insure that your fate will be different from B.W.'s.

Breast Cancer Is Very Common

Breast cancer is the most common cancer in American women: approximately 100,000 develop breast cancer and 30,000 die from it each year. One of every thirteen women will develop breast cancer. This is not a disease of the elderly. Rather, it is the most common nonaccidental cause of death in American women between the ages of forty and forty-four.

Breast cancer can be cured if it hasn't spread beyond the breast. Doctors can usually eradicate all the cancer in the breast. Treatment fails mainly because the cancer has already spread beyond the breast to other parts of the body. The chances of spread increase as the cancer grows. Early detection of small breast cancers that are less likely to have spread, therefore, increases your chance for cure.

Early Diagnosis Is Possible and Can Save Your Life

It is possible to detect breast cancer early and increase your chances for cure. Three methods of early detection are widely used: monthly self-examination, periodic examinations by a physician or trained nurse, and periodic mammograms, or x-rays of the breast. These procedures allow the detection of early cancers—cancers that are more likely to be curable. We cannot overemphasize the importance of early detection. It is the best tool for fighting breast cancer successfully at present.

By age thirty-five, you should be seeing your doctor for a breast examination each year. If possible, you should see the same doctor each year. You should also begin examining your own breasts each month. At least one-half of breast cancers are discovered by women themselves. For self-examinations to be most useful, they must be done correctly. Therefore, your doctor should teach you how to look at and feel your breasts. He or she should also watch you do the self-examination to make sure you do it correctly. If you are not satisfied with the instructions you have received, the American Cancer Society in your area will refer you to a clinic to learn breast self-examination. The American Cancer Society also has a pamphlet and a film that illustrate these examinations.

If you are still menstruating, you should examine yourself seven days after your period. Your breasts change in size during the menstrual cycle and are easiest to examine at this time. If you have gone through menopause and are not menstruating, you should pick one day of the month and examine your breasts on the same day each month.

Mammography or Xerography Mammography, a special x-ray of the breast, is also useful in detecting cancers that are too small to be felt by even the most experienced doctor. It can detect cancers that are likely to be cured. However, mammography exposes the breasts to radiation, and radiation is a carcinogen—it can promote the development of cancer. Therefore, the benefits of mammography must be weighed against the risks.

At the present time, we recommend mammograms yearly for women over the age of fifty. Yearly mammograms should not be performed on a woman under fifty unless she is at high risk (because of family history, etc.). This age limitation will be lowered as new x-ray machines are built to take mammograms with less radiation exposure, thereby decreasing the risk of radiation-induced cancer. Mammograms are also indicated regardless of age if your doctor feels a suspicious breast lump. The radiation exposure from an occasional mammogram is extremely low and is not dangerous.

What Can You Do to Protect Yourself from Breast Cancer?

You should do monthly self-examinations and have yearly physical examinations by a physician or nurse by age thirty-five. Yearly mammograms should be started at age fifty. You must take the responsibility and the initiative to protect yourself by catching a breast cancer when it is still curable.

Are You More Likely to Develop Breast Cancer Than Most Women?

Some women are much more likely to develop breast cancer than others. They need greater protection and should make an even greater effort to detect breast cancer early. Women with cancer in one breast are at high risk for the development of cancer in the other breast.

Women with a family history of breast cancer are also at increased risk. For example, if your mother, sister, or aunt had breast cancer, your risk is greater. In women with a family history of it, breast cancer also occurs at a younger age. Therefore, you should begin monthly self-examinations and yearly physical examinations by age twenty-five, and begin yearly mammography by age thirty-five. The following case history illustrates the usefulness of periodic breast examinations.

A.M., a twenty-seven-year-old lawyer and mother of three, went to her doctor for her yearly Pap smear. She told him her mother had died from breast cancer at age thirty-five. Her physician said that she was more likely than the average woman to get breast cancer and periodic breast examinations were needed even though she was under thirty. He examined her breasts, which were normal, and taught her how to examine herself. For the next seven years, the examinations were normal. At age thirty-five yearly mammography was begun.

At age thirty-eight, A.M.'s mammogram showed a suspicious area in her left breast. The doctor carefully examined her but couldn't feel any lumps. A biopsy revealed a very small cancer only an eighth of an inch in diameter. Her surgeon told her she had breast cancer, but the chances for cure were excellent. Tests, including a chest x-ray, showed no metastases.

The surgeon told A.M. and her husband there were two reasonable treatment alternatives. A radical or modified radical mastectomy was the time-honored treatment. It would involve removal of her breast, the superficial muscle on her chest wall, and the lymph nodes under her armpit, and offered her an excellent chance for cure. However, she would lose her breast and would have to adjust to this major change in her appearance.

Because she had a very small cancer and the lymph glands under her armpit were not enlarged, high-dose radiation to the breast and the lymph nodes under the armpit would offer her the same chance for cure. She would also need the lymph glands removed from under her arm to see if they contained microscopic deposits of cancer. The surgeon told them that recent studies had shown that this was good treatment for small breast cancers without enlarged lymph glands. He also told them there was much less experience with this treatment than with mastectomy.

The obvious advantage with this treatment was she would not lose her breast.

A.M. and her husband thought about the two alternatives for several days and decided to see a radiation oncologist. He explained the treatment and answered their questions. She decided to have her lymph glands removed and then have radiation. The results with radiation for early breast cancer seemed as good as with mastectomy.

The lymph glands under her arm were removed by her surgeon and were free from cancer. She then had cobalt radiation to her breast and lymph glands, and radioactive needles were implanted into the cancerous area of the breast under local anesthesia. The radiation treatment took six weeks. There were some side effects. She felt tired, had soreness on swallowing, had a dry cough, and had skin irritation in the area of radiation. However, all these problems were temporary.

It is now five years since A.M.'s treatment and all is well. Both she and her husband are happy they chose radiation rather than mastectomy. Even naked, her breast appears quite normal. She is thankful her surgeon offered her a choice. Her chances of being cured are better than 95 percent and she has both her breasts.

This case illustrates three important points. (1) Periodic examinations should begin early for a person with a family history of breast cancer. A.M. developed cancer at age thirty-eight. (2) The advantages of mammography are well illustrated. A.M.'s cancer was detected when it was still too small to be felt by the doctor. Without the mammogram, it would have been diagnosed later and possibly might not have been cured. (3) Early breast cancer can be treated with high-dose radiation. A.M. was cured and did not have to lose her breast. The detection of early breast cancer, therefore, has two advantages: the chances for cure are high, and it can be treated without losing the breast.

If You Feel a Lump in Your Breast, Go See Your Doctor

Discovering a breast mass is frightening. Most breast lumps are benign, but you can't be sure. A breast lump, therefore, dictates a visit to your doctor. He should first examine your breasts. If he feels a lump in your breast, he will probably obtain a mammogram. The appearance of the lump on the mammogram helps the doctor decide what to do next. However, a negative mammogram does not mean a lump is not cancerous. Regardless of what a mammogram shows, a persistent firm lump must be biopsied. If he thinks the likelihood of cancer is high, because the lump is hard, because the mammogram is suspicious for cancer, or because you have a family history of breast cancer, he should obtain a biopsy immediately. A biopsy involves removing part of the lump, so that it can be examined under a microscope. This can be done in a physician's office with local anesthesia or in a "day surgery" unit. It is safe, takes only a few minutes, and is relatively pain free.

If your doctor strongly suspects cancer, he may prefer to do the biopsy in a hospital operating room under general anesthesia. If the biopsy, a frozen section that can be checked in a matter of minutes, shows breast cancer, he then performs a mastectomy while you are still asleep. You do not need to sign a consent form to allow your surgeon to proceed immediately with a mastectomy, the so-called "dual consent." Give the matter some thought. We feel there is no advantage to this approach over having a biopsy first and then proceeding with definitive treatment if it shows cancer. The second way will allow you a few days to adjust to the situation and to think about the treatment—to ask questions and, if you wish, to get a second opinion.

You should make the decision that seems most comfortable for you. However, it is important that you trust your surgeon and that you have the opportunity to discuss the planned operation beforehand.

If your doctor feels the breast mass is probably benign, he will examine you several times during your menstrual cycle. If the mass gets smaller or disappears, it is almost certainly not cancer, and you and your doctor can relax. However, if the lump does not get smaller, it should be biopsied. A doctor cannot be sure a persistent breast mass isn't cancer. It you have a cyst (a fluid-filled sac), he will put a needle into it and remove the fluid. If the lump then disappears it is not cancer.

Each New Breast Lump Must Be Examined by a Doctor   Breast lumps are common, and some women develop many lumps. Therefore, it is not unusual for a woman to have many biopsies in her lifetime. Each new breast lump must be checked by a doctor. Six previous negative biopsies do not exclude cancer in the seventh. The following case illustrates this very important point.

M.V., a fifty-nine-year-old housewife, had been troubled for years with breasts cysts and lumps. She had what is known as fibrocystic breast disease. Four previous biopsies had all been benign, and she was tired of repeated cancer scares and biopsies. When another lump appeared, she ignored it. Many of the others had persisted and even grown larger and weren't cancer. Unfortunately, this one was. When M.V. finally saw her doctor, it had spread and was incurable. She received various treatments, but died two years later.

It is unpleasant to have to go to your doctor repeatedly for breast lumps, but it is very necessary. Each new lump might be cancerous. Also, as you get older, you are more likely to get cancer. Therefore, you cannot assume that lumps are benign even if you have had many previously negative biopsies.

If You Are Worried about a Lump and Your Doctor Isn't, Ask to See Another Doctor   What should you do if you have a breast lump but your doctor tells you not to worry? This does not happen frequently. More often a woman will ignore or decide not to worry about a breast mass. Although your doctor is probably correct, you will continue to worry until the lump is biopsied. It is also possible that your doctor is wrong. There may be a lump that should be biopsied.

In this situation you should ask to see another doctor for a second opinion. Whenever you are not happy with your doctor's advice, you should ask to see another doctor. A second opinion is not a snub of your doctor. If he is confident and interested in you, he will understand and even help you find an expert. A second opinion can only benefit you. If both doctors agree, you will probably be reassured. If the second doctor feels a lump, the biopsy he does may show a curable breast cancer.

Treatment

A Team Approach Is Important   The treatment of breast cancer is complicated and potentially involves several doctors—a surgeon, a radiation therapist, and a medical oncologist. The initial therapy may be surgery alone, surgery and radiation, a surgical biopsy followed by radiation, or surgery with or without radiation followed by chemotherapy. Treatment decisions are based on the size of the breast lump and whether or not lymph nodes are involved, and should include consideration of the patient's preference. For these reasons, we strongly recommend that each patient be evaluated by both a surgeon experienced in breast cancer and a radiation oncologist before treatment begins. The patient should have all treatment options explained to her and should consider the benefits and drawbacks before making a decision.

Surgery   Cancer specialists are often uncertain as to the best treatment for different stages of potentially curable breast cancer, and are carefully studying treatment alternatives. One extremely critical question is whether lumpectomy and radiation, which preserves the breast, is preferable to the proven treatment—a mastectomy—for early breast cancer.

Mastectomy.   The standard operation for breast cancer is a radical or modified radical mastectomy: the breast and some of the underlying muscles are surgically removed, along with the lymph glands under the arm. Radiation is sometimes given after surgery to kill any remaining cancer in the area. For example, women with inner quadrant cancers in which some of the lymph nodes cannot be removed often receive radiation. Surgery with or without radiation is very effective in removing all cancer in the local area and will cure you if the cancer has not already spread to other parts of your body. The operation is relatively safe, but is disfiguring. Some women have swelling of their arm or some limitation of use on the side of the mastectomy.

Most American surgeons currently insist that the radical or modified mastectomy is the only acceptable treatment for curable breast cancer. However, their long-accepted view is now being questioned, both by other physicians and by nonmedical women. The popular media almost weekly quote "experts" who question the need for disfiguring surgery for early (small) breast cancers. The suggested alternative is "lumpectomy" or lumpectomy followed by radiation. This treatment will leave the patient with both her breasts. The surgeons answer that women can undergo mastectomy and still have two breasts. After mastectomy, a plastic surgeon may be able to reconstruct the breast. Material is inserted under the skin of the chest wall to form the shape of a breast and a nipple is constructed from part of the nipple from the remaining breast. Though many women are satisfied with the cosmetic results of a reconstructed breast, all would prefer having their own breast.

The major controversy currently under discussion and study is whether lumpectomy (alone or with radiation) is a reasonable alternative for women with small breast cancers.

Lumpectomy without radiation will spare your breast but may cost you your life. Lumpectomy means removing the lump or cancer with only a small amount of surrounding normal breast tissue. The breast is left intact and the lymph glands under the arm are not removed. Lumpectomy will leave a woman with two breasts. She will look normal. Unfortunately, we do not believe it to be adequate treatment for small breast cancers.

There are two problems with lumpectomy. First, breast cancers are frequently multiple in the same breast. Lumpectomy could leave a smaller cancer untreated. A bigger problem is the possibility of not treating lymph glands under the arm that contain cancer. The glands may feel normal yet still contain cancer cells. Quite simply, we cannot tell by examining a woman whether her cancer has spread to these glands. If we do not remove or irradiate them and they contain cancer, it will spread to other parts of the body and eventually prove fatal.

Lumpectomy alone may rob you of your chance for a cure. It will not reliably eradicate all the cancer in the breast or lymph glands. However, the risk of lumpectomy varies with the size of the cancer. The smaller the cancer, the greater the chance that the tumor is really localized to the breast. If you have an extremely small tumor—for example, one detected only by mammography—the chances of spread to the lymph glands are only about 5 percent. Therefore, lumpectomy will only decrease your chances for cure by about 5 percent. If, however, you have the more usual size cancer, which is one-half to one inch in diameter, you have one chance in four of having cancer in the lymph glands. Thus, a lumpectomy alone will substantially decrease your chances for cure.

Our advice is to not have a lumpectomy alone unless you have a very small tumor and also feel that the decrease in your chance for cure is more than balanced by the cosmetic effect. At the present time, simple lumpectomy is inadequate treatment for most women.

A lumpectomy with radiation is an acceptable alternative to mastectomy for small breast cancers. While lumpectomy carries the risk of leaving behind untreated cancer in the breast and the lymph glands, the combination of lumpectomy and high-dose radiation to the breast and lymph glands does not. Clinical trials have shown that lumpectomy with high-dose radiation for small breast cancers without enlarged lymph nodes under the arm is as good as a radical mastectomy. Therefore, we feel that this approach is reasonable for women with early breast cancer. Lumpectomy with radiation for breast cancer with enlarged lymph glands under the arm may also be as good as radical surgery, but is still unproven and experimental.

We do have two reservations about lumpectomy and radiation. First, you must receive the radiation from a board-certified radiation oncologist who has experience in treating breast cancer with radiation. This is a relatively new treatment for breast cancer, and not all radiation oncologists are experienced with it. You should ask the doctor about his or her training and experience. You may have to travel to another city if you want radiation instead of a mastectomy. Secondly, it is important that the lymph glands be removed by a surgeon to see if they contain cancer. If they do, you should consider taking chemotherapy. (This will be explained later in this chapter.) With these reservations, lumpectomy with radiation is good and a reasonable alternative treatment for early breast cancer.

We recommend that you ask your surgeon to send you to a radiation oncologist to discuss the advantages and disadvantages of lumpectomy and radiation if you have a small breast cancer without enlarged lymph glands. Then you should be able to make a well-informed decision about which treatment you want.

Who should be your surgeon?   You need a well-trained, board-certified surgeon who is experienced in breast cancer surgery. A doctor who has completed four years of formal training in general surgery in an approved program becomes eligible to take a test for board certification. You can find out if your surgeon is board certified by looking for his certicate on his office wall. If you do not see one, ask him if he is board certified. If you are uneasy about asking him, you can obtain this information by calling the state or county medical society or checking the AMA *Directory of Physicians* or the *Directory of Medical Specialists*, both of which are in your public library. If your surgeon is not board certified as a general surgeon, you should find another surgeon.

Once you have found a board-certified general surgeon, you should find out if he has experience in breast cancer surgery. Ask him how many mastectomies he has done. If he performs ten or more per year and you trust him and like him, you've found your surgeon. There is no need to travel to a major cancer hospital or center for a mastectomy.

Chemotherapy   *Do you need chemotherapy?* If the lymph glands under the arm are free of cancer, your chances for cure are good. However, if they contain cancer, spread to other parts of the body is probable, even if you feel well and all laboratory tests are normal. These metastases are microscopic, and they cannot be detected, even by the most sensitive tests.

Until recently, regardless of your chances for cure, nothing further was done. However, in the past several years, doctors have evaluated the effectiveness of using anticancer drugs in conjunction with surgery and radiation for several different cancers. Surgery and radiation are directed at the obvious local cancer. Chemotherapy drugs circulate throughout the body and attack the small microscopic deposits of cancer that are in other organs.

Clinical trials of chemotherapy after surgery for breast cancer have been in progress for several years. While it is too early yet to know if this approach will cure more women, we do know that it definitely delays recurrences in menstruating women with breast cancer that has spread to the lymph glands. The results in women who have gone through menopause and are no longer menstruating are unclear at present. Some studies show that chemotherapy delays recurrence and some do not.

Should you take chemotherapy after mastectomy if your lymph glands are involved with cancer?   If the cancer has spread to your lymph glands, your surgeon should refer you to a medical oncologist, a specialist in the use of drugs to treat cancer. The oncologist should discuss the pros and cons of starting anticancer drugs as soon as you recover from your operation. There are many factors to consider in making this decision. Our advice at this time is to take chemotherapy if you are still menstruating. Current studies show a decrease in the recurrence rate with chemotherapy. If you are postmenopausal, we can't make any strong recommendations, as the results of the studies are unclear. Ask your oncologist about these studies. Perhaps in the near future clinical trials will show whether chemotherapy is helpful in postmenopausal women.

Chemotherapy need not make you sick. Although we include an entire chapter on cancer chemotherapy, a few words about chemotherapy in breast cancer are called for. Although anticancer agents have many undesirable side effects, individuals vary in their response. Side effects also depend on your condition and the types of drugs used. Most people who receive chemotherapy are sick from advancing cancer. In contrast, women who take chemotherapy after mastectomy are feeling well and generally have fewer side effects. Most women can continue their normal activities. They may experience fatigue, loss of appetite, and occasional nausea and vomiting. Most do not have all these symptoms. Some do not have any noticeable side effects. Perhaps the most distressing problem is temporary hair loss. Most women will need to wear a wig during therapy and for several months afterward.

You Do Not Have to Face Breast Cancer Alone

To have cancer is to face death. Merely reassuring someone, telling her she is probably cured, will not dispel her realistic fears of death and suffering. Most patients need to recognize and share their fears if they are to deal with them effectively. The breast is also a sexual organ—one especially stressed in our society. It is unnatural for a woman not to be upset by the loss of a breast. Most fear loss of sexual appeal and loss of one's husband or boyfriend. Few if any women can face these problems alone.

Some surgeons take the time and have the ability to help women handle their fears. They should include the husband in any counseling they do. His acceptance of the woman's altered physical and sexual appearance is necessary for her to adjust and live with it.

Many physicians don't have the time or the aptitude needed to help women adjust. Fortunately, there are other alternatives. If you are religious and have a close relationship with your clergy, they may be able to help you. For some women a psychologist or psychiatrist is helpful. Occasionally, although not often, a woman can resolve her fears with the help of her friends or family without trained help. For many, however, talking with other women who have gone through the same experience is the most rewarding approach. The American Cancer Society sponsors the Reach to Recovery program. Through this program women who have had a mastectomy themselves help other women deal with their cancer. A Reach to Recovery volunteer can visit a patient only if her doctor requests it. Therefore, if you have had a mastectomy, ask your doctor to request that the American Cancer Society send a volunteer. If a relative or close friend has had a mastectomy, suggest that she ask her surgeon for a volunteer.

What Does the Reach to Recovery Volunteer Do?

The Reach to Recovery volunteer, who is always a former mastectomy patient, visits the new cancer victim while she is still in the hospital.

The volunteer is living proof that life can go on after a mastectomy. To see a woman alive and well many years after breast surgery means much more to a patient than the reassurance of a (usually male) physician. The volunteer can answer questions. She will give out a breast pad to be worn under a bra and a list of stores that sell breast prostheses and special clothes for women who have had a mastectomy. Finally, she will give out a kit that includes instructions on how to exercise the arm and shoulder to reduce swelling and improve shoulder motion and a manual that answers many questions about life after a mastectomy.

There is no need to suffer alone in silence. Most women need help to face breast cancer and live a meaningful life again. If you try to face it alone, you will probably extend the normal period of depression and anxiety. Let your doctor and your family know about your suffering and reach out for the help you need.

Metastatic Breast Cancer: You Can Live for Years with Widespread Disease

After initial treatment for breast cancer, you should see your surgeon or radiation therapist on a regular basis. Cancer recurs in 50 percent of women with breast cancer. Most relapses occur in the first two years after surgery, but cancer can recur even after five years. Only a minority of women have recurrent breast cancer in a vital organ such as the liver, do not respond to therapy, and die within months. Many women live for years with widespread breast cancer.

A Team of Experts Is Needed to Treat Metastatic Breast Cancer

The management of metastatic breast cancer is complicated. The course of the disease varies considerably, and there are several effective treatment alternatives. Hormonal alterations (either removing glands that produce female hormones or administering hormones), chemotherapy, and radiation are all used. To receive the best treatment, you need a team of specialists to consider your case individually and map out a plan of therapy that will utilize each of these treatments most effectively. We recommend that a medical oncologist, a radiation oncologist, and a surgical oncologist be involved in planning your care. The medical oncologist is an expert in the use of hormones and chemotherapy, and the radiation oncologist is an expert in the use of radiation therapy. These specialists together can best plan treatment for widespread disease.

It pays to travel to a large center where specialists are available to plan your treatment. This does not mean that all the treatment need be given by specialists. Good care can be delivered by using the experience and expertise of cancer specialists to plan therapy and having your own family doctor administer it. You can then benefit from a close personal relationship with your family doctor and also from the experience and training of cancer specialists. Your family doctor, for example, can administer hormone treatments and low-dose chemotherapy. However, if you need radiation therapy, it must be given by a radiation oncologist. More complex or toxic chemotherapy should be given by a medical oncologist.

If you have widespread breast cancer, we recommend that you ask your doctor to refer you to a medical center that has a team of cancer specialists to plan your therapy. We feel that every case deserves a team approach. It is surprising how often a different treatment decision is made after discussion with several different specialists.

S.R., a forty-three-year-old real estate agent, felt a lump in her right breast. She saw her family doctor, who sent her to a surgeon. A biopsy showed cancer, and she had a modified radical mastectomy. Unfortunately, the cancer had spread to the lymph glands. She was not referred for chemotherapy, since it was not then known to be of benefit.

S.R. felt well for four years, but then developed back pain. Bone x-rays were normal, but a bone scan showed the cancer had spread to the spine in the painful area. She was given radiation therapy to her spine, and the pain disappeared. She had no further problems for three and a half years. Then she developed pain in her hip. A bone x-ray showed bone destruction by cancer. She was again treated with radiation and had complete pain relief.

S.R. felt well for two additional years, but then she developed pain in her ribs and left arm. Her cancer had spread to several bones, and she had fluid in her left lung. Her surgeon presented her case to a tumor board, which suggested removal of her ovaries because she was still menstruating. She had the operation, and her pain and the fluid in her lung disappeared. She was well for eighteen months. During this entire period of time she missed only three weeks of work and was able to care for her family.

When she was fifty-four, eleven years after mastectomy and seven years after her first recurrence, S.R. lost her appetite, lost ten pounds in a month, and became short of breath. She had developed further metastases to her lung and bones. Her adrenal glands were surgically removed, but she did not improve. She was referred to a medical oncologist, who started her on anticancer drugs. Her appetite returned, she gained weight, and her shortness of breath improved. A chest x-ray showed tumor shrinkage. She felt well, returned to work, and received chemotherapy for sixteen months. Her only side effects were mild nausea on the day she got the shots and hair loss. Then the shortness of breath returned and an x-ray showed renewed tumor growth. She died six months later. During her last months, she again developed more bone pain. This was well controlled, first by radiation and later by oral narcotics and tranquilizers.

S.R.'s case is representative of many others we have seen. Some of our patients have lived twenty years after breast cancer recurrence and feel well most of the time. Recurrent breast cancer does not mean a quick, painful death. Doctors cannot cure women with widespread breast cancer, but they can help them have years of symptom-free life.

S.R.'s case also illustrates the complexity of modern treatment for metastatic breast cancer. At different times, she received radiation therapy, hormonal treatment (oophrectomy and adrenalectomy), and chemotherapy. There is no single best treatment for metastatic breast cancer. It needs to be individualized by experts.

SUMMARY

1. Seven percent of American women, or one in thirteen, will develop breast cancer.

2. Regular checkups for breast cancer increase your chance for cure. Women should be properly instructed to examine their own breasts. Women should start monthly self-examinations and yearly examinations by a physician or trained nurse by age thirty-five.

3. Mammography, or x-rays of the breast, should be done yearly after age fifty. You should start monthly self-examinations and yearly examinations by a physician by age twenty-five and yearly mammograms by age thirty-five if you have a family history of breast cancer. Regular examinations and mammography are indicated regardless of age if you have had one breast cancer.

4. If you feel a breast lump, go see your physician. He or she should biopsy any lump that persists longer than one menstrual cycle. If you think a lump is still present or growing and your doctor has not biopsied it, ask for a second opinion.

5. The standard treatment for breast cancer is a radical or modified radical mastectomy. You should see a board-certified general surgeon who has experience with breast cancer surgery.

6. Lumpectomy alone is inadequate treatment for breast cancer. It decreases your chance for cure. Lumpectomy with high-dose radiation to the breast and lymph glands is a reasonable alternative treatment for early breast cancer. The lymph glands under the arm should also be removed before the radiation to be sure they are not involved with cancer.

7. If you decide to have a lumpectomy and radiation, the radiation should be administered by a board-certified radiation oncologist who is trained and experienced in treating breast cancer with radiation. At present only a minority of board-certified radiation oncologists are trained and experienced in this technique, so you may have to travel to a medical center to receive adequate treatment.

8. The course of metastatic breast cancer is unpredictable, and there are many treatment alternatives. Therefore, treatment should be planned by a team of cancer specialists. A surgeon, a medical oncologist, and a radiation oncologist should be involved. Much of the treatment can be given by your family doctor in consultation with these specialists.

9. People need help to adjust to breast cancer. All cancers arouse fear of suffering and death. Breast cancer in addition arouses fear of loss of love and self-image if the breast is removed. You should not try to face these very difficult problems alone. We recommend that you ask your doctor to request the American Cancer Society to send a Reach to Recovery volunteer to see you.

10. Be sure that your surgeon sends a sample of your cancer for hormone (estrogen and progesterone) receptor determination. The results may influence your further treatment.

13

Cancers of the Gastrointestinal Tract

The digestive system of the human body is a series of hollow tubes, glands, and organs located between the mouth and the anus with the primary function of digesting food. As a group, cancers of the gastrointestinal tract (in which we include cancer of the esophagus, stomach, pancreas, colon, and liver) are extremely common, and are responsible for approximately one-quarter of the cancer deaths of men and women in this country. Approximately 175,000 Americans develop and 100,000 die of cancers of the digestive tract yearly.

The gastrointestinal tract, with the exception of the liver and pancreas, is in direct contact with the environment, and is exposed to carcinogens in the form of foods and contaminants in the foods we eat. Thus, it is not surprising that there are wide geographic variations in the incidences of gastrointestinal cancers that are probably diet related. Unfortunately, the components of the diet directly responsible for cancers of the gastrointestinal tract have not as yet been totally identified, and most information is still speculative. However, certain factors are quite clear: (a) excessive intake of alcohol is associated with cancer of the mouth, larynx, esophagus, and stomach, (b) the diet consisting of high animal fat and protein and low roughage intake unique to the Western world (including northern Europe, North America, Australia, and the Caucasian populations of countries such as South Africa) is associated with a high incidence of large bowel cancer, and (c) certain chemical carcinogens, such as vinyl chloride and contaminants of molding food called aflatoxins, cause liver cancer.

One of the areas where progress can be expected over the next decade is in defining the dietary causes of gastrointestinal cancer and altering our diets accordingly. In chapter 2, "Carcinogens in Our Environment," we make certain common-sense recommendations about diet and cancer and also refer to books that have more detailed information about diets and cancer.

CANCER OF THE ESOPHAGUS

The esophagus is a muscular tube connecting the mouth with the stomach. Regular, sequential contractions of the muscles making up the esophagus are responsible for swallowing and passing food from the mouth to the stomach. Cancer of the esophagus, almost certainly an environmentally caused cancer, is not as common in the United States as it is in some other countries, such as Japan. In societies with high incidences of esophageal cancer, such as Japan, Finland, and Iran, the disease is caused by dietary rather than genetic factors. Japanese who emigrate to the United States and adopt American-type diets do not have the high incidence of esophageal and stomach cancer observed in their native countries. The major factor predisposing to esophageal cancer in our society is alcohol abuse. Several noncancerous diseases of the esophagus can also predispose a person to develop esophageal cancer by causing chronic irritation.

If esophageal cancer can be diagnosed prior to the onset of symptoms, cure is more likely to be achieved. But testing for early esophageal cancer is useful only in a population known to have a high incidence of the disease and is unwarranted in this country. However, if you have one of the esophageal diseases that is associated with an increased incidence of esophageal cancer (Plummer-Vinson syndrome, achalasia, stricture secondary to ingestion of lye, or Barrett's esophagus), frequent examinations of your esophagus are justified. If you have one of these diseases, you may wish to discuss with your physician the benefits of yearly examinations of your esophagus by either x-rays or endoscopy.

Symptoms

Unfortunately, most people with esophageal cancer go to their physicians with large tumors that cause difficulty in swallowing. These people are rarely curable. Fewer than 5 percent will be alive five years after their diagnosis. The problem is, there are no early symptoms with esophageal cancer. Only large cancers cause the symptoms for which people see their doctor. These symptoms include weight loss and greater difficulty swallowing solid foods than liquids. In very late cases, total obstruction of the swallowing mechanism may occur and the patient may have difficulty even swallowing saliva. Occasionally, inhalation of saliva and food into the lungs causes a type of pneumonia termed aspiration pneumonia.

Diagnosis

X-rays   If cancer of the esophagus is suspected, an x-ray of the esophagus will be obtained while you are swallowing barium, a white liquid that outlines the esophagus on an x-ray. This x-ray study will show whether there are any abnormalities suspicious of cancer. If the x-rays indicate the possibility or probability of esophageal cancer, you should then be referred by your doctor to a gastroenterologist, who specializes in the diagnosis and treatment of the diseases of the gastrointestinal tract and is experienced in performing endoscopy.

Endoscopy   Endoscopy of the esophagus is performed when you are awake but lightly sedated. A throat spray is used to prevent gagging. You are asked to swallow a flexible tube about one-half inch in diameter. With this tube, the endoscopist can look at, take pictures of, and obtain small biopsies of any suspicious areas. The whole procedure takes about a half hour and can be done in a doctor's office. Although endoscopy is not a painful procedure, it can cause some gagging. However, it is safe when performed by a trained gastroenterologist.

Evaluating the Extent of the Disease

Once the diagnosis of esophageal cancer is established by a biopsy through an endoscope, the next step is to determine if the cancer has spread. Tests or procedures that your physician will order include looking down your throat and bronchial tubes with another instrument called a bronchoscope to determine if the cancer has spread to the breathing passages, and a chest x-ray, a blood test for liver function abnormalities, a liver scan, and a bone scan to determine if the cancer has spread to other organs. After these tests have been obtained, it is time to decide upon a course of treatment.

Treatment

Treatment options for esophageal cancer include surgery, radiation, a combination of both, or, as a last resort, placement of a plastic tube through the obstructed area of the esophagus. Unfortunately, the aim of therapy for the vast majority of patients with cancer of the esophagus is palliation, or relief of symptoms, rather than cure. By the time symptoms of esophageal cancer appear, the cancer is usually far advanced; that is, it has spread beyond the esophagus to lymph nodes and tissues adjacent to the esophagus or to other organs. Only about 5 percent of patients with cancer of the esophagus can be cured.

If tests show no spread beyond the esophagus, surgery or radiation can offer a chance for cure, though it is small. In any case, treatment is indicated to relieve the obstruction of the esophagus and thereby allow the patient to eat solid foods again. Treatment for esophageal cancer can be very effective in relieving symptoms.

The choice of treatment is determined by the location of the cancer. Surgery is the standard treatment if the cancer is located in the lower portion of the esophagus, and radiation is standard when the cancer is located in the upper and middle portions of the esophagus. Surgery for esophageal cancer located in the middle and upper portions is extremely difficult and has a high mortality rate even when performed by a well-trained expert surgeon. In general, we suggest radiation therapy for these cancers.

Surgery   Surgery for cancer located in the lower portion of the esophagus is technically difficult and rarely curative. However, if successful it can restore normal swallowing. If the cancer is in the lower third of the esophagus and is not too large, the surgeon will attempt to remove it and bring the stomach into the chest to connect with the remaining esophagus. If the cancer is higher, a complicated series of operations is necessary to bring a segment of the large bowel into the chest to construct a new swallowing tube. In either case, the surgeon must open both the chest and the abdomen to remove the tumor. This is a major operation, and it may take several weeks to recover. Since surgery for esophageal cancer is so difficult, it should be performed by a board-certified general surgeon who is experienced in such surgery. Be sure to ask your surgeon about his experience in operating for cancer of the esophagus. Remember that, even in the best of hands, it is a risky operation.

Radiation   When cancer is present in the middle or upper third of the esophagus, radiation therapy is the standard form of treatment. This also is seldom curative, but it can alleviate symptoms such as pain and difficulty in swallowing. Radiation therapy to the esophagus is usually given in daily treatments over four to six weeks. Side effects from radiation vary, but usually include some nausea, loss of appetite, and reddening or irritation of the skin over the area that is irradiated. Radiation should be administered by a board-certified radiation oncologist.

If there is no chance for cure because the cancer is too advanced, a third therapeutic option is to put a plastic tube through the obstructed area of the esophagus either surgically or through the mouth. This approach has the advantage of rapidly relieving symptoms or difficulty in swallowing. Dangers of tube placement include perforation of the esophagus, which usually leads to death from infection. Once the tube is in place, it is possible to eat again, and often the person can gain weight and feel stronger. Since most people with esophageal cancer die from starvation and lung infections due to an inability to swallow, life can be prolonged by up to several months if swallowing is restored using this relatively simple but dangerous procedure.

Chemotherapy Chemotherapy for cancer of the esophagus is relatively ineffective. At best 10 percent of patients will have relief from symptoms for a short period of time. Therefore, most patients either receive no chemotherapy or relatively nontoxic, low-dose chemotherapy. However, any cancer patient may benefit from chemotherapy. Physicians can only give advice based upon the odds of a particular treatment's helping a patient. They can never be completely sure that treatment will fail. The last of the three case histories in this section, that of a man (L.R.) with esophageal cancer who was helped by chemotherapy, illustrates this point.

Adequate treatment for esophageal cancer can be obtained in most middle-sized and large American cities. Well-trained, experienced surgeons and radiation oncologists are available in most areas of the country. There is no advantage in traveling to major cancer centers for treatment of esophageal cancer, since there are no promising experimental approaches at the present time.

C.H., a twenty-eight-year-old Iranian student in chemical engineering, had had difficulty swallowing solid food for several months and was referred by the student health service to a specialist in gastrointestinal diseases. He had lost twenty-five pounds but otherwise felt well. He did not smoke cigarettes and, as proscribed by his religion, did not drink alcohol. An upper gastrointestinal x-ray examination was obtained. This is an examination where you are asked to swallow a white liquid—barium—that outlines the hollow tubes of the esophagus and stomach; C.H.'s x-ray showed an obstruction above the level of the stomach. A fiberoptic endoscopy examination also showed obstruction, and biopsies taken at the site of the obstruction showed cancer. Tests done to detect spread of the cancer were all negative.

Since the cancer was in the lower third of the esophagus, C.H. was sent to a general surgeon, who performed an abdominal exploratory operation three days later. Widespread cancer involving the liver, stomach, and many lymph nodes was found. Therefore, the esophageal cancer was not removed surgically. Instead, a tube was placed through the cancer, relieving the obstruction between the esophagus and stomach, to allow him again to eat solid foods.

When his doctor told C.H. that he had cancer, that it was incurable, and that treatment was not very effective, C.H. replied that he wished to return home to Iran rather than stay in school and receive further therapy. Physicians in Iran offered him no further therapy, as his difficulty in swallowing had been relieved by the operation, and they felt that chemotherapy probably would not prolong his life.

The decision by C.H. and his physicians not to try chemotherapy was very reasonable in view of its general ineffectiveness in treating cancer of the esophagus. Three months after returning to Iran, C.H. died of progressive esophageal cancer. Although he was the youngest patient we know of with this cancer, in certain parts of the world, especially in the Middle East, it is not uncommon for the disease to afflict young people.

This case illustrates how simple placement of a tube through the obstruction will allow a person to eat solid foods again. If cure is impossible, as was the case with C.H., the tube may be preferable to radiation or surgery to relieve symptoms since it is simple and inexpensive and does not involve prolonged treatments. C.H. accepted his death and spent his remaining months with his family. Unfortunately, not many Americans can accept impending death without trying some sort of therapy. Chemotherapy is relatively ineffective for esophageal cancer, and if you try high-dose therapy, your chances of being made worse or even having your life shortened are greater than your chances for benefit.

C.F. was a forty-eight-year-old married secretary with two children who drank heavily. She developed difficulty eating, and she felt full after only small amounts of food. She belched excessively and had pain in her upper abdomen that she called indigestion. She went several times to her family physician, who examined her and eventually ordered an upper gastrointestinal x-ray. This x-ray showed a hiatus hernia (a condition where part of the stomach slips through the diaphragm into the chest and may cause some symptoms of heartburn).

C.F. continued to feel ill and was not satisfied with her physician's explanation that the hiatus hernia was causing all of her problems. She wanted a second opinion and, through a physician friend, she was sent to a specialist in the diseases of the esophagus and stomach (a gastroenterologist). The specialist decided that the quickest and easiest way to find out what was wrong was to examine the esophagus with an endoscope. A small, crusted, raised lesion of the lower esophagus was seen that on biopsy was cancer.

A series of tests, including a chest x-ray, liver function tests, and a liver and bone scan, were all normal. Therefore, C.F. underwent an operation in which the surgeon removed the lower esophagus and upper part of the stomach and connected the remaining stomach to the remaining esophagus. Microscopic examination of the cancer showed that it extended to the edges of the surgically removed specimen. When cancer cells are present at the edge of a specimen, surgery is usually not curative. Despite this, C.F. felt well. She ate normally and regained her previous weight. She and her husband decided to retire and spend the remaining time together in an isolated island home they had always wanted. After two years, C.F.'s cancer recurred. Although she was treated with chemotherapy, the cancer continued to grow and she died four months later.

When C.F. retired, she had not been able to keep her previously excellent group health insurance and was too young to qualify for Medicare. Her only option was an individual health insurance policy that specifically excluded her preexisting cancer-related health problems. Unfortunately, this is an all too common occurrence. The staggering expenses of cancer treatment and terminal care can leave the remaining members of a family with large debts to pay. C.F.'s husband had $17,000 in unpaid bills accumulated from his wife's four-month terminal illness. He had to deal not only with the death of his wife but also with the loss of his hard-earned financial reserve. (The financial impact of cancer care is discussed more fully in chapter 6, "Four Problems Common to People with Cancer.")

L.R. was a fifty-two-year-old house painter whose esophageal cancer developed from a premalignant condition called Barrett's esophagus. He had difficulty swallowing, and esophageal cancer was diagnosed by an x-ray examination and an endoscopic examination and biopsy of his esophagus. The cancer was in the upper third of his esophagus, so he was treated with radiation therapy over six weeks. L.R.'s symptoms were relieved. He felt well for eight months, continuing to work and regaining the ten pounds he had lost. His physician then noticed several lumps under the skin on his chest and scalp. A biopsy of one of these lumps showed cancer. L.R. was referred to a medical oncologist, who explained to him that chemotherapy was not very effective for esophageal cancer. Nevertheless, L.R. decided to try experimental chemotherapy because he wanted something done.

Treatment was started with high doses of an experimental drug, and within two weeks the skin tumors disappeared. Although this result was very unusual, as less than 15 percent of patients with esophageal cancer respond even to high-dose experimental chemotherapy, L.R. was one of those 15 percent. He continued to receive the experimental drug for ten months, during which time he felt well. Then he developed pain in his hip, which was found by x-ray examination to be due to the spread of his cancer. His pain was completely relieved by radiation therapy to his hip, but the cancer spread to his liver and he died two months later of liver failure.

L.R. did die of esophageal cancer, but his case illustrates what treatment can offer people. Radiation therapy relieved his obstruction and allowed him to eat normally again, and later it also relieved his bone pain. Chemotherapy controlled his cancer for almost one year. Without treatment he would have died within a few months. With therapy he lived and felt well for nearly two years.

Medical oncologists are unable to determine which patients will be helped by cancer chemotherapy. Therefore, where only a small percentage of patients will benefit from chemotherapy, as is the case with esophageal cancer, oncologists routinely offer no chemotherapy or low-dose, nontoxic chemotherapy. The odds are that high-dose, toxic therapy is more likely to harm the patient than help. But in the final analysis, you, the patient, must decide. L.R. gambled against heavy odds, took experimental chemotherapy, and gained almost a year of life.

These three cases illustrate many of the important facts about esophageal cancer, including the usual symptoms, how it is diagnosed, and the usual results with treatment. While none of the patients were cured, all were helped by treatment; treatment relieved symptoms and prolonged life in all three patients.

CANCER OF THE STOMACH

The stomach is the first portion of the gastrointestinal tract to have prolonged contact with food. Food may stay in the stomach for up to three hours normally, and longer if there are any abnormalities in stomach function. It is tempting to correlate the marked geographic differences in the incidence of stomach cancer with differences in diet. Factors in the diet that have been suggestively implicated include diets high in pickled vegetables, salted fish, abrasive food grains, and smoked meats. Some authorities have suggested that the lining of the stomach can be damaged by such irritants early in life and that cancer can result many years later.

The incidence of stomach cancer in Japan is so high that Japanese physicians have effectively instituted screening programs designed to diagnose the disease early, and Japan has a higher cure rate than other countries. Mobile vans are sent out into the communities to perform screening for stomach cancer with a technique known as fiberoptic endoscopy. Patients undergoing this procedure are given a drug to relax them and then they swallow a thin tube composed of glass fibers through which the physician can see, take pictures, and take small pieces or biopsies of any suspicious areas. Although not pleasant, this procedure is safe, and an experienced operator can perform an examination of the stomach and esophagus in about thirty minutes.

Cancer of the stomach, for totally unknown reasons, has been declining in Western societies for the past three decades, and now has an incidence only half that of twenty-five years ago. The disease occurs more often in men than in women and is usually seen between the fifth and seventh decades of life. Two predisposing factors in our society include excessive alcohol intake and a relatively rare disease called pernicious anemia that primarily affects people of Northern European descent.

A somewhat unusual course of diagnosis and treatment of stomach cancer is represented by C.R., a forty-two-year-old insurance salesman who went to his doctor for persistent, gnawing pain in his upper abdomen. The pain was somewhat relieved when he drank milk but was made worse by alcohol and spicy foods. He had never had an ulcer previously and had been in otherwise good health.

His doctor found nothing abnormal on physical examination, but a stomach x-ray showed a small (less than one inch in diameter) shallow ulcer in his stomach. (An ulcer is a hole in the wall of the stomach or duodenum.) The radiologist who interpreted the x-ray felt that C.R.'s ulcer was most likely nonmalignant. Despite the x-ray findings, C.R.'s physician felt that cancer should be excluded by endoscopy, and, surprisingly, on endoscopic examination and biopsy, a small cancer was indeed found. An operation was performed, and three-quarters of C.R.'s stomach was removed. C.R. was cured. He continues smoking and drinking to excess seven years after his cancer was removed.

C.R.'s cure with stomach cancer was fortuitous. His stomach symptoms may not even have been from his cancer but instead from a completely noncancerous gastritis from excessive drinking.

A Stomach Ulcer May Be Cancer

Stomach ulcers, unlike the more common duodenal or peptic ulcers, can be either benign or malignant. Most stomach ulcers are benign. If a stomach ulcer is found to be noncancerous, it does not become malignant. An early and thus small, malignant ulcer is virtually the only gastric cancer that can be cured. Duodenal ulcers are almost never malignant. Therefore, if you have duodenal ulcers or a gastric ulcer that is found to be noncancerous with endoscopy, you need not fear that you will get cancer.

Symptoms of stomach cancer are similar to those of duodenal ulcers and benign gastric ulcers. Usually people get a gnawing pain that often improves after eating or taking antacids. When you see your physician with symptoms such as these, he will commonly perform an upper gastrointestinal x-ray examination.

If a duodenal ulcer is found, most physicians will try diet modification, drugs, and antacid therapy. However, if a stomach ulcer is found, endoscopy should be performed. We favor this approach because: (a) treatment with antacids will often relieve the symptoms of stomach cancer and, therefore, delay the diagnosis; (b) with antacid therapy cancerous stomach ulcers may even show some healing on x-ray examination; and (c) only by endoscopy can the physician really be certain whether an ulcer of the stomach is benign or cancerous.

It is possible for an experienced endoscopist to be almost entirely certain, without surgery, that a stomach ulcer is or is not cancerous. So when you have symptoms of ulcer pain without having had previously proved peptic ulcer disease, see your doctor. Self-treatment for malignant stomach ulcers may result in significant delay, which may cost you your life. We strongly recommend that you request a referral for endoscopy if your physician tells you that you have an ulcer of your stomach. The only situation in which this may not be required is if your stomach ulcer resulted from drugs such as aspirin and heals quickly once the drug is stopped.

Unlike C.R., who was exceptionally lucky in having early symptoms of cancer, most symptoms occur quite late, and by the time they do occur, stomach cancer is usually incurable, as illustrated by the following case history.

L.N., a sixty-two-year-old heavy construction worker, had never seen a physician since childhood. He began to be troubled by a burning pain in his upper abdomen that he partially relieved for several months with antacids and milk. Eventually, when he could no longer stand the pain and was not able to sleep, he went to a doctor. By that time he felt full after eating only small amounts, had lost twenty-five pounds, and was unable to work without becoming completely exhausted.

His physician performed an upper gastrointestinal examination, which showed a very large ulcer and tumor in his stomach. The radiologist felt sure this was a stomach cancer. Laboratory tests showed no spread to other organs. Therefore, L.N. was sent to a board-certified general surgeon, who operated upon him within three days. At operation, the cancer was found to be incurable. It involved the liver as well as many lymph nodes in the region of the stomach.

After he recovered from surgery, L.N. was sent to a medical oncologist and treated with a combination of three toxic drugs. He developed severe nausea and vomiting from the chemotherapy, and continued to lose weight rapidly. The chemotherapy was stopped after six weeks because his liver continued to enlarge. He next developed severe abdominal pain that could not be controlled by pain medication. Therefore, a nerve block was performed, which controlled the pain completely. L.N. died several weeks later of widely spread stomach cancer.

Unfortunately, the case of L.N. is all too typical. Symptoms of stomach cancer are often treated with antacids by the patient himself as well as by physicians who see many patients with similar complaints who have no serious ailment. By the time the diagnosis is made, the cancer has usually spread and cure is impossible. Only 10 percent of Americans with stomach cancer are currently being cured. Ninety percent, or approximately 13,000 Americans, die yearly of stomach cancer. Also typical is the lack of response to chemotherapy even when high-dose combination chemotherapy is used. Indeed, L.N. was probably hurt by aggressive chemotherapy.

It is difficult at times not to try to control cancer with drugs, but too often we have seen people harmed by toxic chemotherapy when the chance of helping was very small. The medical oncologist can only give a cancer victim the facts, and L.N. was told that combination chemotherapy most likely would not help and might hurt him. Nevertheless, he decided to take a chance with combination chemotherapy rather than receive no chemotherapy or a relatively nontoxic drug called 5-Fluorouracil because he hoped that he would be one of the few people who would respond well.

Diagnosis

Cancer of the stomach is usually symptom free (asymptomatic) until it is quite advanced and interferes with the normal functioning of the stomach. Furthermore, symptoms often are much like those of less serious gastrointestinal illnesses and include vague abdominal discomfort, indigestion, stomach pains, loss of appetite, and fatigue. The diagnosis is often made months after symptoms appear because the same symptoms are often due to such common problems as anxiety or heartburn. If you have persistent abdominal pain, your doctor should obtain x-rays of your stomach. This involves swallowing barium, which coats the lining of the stomach so that it can be seen on x-rays. If the x-rays suggest possible cancer, you should be referred to a gastroenterologist, who will perform an endoscopy and biopsy any area that looks abnormal. If the biopsy shows that cancer is present, a few laboratory tests, including a chest x-ray and liver scan, should be obtained to determine if the cancer has spread to the lungs or liver.

Treatment

Surgery   Stomach cancer, like cancer of the esophagus, claims most of its victims, leaving only 10 percent of victims alive five years from their time of diagnosis. However, surgery, the standard treatment, can be quite effective in prolonging life and reducing symptoms and can cure cancer that is still localized to the stomach (such as C.R.'s). Surgery for cancer of the stomach is a major operation and should be performed by an experienced, board-certified general surgeon. It involves the removal of a large part or all of the stomach and nearby lymph nodes. The operation is called a radical, subtotal, or total gastrectomy. Although it is major surgery it is rarely life threatening. After your stomach is removed you may need a special diet consisting of small amounts of food high in protein and fat but low in sugar.

Radiation   Radiation for gastric cancer has no proven value except to treat local problems such as pain from metastases.

Chemotherapy   Chemotherapy is relatively ineffective against cancer of the stomach. Only 25 percent of patients will receive some benefit. Those that do respond to chemotherapy will have relief of symptoms for only a matter of months. Occasionally an individual will respond for a long period of time and will, in fact, live much longer because of chemotherapy. You have three choices when faced with chemotherapy for stomach cancer. You can decide to take nothing, to take low-dose, relatively nontoxic therapy, or to take experimental high-dose therapy, which will have many more side effects. Most oncologists will recommend and most people will choose low-dose, nontoxic therapy as the best alternative. The standard drug used is 5-Fluorouracil (5-FU). The following case illustrates an unusually good response to 5-FU.

J.S., a fifty-five-year-old executive, had stomach cancer, and spread to his liver was found during operation. After he had recovered from surgery and left the hospital, his surgeon sent him to a medical oncologist because of the metastases. The medical oncologist explained that J.S.

could either wait to receive treatment later when he developed symptoms from his cancer or take therapy in an attempt to prevent the cancer from causing problems. J.S. decided that he would take a chance and start chemotherapy as soon as possible.

He was begun on low-dose therapy with 5-FU, and he had no side effects. He was told by the oncologist that his chances for living more than one year were small due to the liver metastases. J.S. decided to move to Palm Springs, California, and continue therapy there. He did not maintain contact with his first medical oncologist. Then three years later, much to the oncologist's surprise, he received a letter from J.S. stating that he was feeling well and still taking 5-FU. Furthermore, his liver scan and liver function tests were completely normal.

Each time a patient is treated with either established or experimental therapy, the physician hopes to achieve results such as those that occurred with J.S. Unfortunately, such occurrences are very rare with stomach cancer. However, these remarkable, if rare, responses give both the physician and the patient hope. Perhaps in the future better drugs and newer methods of determining their effectiveness will enable more patients to benefit from chemotherapy.

PRIMARY CANCER OF THE LIVER (HEPATOMA)

Although primary cancer of the liver is common in some areas of the world, such as Africa and the Far East, it is quite rare in this country. The most common liver cancer is cancer metastatic from elsewhere. Many cancers from the gastrointestinal tract, lymphomas, female reproductive cancers, breast cancer, lung cancer, and testicular cancer, to name a few, commonly spread to the liver. Those cancers are discussed in other chapters. The reason for discussing primary liver cancer in this book despite its rarity is the possibility that we will be seeing increasing numbers of liver cancer due to drugs and environmental carcinogens over the next decades. We wish to alert you to the dangers of these substances.

Vinyl Chloride   The most dramatic story of carcinogen-induced liver cancer is that of vinyl chloride workers. The first evidence that vinyl chloride, a common material in plastic manufacture, might produce liver cancer in man was presented in 1970 at an international cancer congress. It has been known since 1949 that vinyl chloride caused liver disease. The *Wall Street Journal* on 24 January 1974 reported three cases of the exceptionally rare liver tumor called hemangiosarcoma among vinyl chloride workers at the B. F. Goodrich plant in Louisville, Kentucky. It is estimated that 1.5 million Americans have been exposed to polyvinyl chloride at work. Many millions also live close to these chemical plants and may have been exposed.

As with many carcinogens, the period between exposure to vinyl chloride and the development of cancer can take up to twenty years.

Thus, it is impossible to tell how many people who have been exposed to polyvinyl chloride will develop liver cancers. It seems incredible that a substance shown to be toxic to the liver as early as 1949 was allowed to be produced in a totally uncontrolled manner for twenty-five years.

Male Hormone   Certain drugs can also cause liver cancer. Synthetic male hormones (testosteronelike compounds) are some. These drugs are useful treatment for some diseases. However, they are also used as life-long therapy by people who have decided to change from female to male sex. Also, some athletes attempt to improve their muscular development and performance in athletic contests with male hormones. Many body builders, professional football players, and weight lifters use these drugs. Nearly all competitive body builders have taken male hormones. Although these hormones probably have a low risk of inducing liver cancer compared to other agents such as vinyl chloride, we believe the risk outweighs the benefits to athletes.

Oral Contraceptives   In 1973, a possible association of oral contraceptives usage and liver tumors in young women was reported. Most of the tumors were benign; however, some were definitely malignant, and most women who had malignant cancers died. Although at the present time there are only several hundred reported cases, certain factors that increase the risk of liver tumors have been identified; the longer the birth control pills were used, the more likely liver tumors are to develop; and exposure to birth control pills with the synthetic hormone mestranol increases the cancer risk.

We do not suggest that the benefits of oral contraceptives are outweighed by the very small risk of developing a liver tumor. However, oral contraceptives have many other side effects, such as hypertension, heart disease, strokes, and fluid retention, and are as yet far from the perfect birth control method. Oral contraception should be used only under a doctor's direct supervision and its use limited to those women who cannot or will not use other contraceptive methods.

Alcohol Abuse   Perhaps the most common cause of liver cancer in our society is long-term alcohol abuse. Alcoholics develop a liver disease called cirrhosis, which causes the liver to be partially replaced with fibrous tissue. A small precentage of these people, if they live long enough, develop liver cancer. Seventy percent of liver cancer in Americans is associated with cirrhosis. Liver cancer is a rare complication of alcohol abuse. There are many other more common and equally dangerous problems caused by alcohol abuse, such as tragic car accidents, cirrhosis, violent behavior, and brain and nerve damage, which should be sufficient to prevent consistent overindulgence by someone who cares about his health.

Diagnosis and Treatment

Symptoms of liver cancer are often vague and commonly include weakness, loss of appetite, abdominal fullness, and pain. The diagnosis is usually suspected because the physician feels an enlarged, hard liver. The physician will obtain liver function tests and a liver scan. Certain liver scan abnormalities, such as a single large abnormality, are very suspicious for liver cancer. The diagnosis is confirmed by a biopsy of the liver obtained by introducing a needle into the liver through the skin. This is a safe and usually painless procedure, performed in a hospital bed with only local anesthesia.

The prognosis with liver cancer is grim. The only chance for cure hinges on the remote but real possibility that the cancer is localized to one part (lobe) of the liver that can be surgically removed. If tests show that the liver cancer might be only within one part of the liver, surgery for attempted removal of the cancer should be performed. This should be done, however, only by experienced surgeons who have performed this type of surgery before. It pays to find an experienced surgeon and even to travel to a larger center if resection is thought feasible because liver operations are major and very risky. For the more than 95 percent of patients whose liver cancer cannot be resected, radiation to the liver and chemotherapy offer relief of symptoms, especially pain, but death usually occurs fairly rapidly. The average survival is less than six months. Cancer centers do not offer more effective chemotherapy treatment for the person with liver cancer. We, therefore, do not recommend that patients travel long distances for experimental chemotherapy at the present time.

Liver transplantation, currently under study, has apparently cured several young people who have developed liver cancer. This is a highly experimental approach to therapy and may offer some hope for the future.

PANCREATIC CANCER

The pancreas is a glandular organ located behind the stomach and duodenum that produces digestive enzymes that it puts into the intestine through a duct. It also is the organ that produces insulin.

Cancer of the pancreas, like cancer of the esophagus and stomach, is rarely diagnosed when it is localized and curable. This is not unexpected. The pancreas lies hidden deep in the abdomen. Cancer of the pancreas produces few symptoms and is undetected by the patient and his doctor until it is far advanced. Early diagnosis is not possible. In fact, even when the disease is advanced, the diagnosis is often difficult. Approximately 22,000 Americans develop pancreatic cancer each year and 20,000 die from it.

The usual symptoms of this cancer include weight loss, pain in the upper abdomen usually extending through to the back, loss of appetite, and in some cases painless jaundice. (Jaundice is the accumulation of bile in the blood and is manifested by a yellow coloration of the eyes and skin.)

Diagnosis and Treatment

When cancer of the pancreas is suspected, your physician should determine if the pancreas is enlarged. Tests that may demonstrate a pancreatic cancer include a barium x-ray study of the stomach and first part of the small bowel, an ultrasound examination (a scanning examination that uses sound waves) of the abdomen, a CAT scan (a new type of x-ray of the abdomen), or an arteriogram. Arteriograms are performed by putting a catheter through a needle puncture into the major artery of the leg and injecting dye into the artery that supplies blood to the pancreas. A new test called ERCP (endoscopic retrograde cholangiopancreatography, which is now available only in some major hospitals, represents a major advance in diagnosing pancreatic cancer. A special endoscope is swallowed and passed into the duodenum. The endoscopist looks for and finds the tiny entry of the pancreatic duct and places a small catheter into it. X-rays can then be done and also cells from the pancreas can be examined for cancerous changes.

Surgery   If any of these tests is abnormal, exploratory surgery of the abdomen, an exploratory laparotomy, is indicated. At surgery, the diagnosis can be made by biopsy of the cancer. Once the diagnosis is confirmed, the surgeon should assess whether or not the cancer has spread beyond the pancreas. He or she does this by carefully looking at the liver and lymph nodes in the area of the pancreas and obtaining biopsies for immediate examination (frozen sectioning) of any suspicious areas. It is thus during surgery that the diagnosis and extent of disease are determined. In most cases, the tumor will have spread beyond the pancreas, and surgical treatment should consist only of insuring that the bowel and drainage from the liver are not obstructed by the cancer. These connections may need to be altered and enlarged if they are in danger of obstructing. In the rare situation where cure might be possible, the surgeon may attempt to remove the pancreas and nearby lymph nodes (Whipple procedure or radical pancreatectomy), which is a complicated operation that carries an appreciable mortality even in experienced surgical hands.

Radiation   The value of radiation therapy administered to the area of the pancreas is currently under study. There is evidence that it may prolong life and decrease symptoms in some people. Few, if any, will be cured by radiation, since by the time it is diagnosed the disease almost always has spread beyond the pancreas and has involved areas that cannot be radiated.

Chemotherapy Chemotherapy is relatively ineffective against this cancer. Approximately 25 percent of patients respond and improve, but the response is short-lived, often under twelve weeks. The options for chemotherapy are the same as those discussed for stomach cancer. The usual approach is to try treatment with 5-FU, a relatively nontoxic drug. With this drug most people are not harmed and some will benefit from treatment. As with the other gastrointestinal cancers, high doses and experimental drugs will hurt more often than help. Occasional people do benefit, so you must make up your own mind what is best for you.

Pain Relief

Abdominal pain is the most common severe problem with cancer of the pancreas. Fortunately, the pain can often be relieved by blocking nerves to the area of the pancreas. This can be done without surgery by injecting a drug that anesthetizes the nerve that supplies the pancreas.

There is little cause for optimism at present in the treatment of cancer of the pancreas. There are no promising experimental approaches. Therefore, we do not recommend that you travel to a cancer center for the treatment of pancreatic cancer. The following case history is all too typical of this cancer.

M.R. was a sixty-four-year-old physician who had been in general practice for forty years. He went to a hospital because of abdominal pain, weight loss, and a swollen abdomen. A small needle was inserted into the abdominal cavity, and fluid was removed and sent for pathologic examination. The fluid contained cancer cells. An ultrasound radar examination of his abdomen suggested that he had a large tumor involving part of his pancreas. The physician-patient suspected that he had pancreatic cancer, and his doctor confirmed his impression. He was told that treatment had little to offer except the possibility of pain relief by nerve block. He requested this, and a successful nerve block was performed by an anesthesiologist specializing in pain control. Both the patient and his family requested that his doctors do nothing to prolong his life. His wife took him home and cared for him there. He died at home four weeks later of malnutrition.

This physician, once he realized the inevitability of his death, wanted to spend his remaining time with his family and not isolated in a hospital room. It is probable that if intravenous feedings, diet supplements, and chemotherapy had been used, his life might have been prolonged by one to three months. However, the little additional time would have been bought at the price of hospitalization. Instead, he spent his remaining time with his family and friends and in his own home.

It is one of the responsibilities of a physician caring for cancer patients to assist the patient and his family in coping with death, and to allow patients to determine, as much as possible, how they die. If cure is impossible, the physician and his patient should talk about how the patient wishes to die. These discussions should usually include the spouse and often older children. Realistic plans should be made. Most people do not wish to spend their last days in the hospital, and a good doctor can do much to help the patient spend his or her remaining days at home in comfortable and familiar surroundings.

Organizations such as the American Cancer Society and the Visiting Nurse Association provide valuable assistance to a family coping with the physical needs of a bed-ridden person. Spouses or friends can often be trained to give injections for pain relief should it become necessary. If the cancer victim and his family feel that hospitalization only offers a sterile place to die, every effort should be made to allow the patient to go home. We always offer families the option of hospitalization if they change their mind. In several instances, patients were brought back to the hospital only hours before they died, having spent all their remaining time at home.

It has been our experience that acceptance of the death of a spouse, a parent, or even a child is dependent upon the physical closeness to the dying person during the last few weeks of life, and often this is best accomplished at home. Some people and/or their families need the security of the hospital while preparing for death. It is most important that the physician listen to his patients and their families and try to help them die in the manner that best suits them.

CANCER OF THE LARGE BOWEL

The large bowel, or colon, is a muscular tube that reduces the water content and thus the volume of stool. It is about five feet long, starts at the cecum in the right side of the abdomen, and includes the sigmoid colon and the rectum, the six inches above the anus.

The Relationship between Bowel Cancer and Diet

Cancer of the large bowel is a disease of affluent Western man. Seventy thousand Americans develop colon cancer each year and 40,000 die from it. Only lung cancer claims more cancer victims in this country. The disease is virtually nonexistent among the poor in the Third World. Studies show that colon cancer is more frequent in people with diets high in animal fat and protein and low in roughage or fiber. Conversely, diets high in vegetable protein and unrefined starches and sugars (which make up much of the diet in the Third World) are associated with a low incidence of colon cancer.

Western man eats little bulk and has a stool volume about one-fifth that of African natives, who rarely develop colon cancer. The African diet consists of bulk foods (high fiber) and is also low in animal fat and protein. Further confirmation of the effect of diet in colon cancer is the remarkable increase of the disease in people who move from areas of low risk such as Africa to areas of high risk such as the United States if they change to an American diet.

There are two common current theories about how dietary habits may influence the development of colon cancer: (1) if a carcinogen was either eaten or produced in the bowel, a small stool volume such as is common among Americans increases the time between defecations and prolongs contact between the carcinogen and the bowel wall, and (2) bacteria present in the digestive tract of people eating high animal protein and fat diets are capable of converting substances present in the diet into carcinogens, which can then act on the lower bowel. Studies have shown that the bacteria in the lower bowel of Africans is quite different from that of Europeans and Americans.

Although all the factors associated with the development of colon cancer are not known, a few common sense recommendations seem in order. For those of us eating a Western diet, until more information is available, little harm and some benfiet may result from eating more fiber-rich, high-bulk foods. We should also reduce our excessive intake of animal fat and protein. This can be done simply by substituting fish or chicken for red meat and eating only nonmeat products two to three days a week. Since carcinogens act over many years, we should especially try to influence our children's diet. Many people near or over age forty are already at risk for developing colon cancer, and it is quite improbable that a change in diet will be of any benefit. Perhaps, however, encouraging healthy eating habits among our children may protect future generations from this common cancer.

Early Diagnosis

Unlike cancer of the esophagus, stomach, liver, and pancreas, almost half of all cases of colon cancer can be surgically cured. Despite the large number of cured patients, cancer of the colon is so common that it is one of the leading causes of death in our society. Approximately 40,000 Americans die each year from colon cancer, many in their fifties and early sixties. This is unfortunate because it is a cancer that can be diagnosed early, simply by checking the stool for blood. This cannot be done yourself by merely examining your stool: with small amounts of bleeding, the stool appears normal. However, this small amount of bleeding can be detected by simple laboratory test. For people over the age of forty, we recommend that five different stool samples be tested for the microscopic presence of blood each year. If these stools are negative, and if a rectal examination is normal and you have no symptoms such as changed bowel habits, you can be 95 percent certain that you do not have colon cancer. If, however, there is blood in any one of the stool samples, a more thorough investigation of the lower bowel becomes mandatory.

An investigation of the lower bowel should include a rectal examination, a sigmoidoscopy (an examination of the lower twelve to eighteen inches of the bowel by a hollow tube through the rectum), and a barium enema examination (an x-ray examination of the entire lower colon). Many cancers of the lower bowel occur within one foot of the rectum, some occurring within reach of an examiner's finger. If no cause for the bleeding is found with these examinations, a fiberoptic colonoscopy (a visual examination of the entire colon performed with a tube similar to that used for the examinations of the stomach and esophagus described earlier) should be performed as well. You have not had an adequate physical examination unless your doctor at least performs a rectal examination and checks your stool for blood. This should be done on a yearly basis if you are over forty years of age.

None of these examinations is pleasant, but none of them is unduly painful, none is dangerous, and all can be life saving. You may say to yourself that all of these tests are a bother. However, if cancer of the colon is diagnosed when it is asymptomatic because there was a trace of blood in your stool, your chances for cure are aproximately 80 percent, or twice that of patients diagnosed with symptoms of colon cancer. The following case history illustrates the value of looking for blood in your stool on a yearly basis.

J.H., a fifty-year-old tax collector, became worried about colon cancer when his best friend developed and eventually died of it. He called the American Cancer Society and was sent literature about colon cancer and about the value of testing stools for blood on a yearly basis. He then went to his family doctor and asked to be checked. All went well for eight years, but at age fifty-nine his stool contained blood in two of five samples. Sigmoidoscopy showed a small cancer, which was removed several days later at surgery. Ten years have passed and J.H. is alive and well. He roughly doubled his chance for cure by having his stool checked yearly, a simple, painless, and inexpensive test.

Conditions Predisposing to Bowel Cancer

Certain people have a greater likelihood of developing colon cancer. If you have had a nonmalignant disease called ulcerative colitis for more than ten years, not only may you get this cancer but it can happen in your thirties. Several genetic or inherited diseases (discussed in the chapter on heredity), such as familial polyposis, can lead to colon cancer in your twenties. Most physicians advocate removal of the colon to prevent incurable colon cancer in patients with these diseases. With either disease, you need to be under the care of a board-certified gastroenterologist.

Polyps, a type of benign colon tumor, can lead to cancer. If you have one polyp, you are likely to get more. Many gastroenterologists feel that most colon cancer starts in polyps. These can usually be removed nonsurgically with a colonscope. If you have had any colonic polyps removed, you need to be checked for more polyps yearly and should consult a gastroenterologist.

Symptoms

Symptoms from colon cancer include changes in bowel habits such as difficulty in evacuating the stool, a feeling of fullness in the rectum, a decrease in the diameter of the stool (pencillike stools), lower abdominal pain, or frank blood in the stool. Most of these symptoms will be observed only if the cancer is in the lower part of the colon. If the cancer is in the upper colon, symptoms may not occur until the cancer is very widespread. However, almost all colon cancers bleed. The diagnostic approach in a patient with symptoms of colon cancer is exactly like that of the patient with blood in his stool, and consists of a rectal examination, sigmoidoscopy, a barium enema, and, if needed, colonoscopy. If these tests demonstrate probable cancer, a chest x-ray, blood tests for abnormalities, and a liver scan should be done before surgery. An unfortunate common error made by many physicians is illustrated in the next case.

A fifty-nine-year-old tool and die maker saw his family physician because he felt weak. His physical examination was normal; however, he was found to have iron deficiency anemia. His physician placed him on iron tablets, and over the next six weeks his iron deficiency anemia responded to treatment and his blood count returned to normal. Several months later he developed abdominal pain and had emergency surgery. A large incurable colon cancer was found.

In any adult male and in any postmenopausal or posthysterectomy female, signs and symptoms of iron deficiency anemia mean that you have been bleeding. The most common site of the bleeding is the gastrointestinal tract. If you have iron deficiency anemia, your physician should thoroughly investigate your GI tract for bleeding. At the very least, several stool samples should be examined for the presence of blood. If blood is present, your doctor should find out what is bleeding. We have seen numerous instances similar to the case described above of patients with iron deficiency anemia who had been treated with iron and recovered from their anemia only to have a late-stage colon cancer discovered several months later.

Treatment

Surgery Surgery is the standard treatment and cures about 50 percent of people with colon cancer. If the cancer is within the bowel wall, more than 60 percent of patients will be cured. If the cancer extends through the entire bowel wall to what is called the serosal surface, cure is much less likely. Finally, if the cancer involves the lymph nodes removed at the time of surgery, cure is rare. The surgeon you choose to perform this operation should be highly qualified; specific criteria for evaluating surgeons are suggested in chapter 8, "The Surgical Treatment of Cancer." He or she should be certified by the American Board of General Surgeons or the American Board of Colon and Rectal Surgery, and should perform this operation with some regularity.

The type of surgery necessary to cure colon cancer depends upon the location of the cancer. When colon cancer occurs more than six inches from the rectum, it can be surgically cured without the necessity of colostomy. The cancerous section of the colon is removed and the upper and lower sections are sewn together. For cancers close to the rectum, the surgeon must remove the rectum and create what is termed a colostomy. A colostomy is an artificial rectum usually placed on the lower abdominal wall that is covered with a bag to collect stool. The reason this procedure is necessary is that only by removing all of the cancer can it be cured. It is impossible to remove cancer close to the rectum and leave the rectum intact. If the surgeon attempts to leave the rectum intact and fails to remove all the cancer, the chance for cure is lost.

Adjusting to a colostomy is difficult. Most patients have a very difficult time adjusting to a colostomy. But after an initial period of severe depression and fear, most people I have seen have adapted quite well. Almost all people feel that they will smell bad and that other people will avoid them. A large part of the fear is sexual in nature. One of the most useful ways to assuage such fears is to have patients talk to other patients who have had colostomies and are leading normal, active lives.

The American Cancer Society in conjunction with the United Ostomy Association runs a volunteer organization that has over 20,000 members located in all states. All the volunteers have had colostomies themselves. You should ask your surgeon to request that a volunteer visit you. The volunteer will see you soon after your operation, teach you to care for your colostomy, and answer any questions that you have about it. The volunteer will also be an example of how life can go on fairly normally with a colostomy. The volunteer will invite you to join the local organization where you can meet other people with colostomies and help similar patients to adjust.

We strongly recommend that you utilize this valuable resource. Ask your surgeon to call and have a volunteer help you who has experienced what you must face. There are also trained therapists who teach people to take care of their colostomies. Group therapy is often available in larger hospitals to help people adjust to their body image. Learning to live with a colostomy is a major adjustment, but most people eventually do so and live fairly normal lives.

M.J. had a disease called ulcerative colitis. Her disease started when she was thirteen and had been active for most of the next fifteen years. People who have severe ulcerative colitis have a high incidence of colon cancer. Therefore, her gastroenterologist recommended an operation to prevent cancer from developing. He told her that they would be unable to prevent her from dying of colon cancer unless they removed her entire colon. She became severely depressed at the thought of living with a permanent ileostomy. (An ileostomy is similar to a colostomy except that the end of the small bowel is brought out through the abdominal wall, as the entire colon is removed.) However, due to her fear of colon cancer she consented to the operation. The operation went well and pathologic examination of the colon revealed several small cancers, none of which had penetrated the colonic wall. The operation had indeed prevented her death from colon cancer.

Before surgery, M.J. was visited by three American Cancer Society volunteers who had ileostomies and were living normal lives. This did much to allay her fears. Following the operation, she went through a period of severe depression related to the change in her body image. Finally, however, she adjusted and she entered graduate school one year after the operation, met a fellow graduate student, and married him six months later. Four years have passed since her operation, she has had a child, and she continues to lead a normal existence despite her ileostomy.

Radiation   The value of radiation in addition to or in combination with surgery for rectal cancer or cancer of the colon near the rectum is currently being tested. Several studies have suggested that radiation decreases the incidence of recurrences in the area of the rectum and also increases the cure rate. Therefore, after surgery, if the cancer is found to penetrate the bowel wall, your surgeon may send you for radiation therapy. Side effects from radiation include some diarrhea, loss of appetite, and tiredness. The diarrhea can usually be controlled by medications. Radiation therapy given after surgery generally takes three to four weeks of treatment given five days a week.

After surgery, your surgeon will usually see you on a regular basis to insure that all is going well. He or she will also obtain tests to find out whether or not the cancer has recurred. One of the more recent advances that helps the surgeon assess your status has been the development of a blood test called carcinoembryonic antigen, or CEA, which is sometimes useful in detecting recurrences of colon cancer. It is also often used as a guideline for responsiveness to chemotherapy. Other tests that your physician may order on a regular basis include a chest x-ray, liver scan, sigmoidoscopy, and barium enemas.

Chemotherapy   Chemotherapy for colon cancer that has metastasized, or spread, is relatively ineffective and only benefits approximately 20 percent of patients; most of the 20 percent who benefit do so for only a short period of time. The status of chemotherapy for colon cancer is much like that for stomach and pancreatic cancer. Most patients with colon cancer are treated with relatively nontoxic drugs such as 5-FU.

This allows the physician to do something for his patient with little chance for harm. There is no evidence at present that using toxic, high-dose combination chemotherapy helps more patients than 5-FU alone.

We recommend that you take either 5-FU or no chemotherapy if you have metastatic colon cancer. Although it is difficult to accept, there is no promising experimental chemotherapy for colon cancer.

Adjuvant chemotherapy.   Many physicians are giving chemotherapy to colon cancer victims who have a high likelihood of developing recurrent disease because of lymph node involvement with cancer or spread through the colon wall. This is called adjuvant chemotherapy. Oncologists hope that these drugs will prevent the growth of small deposits of tumor cells not removed during surgery. There is no clear-cut evidence that this works for colon cancer, but it is still widely used.

It is very difficult for a patient to decide whether he should receive such therapy or not. Many patients choose it in the hope that it will help. It is indeed difficult for patients to accept that not receiving therapy may be better than receiving therapy. Patients very often feel that nothing is being done for them if they are not receiving some form of therapy. However, in all honesty we must state that the probability that adjuvant or preventive chemotherapy will be effective in colon cancer is rather low, since the drugs are relatively ineffective against colon cancer that has metastasized.

Currently, many physicians are participating in cancer-cooperative groups that offer experimental chemotherapy for colon cancer as well as other cancers. Experimental chemotherapy generally involves more side effects for the patient, since combinations of drugs and high doses of drugs are generally used. If you decide to enter into experimental chemotherapy, you should understand that few experimental regimens are better than the drugs we generally use. In the case of colon cancer, experimental chemotherapy is not very promising at the present time.

Your decision about whether to try experimental therapy is mainly determined by how you feel when this is discussed with your medical oncologist. Your oncologist should inform you as thoroughly as possible of the purpose of the studies, the real hopes of the studies, and the possible consequences or side effects. In the end, however, you must decide.

The following case illustrates the dangers of taking experimental therapy.

C.R., a sixty-three-year-old truck driver, had had surgery for colon cancer six years earlier and was cured. He saw his physician for a routine examination, and his physician again discovered blood in his stool. A barium x-ray examination of his large bowel disclosed a large new cancer in the right side of his colon. He was operated on, the cancer was removed, and microscopic examination showed that cancer cells had spread to nearby lymph nodes. C.R. was sent to a medical oncologist, who explained that, unlike his first surgery for colon cancer, the second cancer was probably not curable with just surgery.

The oncologist was participating in a study using experimental drugs to prevent recurrence of colon cancer in patients at high risk for recurrence, such as C.R. C.R. was offered the opportunity to participate in this study. The possible side effects were explained and he was informed that treatment might do nothing to prevent recurrence of the cancer. C.R. decided to participate in the study and stated that he wanted to "try anything" that might cure his disease. Unfortunately, he developed a severe reaction to one of the drugs. It affected his bone marrow to such an extent that he was unable to produce cells needed to fight infections. He died from pneumonia six months after surgery, and ironically had no evidence of recurrence of his cancer at that time.

C.R. was not angry with his physicians, even though he had lived for a shorter rather than a longer period of time as a result of the treatment offered him. Perhaps this was because he felt comfortable with having made his own decision to try treatment.

People often find it difficult to refuse an opportunity to try a treatment that may lead to longer life. Doctors who deal with cancer patients use the term *cure* very rarely, yet patients often think of cure from surgery, chemotherapy, and radiation. It is exceptionally difficult to decide rationally which course is best for you when all your doctor can do is tell you what the likelihood of your chances of responding to therapy will be. However, had C.R. decided not to take chemotherapy, he would probably have lived longer. No treatment can be as good as or better than treatment.

Cancer of the colon, unlike other gastrointestinal cancers, can be diagnosed early and cured in a high percentage of cases. Although it is a simple and inexpensive procedure, few people have their stools tested for blood on a regular basis. You should ask your doctor to test your stools for blood yearly after age forty. Only those people with blood in their stool samples need to consult a physician for further tests. It is our hope that stool testing for blood will become a more widespread practice and will lead to an increased number of people with surgical cures. We also hope that by changing the unhealthy dietary habits of our children, we can do much to avert their developing colon cancer when they reach adulthood.

SUMMARY

1. Cancers of the esophagus, stomach, and pancreas usually are diagnosed after they are too advanced to be curable. At the present time the cure rate for each of these cancers is approximately 5 percent.

2. Most cancers of the esophagus are treated by radiation, though some tumors of the lower esophagus can be treated surgically.

3. Yearly endoscopic examinations of the esophagus are recommended if you have one of the following conditions associated with an increased incidence of esophageal cancer: Plummer-Vinson syndrome, achalasia, lye stricture, or Barrett's esophagus.

4. Cancers of the stomach and pancreas usually are not curable by either surgery or radiation, though these treatments can be used for relief of symptoms. Chemotherapy for these cancers can offer a small chance for temporary improvement. Experimental chemotherapy is not promising.

5. You should have an endoscopic examination of your stomach if you have a stomach ulcer diagnosed by x-ray examination.

6. The prognosis with colon cancer is much better than with stomach or pancreatic cancers, because early diagnosis is feasible. Surgery is the standard treatment, and it cures 40 percent of colon cancers.

7. Radiation for rectal and colon cancer, either before or after surgery, is currently being evaluated. The early results are promising.

8. Chemotherapy for colon cancer is relatively ineffective; therefore, we recommend nontoxic chemotherapy, such as 5-FU, rather than combination chemotherapy in high doses. The use of chemotherapy after surgery to prevent recurrences is currently under evaluation, but the chances that it will work are quite small.

9. All persons over age forty should have several stools tested for the presence of blood and have a rectal examination each year. If blood is present, sigmoidoscopy, barium enema, and even colonoscopy are indicated to determine the source of the bleeding. The chance of curing colon cancer doubles to 80 percent if it is detected by such screening.

10. If you have a colostomy, your surgeon can ask the American Cancer Society to send a volunteer, who also has had one, to help you cope with your new colostomy.

14

Cancers of the Female Reproductive Organs

The female reproductive system includes the ovary (the site of egg and hormone formation), the uterus (the womb), the cervix (the part of the uterus that protrudes into the vagina), the vagina, and the labia (the external genitalia). Any of these organs may give rise to cancer and some do so quite frequently. Cancers from these organs tend to strike different women who have different predisposing factors. Many of them are curable if diagnosed early. The purpose of this chapter is to discuss how you can protect yourself from these cancers, what to expect if you develop any of them, and how best to get treated for them.

A thirty-nine-year-old woman has a yearly Pap smear. Her gynecologist tells her it is very suspicious for cancer. In her office the gynecologist performs colposcopy and biopsies the suspicious area of the cervix. The biopsy confirms the Pap smear: she has *in situ*, or very early, cancer of the cervix. She is admitted to the hospital for hysterectomy, or surgical removal of the uterus and cervix, and she is cured.

Another woman, forty-five years old, saw her gynecologist because she had been spotting blood after sexual intercourse. She had not had yearly Pap smears. On examination her gynecologist found that her cervix was hard and that it had a large ulcer. This woman also had cancer of the cervix but her cancer could not be cured. She was treated with intensive radiation therapy, which failed to control the cancer, and she died two years later from metastatic cancer from her cervix. If she had had yearly Pap smears, the cancer probably would have been detected early enough for her to be cured. Once cervical cancer becomes symptomatic, it is often very difficult or impossible to cure.

A sixty-four-year-old woman saw her physician because of bleeding from her vagina. She had stopped menstruating ten years earlier. Her physician found that her uterus was enlarged and admitted her to the hospital for a dilatation and curettage (D&C), which is a scraping of the inside of the uterus. This is performed under anesthesia, but takes only a few minutes and is a safe procedure. The tissue removed from the uterus was cancerous. The cancer in the uterus was quite extensive, but tests showed no spread beyond the uterus. Her gynecologist and a radiation oncologist both saw her. They decided that a combination of radiation and surgery would give her the best chance for cure. This woman was first treated with both external cobalt radiation and implants of radioactive material into the uterus, and then had a hysterectomy. Ten years later she is feeling well and is apparently cured.

Vaginal bleeding after menopause (the change of life) should indicate to your physician the possibility of cancer. Without delay, an evaluation for cancer of the cervix, vagina, and uterus is indicated. If a pelvic examination does not show that the bleeding is coming from the cervix or vagina, a D&C should be done to see if there is cancer in the uterus.

A forty-year-old woman who had always been very healthy saw her physician for abdominal swelling. She had a large amount of fluid in her abdomen and, when a pelvic exam was done, the doctor found several masses surrounding her ovaries and uterus. Her family doctor suspected cancer and therefore referred her to a gynecologic oncologist. After examining her, the oncologist suspected cancer of the ovary. She was admitted to the hospital and at operation it was found that she had advanced cancer of the ovary. In contrast to cancer of the uterine cervix or uterine body, cancer of the ovary can rarely be diagnosed early. By the time symptoms occur it is often far advanced and rarely curable. This woman was treated with chemotherapy. Her abdominal swelling disappeared and she felt well for one year. Then the cancer recurred and she died. Cancer of the ovary does respond to both radiation and chemotherapy, but most women with advanced disease still eventually die of the disease.

Despite the ability to detect cervical and uterine cancers early and new treatment approaches for ovarian cancer, more than 20,000 American women still die of cancer of the female genital organs each year. Many of these women die needlessly. If they were better informed, obtained yearly screenings, and saw a physician at the first symptom, many would have early, curable instead of late, incurable cancer. The value of early diagnosis of female reproductive cancers is well illustrated by cancer of the uterine cervix. At present, two out of every three such cancers are diagnosed by Pap smears before they are symptomatic. Cancers diagnosed in this manner are almost 100 percent curable.

The Need for a Team Approach

The treatment of cancers of the female reproductive organs demonstrates the importance and value of a team approach. The use of surgery, radiation, and in some cases chemotherapy is necessary. The proper use of these therapies is extremely important if you are to have the best chance for cure with the fewest side effects. Therefore, specialists trained in each of these areas should be involved in the planning and often the execution of the treatment. The surgeon should be a gynecologist with experience and training in surgery for cancer of the female reproductive organs. The radiation oncologist, a specialist in the administration of radiation therapy, must also be involved early in the planning and administration of therapy. For women for whom chemotherapy is indicated, a medical oncologist or gynecologic oncologist should also be involved. These specialists are often available at better community medical centers.

The Board-Certified Gynecologic Oncologist

Perhaps the hardest specialist for you to evaluate is the gynecologist. Most obstetricians and gynecologists are not specialists in the treatment of cancer. However, many gynecologists have received some advanced training in the treatment of gynecologic cancer. There is also a new specialty called gynecologic oncology. Unfortunately, there are fewer than 100 of these specialists at the present time in the entire country. Obviously, they can't treat all the women with cancers of the female reproductive organs. You should ask your gynecologist if there is a gynecologic oncologist available in your city. If there is, you should be treated by him or her. If not, your obstetrician or gynecologist may wish to call a gynecologic oncologist in another area of the country to review your case. This is not as valuable as seeing the gynecologic oncologist personally, but it can often benefit you since he or she can direct your staging evaluation and treatment. Over the next several years, we expect that more gynecologic oncologists will be trained and that most medium-sized and large cities in the country will have this specialist available to treat you in your own community.

How to Choose a Qualified Gynecologist

Many gynecologists take a special interest in the treatment of cancer. For example, if there are six gynecologists in your town, there may be four who mostly do obstetrics, or deliver babies. One may be interested in fertility problems and one may take a special interest in cancers of the female reproductive organs. Although the gynecologist concerned with cancer may not be formally trained, he or she will have more experience and knowledge in this area than the other five. It is worth asking your physician if anyone in your community has more experience. Also ask if any of the gynecologists has had some formal training in the treatment of cancer. Perhaps one of them has spent six months or a year at one of the large cancer centers such as M. D. Anderson, Memorial, or Roswell Park.

In many communities there is no gynecologic oncologist, no gynecologist with any special training in the treatment of cancer, and no gynecologist you can identify who seems to have a special interest in it. Don't give up. Ask your gynecologist if there is a tumor board conference in the hospital and if so whether he attends it and if he presents his cancer patients at this conference. (Tumor boards are open forums where cases are reviewed by doctors who are interested in cancer.) Many hospitals have tumor boards or tumor board conferences in which patients with cancer are discussed prior to therapy. Usually specialists in the treatment of cancer, such as medical oncologists and radiation oncologists, and other doctors who regularly treat cancer patients go to tumor boards. The tumor board offers some reassurance that you are getting the benefit of more than one opinion. Doctors who attend tumor boards are usually more interested in the treatment of cancer than doctors who don't. Therefore, it is reasonable for you to ask your gynecologist whether he goes to and discusses his cancer patients at a tumor board. If not, is there a gynecologist in town who does?

Another question you may ask your gynecologist or your family doctor is which gynecologist performs gynecologic cancer surgery on physicians or physicians' wives? Doctors generally know which doctors in their community are well trained and are good.

Although all obstetrician-gynecologists are considered technically qualified to perform cancer surgery, your chance of cure and minimal postoperative complications are certainly better if you are cared for by someone, if not with formal training, at least with special interest and experience in the treatment of cancer.

The treatment of cancers of the female reproductive organs often involves a complex choice among surgery, radiation, or both together. This depends on the type of cancer and the stage of the disease. The decision is best made by a gynecologist and a radiation oncologist, and possibly also a medical oncologist, who should each see and evaluate the woman and then together decide upon the best treatment for her. If you have cancer it pays to insure that you see the specialists who can offer you the best treatment and therefore the best chance for cure.

CANCER OF THE UTERINE CERVIX

A.H. had seen a gynecologist each year since she was twenty-one years old. Her initial visits had been concerned with birth control and later visits with pregnancy and the delivery of her two children. Her gynecologist had obtained a Pap smear at least once a year. She had many normal

Pap smears but at age thirty-five, for the first time, the test was abnormal. It was a class 4 Pap smear, that is, the cells looked malignant. A class 4 or class 5 Pap smear is considered definite evidence of cervical cancer. Her gynecologist admitted A.H. to the hospital and performed a cone biopsy of her cervix. This involves removing the surface of the cervix to see if cancer is present and if so how extensively it involves the cervix. The cone biopsy fortunately showed *in situ* cancer of the cervix. The gynecologist next performed a very careful pelvic examination under general anesthesia and ordered several tests, including a chest x-ray, an intravenous pyelogram (see chapter 15, "Cancers of the Urinary Tract and Male Reproductive Organs"), and an ultrasound examination of her pelvis. An ultrasound examination is a painless test using a radarlike device that can detect any masses that might indicate spread of cancer.

The gynecologist then talked with A.H. and her husband, and recommended that she have a hysterectomy, an operation that would remove her uterus but leave her ovaries present. Therefore, she would not go through menopause at age thirty-three. The chance of cure with this operation was almost 100 percent.

If she wanted more children, she could wait and have frequent examinations. Only with *in situ*, or stage O, cancer of the cervix can treatment be safely delayed to have children. She was told she should get pregnant as soon as possible and have the hysterectomy after she was finished having children. There was minimal risk in waiting the additional years. A.H. and her husband discussed whether they wanted additional children and decided they did not want to take even the small risk of waiting one additional year. They already had two children and, although they had wanted a larger family, they were not absolutely sure that it was worth the risk. A.H. had a hysterectomy eight years ago, and has not had any recurrence of the cancer. She is most certainly cured of her cervical cancer.

Early diagnosis of cancer of the cervix is relatively easy. The cervix can be seen and felt during a pelvic examination, and scrapings from the cervix can be evaluated by a Pap smear. If you have a yearly pelvic examination by your physician or a trained paramedical person and a Pap smear, your chances of developing advanced cervical cancer are very small. A.H.'s story is repeated thousands of times a year: a Pap smear is abnormal, a biopsy shows *in situ* cancer, a hysterectomy is performed, and the woman is cured. Almost all women treated in this manner for early cervical cancer are cured. In contrast, if you do not have yearly pelvic examinations and Pap smears, but wait for late symptoms of cervical cancer, such as painful intercourse or bleeding between periods or after intercourse, the picture changes. The chance for cure is much lower, and the therapy will be extensive surgery or high-dose radiation to the whole pelvis. The side effects are greater and the chances for cure are lower.

Cancer of the cervix is the second most common cancer in American women. Fortunately, due to early diagnosis with Pap smears, the death rate from this cancer has decreased almost 50 percent in the past twenty years, although the incidence of the disease has not changed. The improvement in curability is not due to an improvement in therapy, which has not changed in the past twenty years, but is solely the result of early diagnosis. For each symptomatic cancer of the cervix diagnosed in the United States this year, two are diagnosed before symptoms have occurred. The peak incidence for diagnosis of cervical cancer by Pap smear, that is, the diagnosis of early, *in situ* cancer, is age thirty-three. Cervical cancer diagnosed after symptoms are present has a peak age incidence of forty-seven. Therefore, it probably takes over ten years for cervical cancer to progress from early, almost 100 percent curable disease to advanced disease.

Cancer of the cervix can occur in any woman, but some women are at greater risk than others. Black and poor women get cervical cancer more often than white or wealthy women. Studies suggest that women who start having sexual intercourse at a young age and with many men are more likely to get cervical cancer. Recently a virus that causes genital herpes (herpes type 2 virus) has been linked to cervical cancer. Genital herpes can cause painful sores on the external genitalia and asymptomatic sores on the cervix. The virus can be transmitted by sexual intercourse. Another suggestive piece of evidence linking sexual intercourse to the development of cervical cancer is the very low incidence of this cancer in nuns and the very high incidence in prostitutes.

Early Diagnosis: The Case for Yearly Pap Smears

There are no early signs or symptoms of cervical cancer. When symptoms have occurred, cervical cancer is advanced and probably has been present for many years. If not detected early by a Pap smear, cervical cancer will often continue to grow and spread to the vagina, the body of the uterus, and even the ovaries before it will cause symptoms that would send you to your doctor. When symptoms occur they are usually vaginal bleeding, either between periods or after intercourse, or pain in the pelvis. Most women with cervical cancer also have a vaginal discharge that usually smells bad. However, a vaginal discharge due to a minor infection is very common in healthy women and therefore should not make you think you have cervical cancer.

Cancer of the cervix is not common in young women but it does occur. To be safe, you should start having Pap smears and pelvic examinations in your early twenties. Pap smears are performed during the pelvic examination by scraping a small wooden spatula over the surface of the cervix. It is somewhat uncomfortable but is totally safe and may save your life. The spatula is then rubbed on a microscope slide, which is sent to a pathology laboratory. The slides are stained and the cells are examined under a microscope by trained technicians.

The Pap smear is reported as class 1 to class 5 depending upon how the cells look under the microscope. If they look normal, the Pap smear is reported as class 1 and 2, and there is nothing to worry about. A class 3 Pap smear means that the cells are abnormal and dictate that another smear be done. A class 4 or 5 Pap smear means the cells look cancerous or malignant. All women with class 4 or 5 Pap smears must have a cervix biopsy to see if cancer is present—which it usually is—and also to see how extensively it involves the cervix. The biopsy can be done by colposcopy or by a cone biopsy.

Colposcopy is quite simply an examination using a magnifying tool. The gynecologist inserts the colposcope into the vagina and can look at the cervix and see the most suspicious or abnormal areas and biopsy them. The procedure is done in a doctor's office, as it isn't very painful and therefore doesn't require anesthesia. However, only a small percentage of American gynecologists know how to perform colposcopy.

A cone biopsy necessitates hospitalization, as it is too painful to do without general or regional anesthesia. The whole surface of the cervix is removed, or biopsied. Both methods are equally good to evaluate cervical cancer, but obviously colposcopy is easier on the patient.

Many people confuse the Pap smear report with how extensive the cancer is. The Pap smear report depends solely on how the cells look. The more abnormal, the higher the class. It has nothing to do with how far the cancer has spread or the stage of the cancer.

Most often Pap smears are normal. Occasionally, not enough cells are obtained to evaluate whether or not cancer is present. If the Pap smear is unevaluable, the gynecologist will call the woman to repeat the Pap smear. When your doctor asks you to come back to have another Pap smear, most often cancer is not present.

Evaluating the Extent of the Disease

The treatment of cervical cancer is surgery, radiation, or a combination of the two. The first order of business after admission to the hospital is a careful evaluation of how far the disease has spread. In medical jargon this is called staging. Cancer of the cervix often spreads to nearby areas in the pelvis rather than to distant parts of the body such as the liver, lungs, and bones. Thus, the tests physicians use to evaluate pelvic disease are of prime importance. The first staging test is a pelvic examination under anesthesia. Anesthesia is used so that you may be completely relaxed and the examination can be totally reliable. Further tests include an intravenous pyelogram (see the section on kidney cancer in chapter 15), a cystoscopy (see the section on bladder cancer in chapter 15), and a sigmoidoscopy (see the section on colon cancer in chapter 13), all of which are used to assess whether the cancer has spread. A chest x-ray is also obtained since cervical cancer can spread to the lungs. Recently, gynecologists have been obtaining lymphangiograms (see chapter 18, "Cancers of Blood Cells and Lymph Glands") to assess the spread of the cancer to lymph nodes in the abdomen.

Treatment

Stage 0. If all staging tests are negative and the cancer is *in situ*, or limited to the surface of the cervix (stage 0), the treatment is a hysterectomy. If you are young, most surgeons will not remove your ovaries so that you will not go through menopause. The cure for stage 0 cancer of the cervix with a hysterectomy is almost 100 percent.

If you have stage 0 cancer of the cervix and want to have children, you can wait and have surgery later after you have had the children if regular checkups show that the cancer does not progress beyond stage 0. A cone biopsy (explained earlier in this chapter) is done. You will then have periodic Pap smears while you have the children. You should have the hysterectomy as soon as you are finished having your family.

Stage 1. If the cancer has invaded the cervix but is still localized to it (stage 1), more extensive treatment is needed to control it. While radiation is the usual treatment, both radiation and surgery are reasonable treatment alternatives. The principle with either approach is to treat the cancer in the cervix and also in the nearby pelvic lymph nodes. If radiation is used, it is administered to the cervix and the rest of the pelvis; surgery likewise involves removal of the uterus and the lymph nodes in the pelvis.

Surgery *Stage 1.* Surgery for stage 1 cervical cancer is fairly safe. Nevertheless, there can be complications with any surgery. Wound infections and urinary tract infections are two common complications. Also, fistulas between the urinary tract and the vagina or rectum do occur. These are very annoying and often difficult to repair. Surgery does have two advantages over radiation. It will not induce menopause, as the ovaries are left unharmed, and the vagina isn't damaged, so the woman's ability to enjoy sex isn't compromised.

In summary, both surgery or radiation offer the woman with stage 1 cervical cancer approximately an 80 percent chance for cure. If you have stage 1 cervical cancer it pays to see both a radiation oncologist and a gynecologist. You should think about the advantages and drawbacks of each and decide which treatment you prefer.

Stages 2–4. The treatment for cancer of the cervix that has spread beyond the cervix (stages 2–4) to other pelvic organs is even more extensive high-dose radiation than that outlined for stage 1 disease. As with almost all cancers, the more extensive the disease the more extensive the treatment and the less chance for cure. Depending upon the degree of spread, the cure rate ranges from 50 percent to 15 percent.

After treatment for cancer of the cervix, you will need to be followed closely by either your gynecologist or your radiation therapist. If the cancer recurs, it will usually recur within the pelvic organs. Occasionally, a radical operation in which the pelvic contents are completely removed should be undertaken. This operation can be dangerous, but can cure about one woman in four with recurrent cancer. It should only be performed by an experienced cancer surgeon. If you are in this situation and have recurrent cervical cancer following treatment, it would be advisable at least to seek an opinion from a major cancer center.

Radiation   Radiation is usually administered both with a cobalt machine (or a linear accelerator) and by implantation of radioactive pellets or needles into the uterus. Use of local radiation implants enables large doses of radiation to be given to a very small area. The implants are usually positioned in the operating room under anesthesia. Extensive radiation to the pelvis is not without side effects. It will damage the ovaries. If the woman is young she will therefore become infertile and also go through menopause. The radiation may also cause some scarring of the vagina, which may interfere with sexual intercourse. Radiation may irritate the rectum and colon and cause diarrhea. Occasionally, irritation of the bladder or communications between the bladder and rectum (fistulas) can occur. Late complications include strictures, or the formation of fibrous tissue, in the rectum or bladder, which can cause either constipation or problems wtih urination. These complications are rare. Most people receive treatment and have either temporary problems or no major side effects.

Chemotherapy   Chemotherapy for cervical cancer is not very effective. Drugs offer some chance of slowing the cancer growth and can make you feel better for several months to a year. Usually, chemotherapy is only given when cancer has spread beyond the pelvis, and thus cannot be treated with radiation or surgery. At present, there is no promising experimental chemotherapy. Therefore, we do not recommend traveling to a cancer center where experimental chemotherapy is offered. Most likely the experimental drugs will fail and you will have spent time away from home and probably experienced considerable side effects from the drugs. However, experimental chemotherapy programs are available if you want to try them despite their poor track record thus far in cervical cancer.

Cervical cancer, if caught early, is curable. Yearly Pap smears will probably protect you from this disease. If you wait until you have symptoms, your chance of surviving drops significantly. If the cancer is advanced, you will need to undergo extensive surgery or extensive radiation and still will have a high probability of dying from this disease.

CANCER OF THE UTERUS (ENDOMETRIAL CANCER)

The body of the uterus or womb not only is the site where babies develop but also is a common site for both benign and malignant tumors. The benign tumors are called fibroids or fibrous tumors, and although occasionally they cause troublesome symptoms of pain and bleeding and may occasionally require surgery, they usually involute, or grow smaller, after menopause. Cancer of the uterus develops in an older age group than cancer of the cervix: three of four cases occur in women over the age of fifty; the one case of four that develops before age fifty usually occurs after age forty. Cancer of the uterus can occur in any woman but is more common in women who are diabetic, are overweight, have high blood pressure, and have never had children. Also, women who take female hormones, or estrogens, after menopause to control symptoms such as hot flashes and also to prevent softening of the bones (osteoporosis) are somewhat more likely to develop uterine cancer. Although you cannot control most of the risk factors, you should remember that taking female hormones after menopause increases your risk of uterine cancer. There is some suggestion that taking these hormones cyclically, that is twenty-one out of twenty-eight days rather than each day, may be safer.

Early Diagnosis

Unfortunately, unlike cancer of the cervix, which is easily detected by a Pap smear, cancer of the uterus is often missed by a Pap smear. The cancer cells stay inside the uterus and are not present on the cervix. The methods for early detection of uterine cancer are, therefore, not as good as for cervical cancer. Thus, the death rate from cancer of the uterus hasn't decreased, as it has with cancer of the cervix.

Early diagnosis, however, is still possible, as there are methods of obtaining cells or tissue from inside the uterus. Currently several techniques for early detection of uterine cancer are under evaluation. One method is to inject a jet spray of fluid through the cervix into the uterus and collect the cells that are shed with the fluid. Biopsies can also be taken from inside the uterus. The most reliable biopsy of the uterus is accomplished by a D&C. We recommend that if you take female hormones and are postmenopausal your gynecologist should check you for uterine cancer every year using one of these techniques.

The following case illustrates the usual pattern of uterine cancer and provides a contrast with that of early diagnosed cervical cancer.

P.L., a fifty-nine-year-old account executive with a brokerage firm, saw her gynecologist because twice in a month she had noticed blood spotting on her underwear. She was seven years postmenopausal and had both mild hypertension and diabetes. Her gynecologist had given her estrogens to decrease symptoms from menopause. She examined her and found a mildly enlarged uterus. She advised P.L. to be admitted to the hospital for a D&C to evaluate the bleeding. The scrapings from the uterus revealed cancer of the endometrium.

P.L. was referred by her gynecologist to another gynecologist, who specialized in cancer therapy. He performed a series of examinations and tests to determine the extent of the disease. After admitting her to the hospital, he performed a pelvic examination under anesthesia. Then he obtained an intravenous pyelogram, performed a sigmoidoscopy, and had a urologist perform a cystoscopy. P.L. also had a bone and liver scan and a chest x-ray. All tests were normal.

The cancer had deeply invaded the uterine muscle. When this happens, the chances of spread to the nearby pelvic lymph glands increase. P.L. received external radiation to the pelvis. During this radiation her appetite decreased somewhat, and she had some diarrhea. However, she did not feel too ill to work. Following the radiation she had a complete hysterectomy with a bilateral salpingo-oophorectomy, that is, her uterus, ovaries, and fallopian tubes were removed. P.L. is now sixty-four years old and is thinking of retiring. Her cancer has not returned and she is almost certainly cured.

P.L.'s gynecologist was alert and did not dismiss her symptoms of post-menopausal bleedings. Instead, she performed an immediate D&C to determine the cause of the bleeding. She then referred her patient to a specialist in gynecologic oncology who knew how to evaluate and treat her. The oncologist arranged consultation with a radiation oncologist and presented her case at the hospital tumor board. P.L. thus received the benefit of several specialists working together and received excellent care. Several other points are illustrated by this case. Any vaginal bleeding after menopause could be serious. You should see your doctor and he or she should completely evaluate you. This evaluation should include a pelvic examination, a Pap smear, and, if these do not reveal the cause of bleeding, a D&C to evaluate the possibility of uterine cancer.

Treatment

Treatment of cancer of the uterus involves surgery, radiation, or a combination of both. In addition, hormonal therapy can alleviate symptoms and prolong life if radiation and surgery fail to eradicate the cancer. The extent of disease is evaluated by a careful pelvic examination under anesthesia, an intravenous pyelogram, a cystoscopy, and sigmoidoscopy. These tests all help evaluate the spread of the cancer from the uterus to nearby pelvic structures.

Surgery for Very Early Disease   For very early cancer of the uterus, that is, cancer confined to the uterus and not deeply invading the muscle wall, surgery to remove the uterus and ovaries (a hysterectomy with a salpingo-oophorectomy) is the treatment of choice and offers a 90 percent chance for cure.

Radiation and Surgery for More Advanced Disease If the cancer is deeply invading the muscle wall of the uterus but is still confined to the uterus and/or cervix (stages 1–2), more extensive treatment is needed. Approximately 50 percent of women in this situation are cured. Radiation, both external and employing radium implants, with surgical removal of the uterus after the radiation is finished is the treatment of choice.

Radiation for Very Advanced Disease With spread of the cancer beyond the uterus to other structures in the pelvis (stages 3–4), radiation is used alone and the chance for cure is minimal (10 percent). As the disease becomes more advanced, your chance for cure declines and the extent of treatment and therefore the side effects increase. Thus, you should do everything possible to have this cancer detected early.

Hormones Can Control Endometrial Cancer In contrast to cancer of the cervix, cancer of the uterus often responds to hormones. Progesterone, a female hormone, is effective treatment for advanced cancer. This is well illustrated in the following case.

H.C., a sixty-year-old school teacher, received radiation and surgery for advanced cancer of the uterus. She felt well for three and a half years after treatment, but then a chest x-ray showed that the tumor had spread to her lungs. Although she still felt well, the lung metastases grew larger over several months. H.C. was treated with high doses of progesterone, and over several months, all the tumors present on her lung x-rays disappeared. It has been six years since the metastases originally appeared. She currently has no evidence of cancer. She feels completely well except for some mild arthritis that has nothing to do with her cancer.

Progesterone is very effective therapy for some women who have advanced cancer of the uterus. Up to 30 percent will respond to progesterone therapy. Unlike responses to chemotherapy, progesterone responses can last for many years. The side effects of progesterone are minimal and include retention of fluid and occasional nausea. The fluid retention can be controlled with diuretics or water pills and the nausea is usually mild and temporary.

Uterine cancer occurs in older women than cervical cancer and is harder to diagnose. However, careful checkups and immediate medical attention for symptoms of postmenopausal bleeding can lead to earlier diagnosis and curative treatment. Estrogens given for menopausal symptoms are known risk factors for this cancer. Therefore, women should consider the benefits and risks of taking estrogens. Estrogens have been available for only twenty to thirty years, and thousands of generations of women have gone through menopause without them. However, there are definite benefits. Estrogens relieve menopausal symptoms such as hot flashes and also help keep bones from becoming soft as you get older, which is a common problem. But there is the risk of cancer of the uterus to consider also.

CANCER OF THE OVARY

Cancer of the ovary is far less common than cancer of the uterus or cervix, but it is far more dangerous and it accounts for more cancer deaths. It can occur at any age; even teenagers can get this disease. It is less curable than the other tumors because the ovaries lie deep within the pelvis and are inaccessible for early diagnosis. There are no early symptoms or signs of this cancer. It does not usually cause symptoms until it grows to a large size. By this time it has often spread and is difficult or impossible to cure.

Diagnosis

Although it can occasionally be diagnosed in a routine pelvic examination, cancer of the ovary most often presents with symptoms. Women complain of vague pains or discomfort in the pelvic area. They may have constipation from compression of the colon or marked swelling of the abdomen because of accumulation of fluid, called ascites.

Occasionally, your gynecologist may find a cyst on examination of your ovaries. In general, cysts less than two inches in diameter can be watched. Many of these will disappear after your next period. However, cysts larger than two inches require immediate further evaluation, including an examination called laporoscopy. Under local anesthesia, the gynecologist is able to introduce a tube through the abdominal wall and look at the organs in the pelvis. He may see through this tube and examine the ovary and also obtain small biopsies. This is not a very painful procedure. He is often able to tell just by visual examination whether an ovarian cyst is benign. If he is not sure, he may obtain a biopsy, but more often he will perform an abdominal exploration.

If you have gone to your doctor with symptoms and he finds masses in the pelvis or if there is fluid in your abdomen, surgery is almost always indicated. If fluid is present, he may introduce a small needle into the abdomen, remove some fluid, and examine the fluid under a microscope to see if cancer cells are present. Most often an exploratory abdominal operation called a laparotomy is needed for diagnosis, treatment, and also to evaluate the extent of the disease. If ovarian cancer is suspected, it is important to seek the most qualified surgeon available. Qualifications for a gynecologic cancer surgeon were discussed earlier in this chapter.

Treatment

Surgery The laparotomy is very important. The best chance for cure is with complete removal of the cancer, and the extent of disease is best evaluated at surgery. Prior to surgery, a chest-x-ray, an intravenous pyelogram, an abdominal ultrasound examination, and possibly a lymphangiogram are obtained. At surgery, the surgeon should evaluate the extent of the cancer. He should very carefully look at the surface of the abdomen and biopsy any areas that look suspicious for metastases. He should also remove as much of the cancer as possible. The usual operation is a bilateral oophorectomy with hysterectomy. Occasionally in early cancer, and this is rare, the opposite ovary can be left in. As with other gynecologic cancer surgery, the more experienced your surgeon, the more he will be able to do for you. Most critically, the experienced cancer surgeon is better able to evaluate the extent of disease. This is extremely important, as the extent of disease plays a key role in deciding what therapy if any you should receive after surgery.

Ovarian cancer spreads rapidly throughout the abdomen by a seeding process. This is what makes it so difficult to cure. Cells exfoliate, or fall off the surface of the ovary, and spread throughout the abdominal cavity much like seeds falling off a tree. These seeds may take root and continue to grow in any area of the abdomen. The metastases can irritate the surface of the abdominal cavity and cause fluid to be formed that leads to ascites, a common problem with ovarian cancer. More often than not the gynecologist at laparotomy will find spread to the surface of the abdomen, and further treatment is necessary to treat these metastases.

The Role of Radiation and Chemotherapy after Surgery Treatment after surgery involves technically difficult radiation, chemotherapy, or both. Both radiation and chemotherapy are used to treat women whose ovarian cancer has spread beyond the ovaries. However, the optimal treatment for ovarian cancer beyond the earliest stage is still controversial. Both chemotherapy and radiation are effective ways to treat the cancer, and the exact role that each should play in advanced disease is still under study. Therefore, you should be evaluated by a group of cancer specialists including a radiation oncologist and a medical oncologist, in addition to your surgeon. Unlike the other gynecologic cancers previously discussed, experimental therapy may have a role in ovarian cancer. Cancer centers are currently studying new ways of using radiation and chemotherapy to treat advanced disease more effectively. A consultation with such a center may be worthwhile rather than receiving treatment in your home community.

Treatment for the Different Stages of Ovarian Cancer If you are lucky and the cancer is confined to the ovary (stage 1), surgery alone has a high chance of curing you. If the cancer has spread to other structures in the pelvis (stage 2), you will probably receive radiation in addition to surgery and still have a reasonable chance for cure (50–60 percent). Some centers are evaluating the usefulness of chemotherapy for this stage of disease. The question is whether chemotherapy will cure more women than radiation. Doctors still do not know whether chemotherapy is of benefit if the disease is limited to the pelvis.

If the cancer has spread into the abdomen (stage 3), a combination of radiation and chemotherapy is used to control the cancer but the chance for cure is not good (10–15 percent). The best treatment for advanced, or stage 3, cancer of the ovary isn't known yet. It is generally agreed that as much tumor as possible should be removed during surgery. However, the relative roles of radiation and chemotherapy to treat the remaining disease in the pelvis and abdomen are controversial. Current approaches include extensive radiation of the pelvis and abdomen, a combination of radiation to the pelvis and chemotherapy, or chemotherapy alone. Both radiation and chemotherapy are effective treatments for ovarian cancer. Both, in fact, can cure some women whose disease isn't totally removed surgically. Clinical trials are currently in progress to see which approach, if any, is superior.

This type of therapy is both complex to plan and difficult to carry out. It may be best accomplished in larger hospitals or cancer centers. If you do not wish to be treated in such a center, a trip to a large center for a consultation to help plan your therapy may be worthwhile. The following case history illustrates some of the features of advanced ovarian cancer.

A.L., a forty-year-old housewife and mother of three children, began to feel ill and to lose weight. Over several months she lost fifteen pounds, but although she was losing weight, she noticed that her waist size was actually increasing. Slacks and dresses that she used to be able to wear easily no longer fit. At her husband's insistence she saw her family physician. When he examined her he found she had fluid in her abdomen.

He admitted her to the hospital for evaluation. She underwent several tests, including a liver scan (which was normal) and an abdominal ultrasound (which showed multiple pelvic masses and the presence of fluid in the abdomen). The doctor, under local anesthesia, placed a small needle into the abdominal cavity and withdrew half a cup of fluid. He sent this fluid to be examined for the presence of cancer cells. The report from the pathologist said that cancer cells were present and were most likely from the ovary.

A gynecologist with experience in cancer surgery was consulted. A laparotomy was performed and he found a large cancer of the ovary that had spread extensively throughout the pelvis. The surgeon removed as much of the tumor as he could, along with the uterus and both ovaries. Although there was fluid in the abdomen, he did not notice any tumor deposit outside of the pelvis.

After A.L. recovered from surgery, her gynecologist asked both a radiation therapist and a medical oncologist to see and evaluate her.

Together they arrived at a treatment program that consisted of three courses of chemotherapy to be followed by pelvic irradiation and then further chemotherapy.

A.L. was treated with two drugs, Cytoxan and Adriamycin, given every three weeks. The side effects from this therapy included nausea and vomiting for two days after she was given the drug, and she lost her hair. She bought a wig. After recovering from the surgery and starting the chemotherapy, she began to feel better. She gained fifteen pounds, felt stronger, and was able to resume many of her normal activities.

Twelve weeks after the operation, A.L. started a course of pelvic irradiation. During the radiation she felt sick to her stomach much of the time, and again started to lose weight. Radiation took six weeks. She then had a month with no further therapy and was started on lesser doses of the same two drugs, which she continued for two years. At the present time she has been off all treatment for one year and has no evidence of recurrence of disease. We do not know if she has been cured, but her life most certainly has been significantly prolonged.

A Team Approach Is Important for Cancer of the Ovary

Ovarian cancer is a complex cancer to treat. It involves cooperation among physicians skilled in different disciplines. Specialists in surgery, radiation, and chemotherapy must work together to offer you the best chance for a longer life if you have this dread disease. A.L. was treated with all three forms of therapy: surgery to remove as much of the cancer as possible, radiation to treat the remaining cancer in the pelvis, and chemotherapy to treat any cancer cells that had spread to the abdomen.

Other Female Reproductive Tract Cancers

The cancers of the female genital tract other than cancer of the cervix, cancer of the uterine body, and cancer of the ovary are relatively uncommon and will be discussed very briefly.

CANCER OF THE VULVA

The vulva is the external region of the female genital tract. When cancer develops there, patients feel a lump or complain of discharge, bleeding, irritation, itching, and pain. The diagnosis is quite easily made, and the treatment is surgery. The cure rate is high with early cancer of the vulva, but decreases with advanced disease. If you notice any sores, irritations, or lumps in this area of your body, you should see your doctor immediately.

CANCER OF THE VAGINA

This is a fairly uncommon cancer and is usually seen in women over the age of fifty. Vaginal discharge, spotting of blood, and pain are the usual early symptoms. Treatment involves radiation therapy. Approximately one patient in three is presently cured with this cancer.

Exposure to Estrogen Injections in Utero Causes Cancer

In the past several years, for the first time young women have developed cancer of the vagina. These young women all had been exposed to estrogens before they were born (in utero). Their mothers were given large doses of female hormones while they were pregnant to prevent threatened abortions. If you as a mother know that you took female hormones while you were pregnant, or you as a young woman know that your mother received such treatment, you should inform your gynecologist. Vaginal cancer in exposed women occurs very soon after the start of menses. There have been several hundred cases of vaginal cancer in exposed women. We therefore recommend that all women who have been exposed to estrogens in utero be seen by a gynecologist every six months for a thorough examination and a Pap smear. With early diagnosis, treatment often results in cure. This unfortunate occurrence points up the hazards of taking any form of hormones or drugs when pregnant. These hormones did not prevent abortions and only endangered the fetus. Drugs, alcohol, and radiation should be avoided during pregnancy because of the unknown risks they pose to your children.

CHORIOCARCINOMA OF THE UTERUS

This is a very rare cancer that develops in pregnant women from the placenta. (The placenta is the organ that connects the baby in the mother's uterus with the mother so it can receive nourishment and oxygen.) Choriocarcinoma develops in approximately one of 40,000 pregnancies. It is a very malignant cancer. Choriocarcinomas grow fast and metastasize widely. In fact, the first signs or symptoms of this cancer are often due to metastases. For example, a woman may go to her doctor with a persistent cough or trouble breathing because of spread to the lung.

Chemotherapy Can Often Cure This Cancer   Choriocarcinoma is too rare to discuss in detail but we want to get across one important message. The treatment for this disease is chemotherapy, which is very effective. Depending upon the extent of metastases, either one drug or a combination of drugs is used. It is extremely important that you receive the best possible treatment program so that you have the best chance of being cured. Therefore, we strongly recommend that if you have choriocarcinoma you go to a cancer center that has an experienced gynecologic oncologist or medical oncologist and a program for treating this very malignant but highly curable cancer. It pays to travel even a great distance to a large cancer center or medical center to receive treatment or at least to be evaluated for a treatment program that can be given by a doctor in your community.

HYDATIFORM MOLES

A mole is a benign lesion that also arises in pregnant women from the placenta. It is not uncommon, occurring in about one of every 2,000 pregnancies. Though hydatiform moles are benign, about 2 percent do develop into a choriocarcinoma. Therefore, if you have a mole you should either receive chemotherapy for several months, which will almost always prevent a choriocarcinoma from developing, or be followed very closely by your doctor. He or she should do pelvic examinations and also obtain a blood test for human chorionic gonadotrophins (HCG), a hormone secreted by both moles and choriocarcinoma. This HCG level should be normal if all is well. A rise indicates trouble; either the mole has recurred or has developed into choriocarcinoma, both of which need treatment with chemotherapy.

SUMMARY

1. All women over the age of twenty should have a yearly Pap smear to detect cancer of the cervix; when it is detected early, *in situ*, it is highly curable.

2. The routine Pap smear does not reliably detect cancer of the body of the uterus (womb). If you are postmenopausal and have vaginal bleeding or spotting, you should see your doctor and have a complete evaluation for cancer.

3. Optimal treatment for cancer of the uterine body or uterine cervix is best obtained by a team approach; surgery and/or radiation may be required. A gynecologist (if possible, a gynecologic oncologist) and a radiation oncologist should plan the treatment together. There are not enough trained gynecologic oncologists yet, but you should at least have a gynecologist who has had experience in cancer surgery.

4. If you have ovarian cancer, we recommend that you be treated at or at least visit a large medical center for a consultation so your care can be directed by specialists who are trained and experienced in the treatment of this disease. Surgery, radiation, and chemotherapy should all be considered for the initial treatment of ovarian cancer. The treatment should be planned by a team composed of a gynecologist, a radiation oncologist, and a medical oncologist.

5. All young women who were exposed to estrogens in utero should see a gynecologist at least twice a year for an extensive evaluation because of the high probability of developing vaginal cancer.

6. Choriocarcinoma is a very malignant cancer. The treatment for it is

high-dose chemotherapy, which is very effective and often curative. We recommend going to a large cancer clinic or medical center if you have choriocarcinoma, so that you receive the best chemotherapy program, which will give you the best chance for cure.

7. A hydatiform mole may develop into a choriocarcinoma. Therefore, we recommend several months of either chemotherapy or close observation by your gynecologist to insure all is well.

15

Cancers of the Urinary Tract and Male Reproductive Organs

The cancers discussed in this chapter occur mostly in men. These are common cancers that kill 33,000 Americans each year. Although cancers arise from all portions of the urinary tract, they occur most commonly in either the kidney or the bladder. We have also included cancer of the testicle and prostate in this chapter because, like cancers of the urinary tract, they should be treated by urologists. Female genital cancers are under the care of gynecologists and are therefore discussed in the previous chapter.

The Urologist

The cancers discussed in this chapter are all treated by urologists. These are physicians who have been trained in the diagnosis and treatment of diseases of the genitourinary system. A board-certified urologist has had several years of formal training in general surgery and at least three additional years of training and caring for people with diseases of the kidney, bladder, prostate, and male sexual organs. He is a surgeon who is specially trained and usually restricts his practice to problems of the urinary tract and male sexual organs. If you have proven or suspected cancer of the kidney, bladder, prostate, or testes, you should be under the care of a board-certified urologist. He or she is the physician who is best qualified both to diagnose and to direct treatment for these cancers.

KIDNEY CANCER

Cancer of the kidney, often called hypernephroma or renal cell carcinoma, is much more common in men than in women. It most often occurs between the ages of fifty and sixty. Each year, approximately 15,000 Americans develop and 7,000 die from cancer of the kidney.

Causes

Kidney cancer is rare in animals unless they are given carcinogens. Certain chemicals that cause the disease in animals may do so in man. Cigarette smoking is associated with a fivefold increase in kidney cancer and—unlike lung cancer—pipe smoking, cigar smoking, and chewing tobacco also increase the risk. Factors in cigarette smoke leading to kidney cancer may include tars and a trace metal called cadmium. Workers exposed to cadmium have an increased incidence of both kidney and prostate cancers. Heavy exposure occurs in a number of industries, including electroplating, alloy making, welding, and the manufacturing of storage batteries.

Diagnosis

Cancer of the kidney is often difficult to diagnose. Symptoms vary and not infrequently are quite vague. In about two-thirds of kidney cancer victims the first symptoms are related to the local growth of the cancer: blood in the urine or pain in the side or low back. Often the physician can feel a mass in the area of the kidney when he examines the abdomen. In the other one-third of patients, however, the symptoms are nonspecific and include fever, weight loss, or fatigue. It is difficult for even an experienced physician to think of and diagnose kidney cancer with these vague symptoms. They are common problems and are rarely due to cancer of the kidney.

When a physician suspects cancer of the kidney, he or she will order several tests. First, a urinalysis is checked for blood. With kidney cancer, the urine almost always contains some red blood cells even if it appears normal. Next, an intravenous pyelogram (IVP) is done. This examination is performed by intravenously injecting an iodine-containing dye, which is concentrated and excreted by the kidneys. The IVP will show the kidneys containing the iodine and enable the doctor to determine whether there is a mass in one of the kidneys. Another test that may be helpful is an ultrasound examination of the abdomen. This tells whether a kidney mass is cystic, and thus probably benign, or solid, and probably malignant. If the IVP and ultrasound examinations indicate that cancer of the kidney might be present, an arteriogram will be ordered. For this type of x-ray a needle must be inserted into an artery, usually in the leg, and a plastic catheter is passed through the needle into the artery and up into the abdomen to the area of the kidneys. Dye is then injected into the artery by a pump and many x-ray films are taken. This test is safe and gives invaluable information. It is usually diagnostic in renal cell cancer and also shows the urologist the blood supply of the cancer, giving important information on how to approach the cancer surgically.

Staging: Has the Cancer Spread?

Before treatment is decided upon, several tests should be obtained to see if the cancer has spread beyond the kidney. These tests will usually include a venogram, or x-ray examination of the vena cava (the major vein in the abdomen), to determine if the cancer is pressing upon or invading this large vein, a chest x-ray, a bone scan, and a liver scan. Scans are performed by intravenously injecting a small amount of radioactive substance that is picked up either by the liver or by the bone. Then pictures are taken using a large machine called a camera. This camera, instead of seeing light, sees radioactivity. Areas of decreased radioactivity on a liver scan or increased radioactivity on a bone scan may mean that the cancer has spread to these organs. If these studies show no spread of the cancer, there is a chance for cure. Metastases to the lungs, bones, liver, or any other organ mean that cure is impossible and treatment should be directed at preventing symptoms rather than trying to eradicate the cancer.

Prognosis

The prognosis with cancer of the kidney is neither hopeless nor reassuring. Approximately 30 percent of patients are cured. Early diagnosis is not possible at present, and the basic treatment—surgical removal of the kidney—has not changed in the past twenty years. There are no real prospects for any significant improvement in treatment in the near future. If the cancer is still localized to the kidney, it can be removed and cure is possible. In the majority of victims who already have spread of cancer, cure is impossible.

Unlike the situation with most other cancers, the course of metastatic or incurable cancer of the kidney is very unpredictable. Although most people with metastases die within two years, we have seen patients live and feel well for years with unchanging metastases in bones, lungs, and other organs. Rarely, these metastases may even disappear—so-called "spontaneous regressions." Some people can live a long time with widespread disease. Therefore, people with metastatic cancer of the kidney should not give up hope.

Treatment

Surgery The treatment for cancer of the kidney depends upon whether or not the tests show spread to other organs. If the cancer is still localized to the kidney, the standard treatment is to remove the kidney and nearby lymph nodes. Up to 80 percent of people with localized cancer will be cured by such surgery. Surprisingly, 30 percent of the patients with cancer that has spread to the nearby lymph nodes will also be alive ten years after surgery. This surgery should be performed by a board-certified urologist, since it is a difficult operation even for an experienced surgeon.

Radiation   Radiation therapy to the area of the kidney and nearby lymph nodes to destroy cancer cells is administered either before or after surgery. It is being evaluated in clinical trials at the present time, so its value is unknown.

Treatment for the Person with Metastases

If tests show that the cancer has spread to other parts of the body, treatment varies and should be individualized to match each patient's situation or particular problem. For example, if there is extensive involvement of the liver and the patient has lost a lot of weight, chances are he or she will not live long. In this situation, surgical removal of the kidney, a major operation, makes no sense. However, people with metastases may live for months and even years. Therefore, they might need their cancerous kidney removed. If it is not removed, severe problems such as massive bleeding into the urine or acute pain can make life miserable. Here surgery is palliative; it makes the patient feel better so that he or she can more fully enjoy the time left. Surgical removal of the kidney when cure is impossible should be performed only when there are significant symptoms such as pain and bleeding from the kidney, it should not be done unless the person will live at least several months.

The treatment of metastatic kidney cancer isn't very effective at present. Radiation to control bone pain is usually quite effective and has few or no side effects. However, chemotherapy to control metastatic kidney cancer isn't very effective.

Hormones   Two hormones, progesterone and androgens (or male sex hormone), are both given to control metastatic renal cell cancer. Approximately 10 percent of patients are helped. In these 10 percent, the cancer shrinks and the person feels better. Some live longer with hormone therapy. Although only 10 percent benefit, the treatment is relatively free from toxic side effects. These hormones do not make the patient as ill as high-dose chemotherapy. We advise that all patients with metastatic kidney cancer try hormones. A rare person has his or her cancer controlled even for years with this form of treatment.

Chemotherapy   Chemotherapy is relatively ineffective against cancer of the kidney. Therefore, we recommend either not taking chemotherapy for taking a single drug in low to moderate doses, since the chance for being helped is very small. We think it makes sense to avoid the severe side effects of high-dose combination chemotherapy.

The treatment for cancer of the kidney is fairly standard in this country. There is little to be gained by traveling to a large medical center clinic. There are no promising experimental approaches at present. Adequate treatment is available in communities that have a board-certified urologist.

The following case history is typical of kidney cancer and illustrates several important points about it.

L.K., a piano tuner with two grown children, developed bloody urine and pain in the right side of his upper back. He saw his physician, who suspected a kidney stone and admitted him to the hospital. His doctor gave him narcotics to control his pain and performed an intravenous pyelogram. The x-rays showed a large mass in his left kidney that was undoubtedly cancer. His physician referred L.K. to a urologist, who saw him, reviewed the kidney x-rays, and obtained an arteriogram and a vena cavogram (an x-ray that shows the large vein draining the kidney). The arteriogram showed a large tumor in the upper part of the left kidney and the venogram showed that it was pressing upon this vein. The urologist next obtained a chest x-ray, a liver scan, and a bone scan. These tests were negative. L.K. was operated upon five days after he first saw a physician. At surgery his left kidney and nearby lymph glands were removed. The cancer was advanced: it had spread through the kidney into the surrounding fat and through the vein draining the kidney into the vena cava. The urologist told L.K. and his wife that, while he had removed all the cancer he had seen, the chance for cure was not good. Only time would tell whether the cancer would recur.

L.K. had a rapid recovery from surgery. He was home three weeks after first consulting his physician, and he went back to work after three months. L.K. had to face the frightening fact that he had cancer and that it could recur any time and eventually kill him. He dealt with this quite well. However, his wife was terrified. She was very depressed and cried often. She urged him to call his doctor about every minor pain, for every cough or bowel irregularity. She also called the physician frequently, asking for reassurance that she could not be given. She wanted very much to be told that the cancer had been cured. She couldn't cope, and her unre-solved anxiety made L.K.'s existence very difficult. At his wife's insistence, he treated himself like an invalid. L.K.'s physician understood what was happening between L.K. and his wife and tried to help. He never excluded L.K.'s wife from any conference he had with L.K. and he en-couraged her to call if she had any questions about L.K.'s medical condi-tion. However, he could not do what she wanted and needed: he could not predict the future.

It is not unusual for patients who eventually die of their cancer to lose the months or years when they feel well because they or their family can't face the uncertainty of recurrence. Our advice is to get professional psychological help if anxiety prevents you or your family from dealing with your illness. L.K. was physically well during this period of time, but much of his energies were directed to dealing with his wife's unresolved fears and anxieties.

L.K. was very pleased to go back to work. However, nine months after surgery, a routine chest x-ray showed a shadow in the left lung that was almost certainly spread from his kidney cancer. Although L.K. felt well, his physician placed him on progesterones to control the lung metastases. He took one injection every week without any side effects. Over the next two months the shadow on his chest x-ray disappeared completely. His doctor told him he was one of the lucky few whose tumor responded to hormones.

L.K. felt well for two and one-half years, during which time he continued taking progesterone. At that time he began to have pain in his back. An x-ray showed destruction of a vertebra almost surely due to the cancer. He received radiation therapy over a three-week period with complete relief of pain. He felt well for another year, receiving radiation for two additional painful bone metastases, but then he developed spread to his lung and liver and died of shortness of breath.

L.K. had received excellent care. However, his cancer wasn't caught early enough. L.K.'s quick response to radiation was very typical. With almost no side effects, bone pain can usually be quickly and completely controlled, no matter what type of cancer you have. L.K. eventually died of his cancer, but he lived more than three years and felt well during most of that time. Unfortunately, during these years his wife's inability to cope with his cancer made his life difficult. Too often months and even years are wasted because the patient or his family cannot face living with uncertainty.

CANCER OF THE BLADDER

Bladder cancer is the most frequent malignant tumor of the urinary tract. The disease is most common between the ages of fifty and seventy and accounts for 3 percent of cancer deaths in the United States. As with cancer of the kidney, bladder cancer is associated with exposure to several carcinogens. The urinary tract excretes many substances and therefore is exposed to many possible carcinogens. It was reported as early as 1895 that bladder cancer was unusually common among workers in aniline dye factories. As with many other carcinogen-induced cancers, there is a long latent period (maybe twenty years or more) between exposure to carcinogens and the development of cancer. Thus, workers exposed to aniline dyes even for a short period of time may develop bladder cancer much later.

Several other carcinogens have been associated with bladder cancer. These include the tars in tobacco smoke, other chemicals with aromatic amine groups (such as 2-naphtholmine), and chronic irritation from schistosomiasis infestation, a parasitic infection common in the tropics.

The saccharin controversy (discussed in more detail in chapter 2,

"Carcinogens in Our Environment") illustrates the difficulty of evaluating and possibly removing carcinogens from our environment. Saccharin, a coal tar derivative, in huge doses causes bladder cancer in rats. It has been said that a person would have to drink thousands of saccharin-containing soft drinks to get an equivalent amount. However, it is an axiom of carcinogenesis that a noncarcinogenic chemical cannot cause cancer no matter how high the dose. It is almost impossible to say whether saccharin does or does not cause human bladder cancer, but it is suspect.

We feel that if a substance is not absolutely critical to survival and is identified as a carcinogen in animal studies, no matter what the dose, it should be eliminated from the diet and/or environment. Obviously, this is difficult with strongly addicting substances such as tobacco, but is much easier with chemicals that man has lived without successfully for thousands of years, such as saccharin. The person with diabetes may gain from using saccharin, but most people can live without it. One does not have to see many patients suffering or dying with bladder cancer before one develops a strong bias against chemicals like saccharin that may cause this cancer.

Diagnosis

For most people with bladder cancer, the first symptom is painless bloody urine. Occasionally they may also have trouble urinating, with some pain or a feeling that they have to urinate frequently. The bleeding from the bladder is very often intermittent, and some people delay seeing a doctor if their bloody urine stops by itself. Even worse, some physicians will delay an evaluation because the bleeding has stopped. We cannot emphasize too strongly that all people with bloody urine need a thorough medical investigation. Early bladder cancer is easily curable, while advanced disease is difficult or impossible to cure.

The first test your doctor should perform if you think you have seen blood in your urine is a urinalysis. This will show even a small amount of blood in your urine. If blood is present, you should have an intravenous pyelogram and you should be referred to a urologist, who will perform a cystoscopy.

Cystoscopy is an examination done under local anesthesia. A hollow tube allowing both visual inspection and biopsies of the bladder is passed through the penis in the male or through the urethra in the female into the bladder. The urologist will examine the bladder and biopsy and try to remove any suspicious growths that he, or she, sees. These biopsies will show if bladder cancer is present.

If cancer is present, the pathologist will report how malignant the tumor appears under the microscope and how deeply into the bladder wall it has penetrated. Many bladder cancers do not appear very malignant under the microscope and are located on the surface of the bladder wall. These can easily be removed or destroyed by electrically burning out the tissue. This is done by the urologist during cystoscopy. It is painless since it is done under anesthesia. Bladder cancers, in fact, tend to start superficially, recur over many years, and become more malignant. They then invade the muscles of the bladder wall deeply, necessitating radical surgery or radiation for control.

Treatment

Both the prognosis and the treatment of bladder cancer depend upon how deeply the cancer invades the bladder wall and how malignant the cancer appears under the microscope. These two factors usually go hand in hand. Bladder cancers that don't appear very malignant tend to be superficial, and those that appear very malignant tend to invade the bladder wall deeply. The superficial bladder cancers, not surprisingly, have the best cure rate and can be treated merely by removing them during cystoscopy. More than 80 percent of people with superficial tumors live five years or longer with very simple treatment.

In contrast, cancers that penetrate deeply into the bladder wall are difficult to eradicate, even with extensive surgery and/or radiation therapy. Even with aggressive treatment, less than 20 percent of such people are cured because most of these cancers have already spread beyond the bladder.

Early Bladder Cancer

The urologist is the key figure in the diagnosis and treatment of bladder cancer. He or she often consults with other specialists to offer you optimal treatment. If the bladder cancer is superficial and does not appear highly malignant under the microscope, a urologist can treat it adequately by removal or by fulguration through the cystoscope. Since these superficial cancers are almost always localized, no tests are indicated to look for spread of the cancer and no further treatment is necessary.

Early Diagnosis: The Case for Regular Cystoscopy   Bladder cancer tends to recur and recur. Therefore, anyone who develops one bladder cancer should have cystoscopy on a regular basis, even as often as every three months, to detect and remove any new cancers that arise. At least 40 percent of people with one bladder cancer will develop at least one other, and it is not unusual to develop many, many bladder cancers over the years.

While it is not feasible to cystoscope all Americans on a regular basis to detect bladder cancers early, it is feasible to do so in all who develop bladder cancer. It is also possible to do this for all people at high risk, such as workers exposed to aniline dyes. With regular cystoscopies, bladder cancers can be detected at a very early stage, when they are easily curable. The following case history illustrates the usefulness of regular cystoscopies.

M.H., a sixty-one-year-old bus driver, noticed some blood in his urine and went to see his family physician. His physician ordered a urinalysis, which showed blood. M.H. was then sent to a urologist, who obtained an intravenous pyelogram that was normal. He then performed a cystoscopy and found a small lesion, which was biopsied and removed. The lesion proved to be a superficial cancer.

M.H. was told that he had bladder cancer but that it was caught early, and therefore was almost certainly cured. The urologist told him that he should have regular cystoscopies since he was prone to develop more bladder cancers. M.H. agreed and had cystoscopy every three months over the next four years. Six small bladder cancers were removed during that time. All were superficial and completely removed at cystoscopy.

Because bladder cancers were developing so often, the urologist recommended that thio-tepa be instilled in his bladder in an attempt to prevent development of these cancers. Thio-tepa is an anticancer agent that seems to prevent the development of bladder cancers in some patients. M.H. had several of these treatments, and over the next four years did not have another bladder cancer. It is now eight years since his first bladder cancer developed and he is healthy.

If M.H. had not had regular cystoscopies, most probably one of his cancers would have deeply invaded the bladder wall, spread beyond the bladder, and ultimately killed him. Instead, M.H. had regular cystoscopies and is alive and well eight years later.

Advanced Bladder Cancer

If the biopsy done during cystoscopy shows that the cancer penetrates deeply into the bladder wall, the story changes dramatically. Deep invasion signals a very malignant tumor that probably has spread beyond the bladder. A series of tests is done to determine if and to which organs the cancer has spread. A chest x-ray, a liver scan, and a bone scan should be obtained. If these do not demonstrate metastases, curative treatment can be tried. Cancer must be eradicated in the bladder and nearby lymph nodes.

Extensive surgery, intensive radiation, or both are used. Even with this aggressive therapeutic approach, only 20 percent of people are cured. The other 80 percent die. Despite negative tests, the cancer had already spread to other parts of their bodies.

A Team Approach Is Needed for Advanced Bladder Cancer   Therapeutic options in advanced bladder cancer include surgery, radiation therapy, or both together. Therefore, optimal treatment can be obtained only when a urologist works closely with a radiation oncologist. The patient should be seen by both specialists, so the advantages of either therapy alone or both together can be evaluated for each individual. Often an internist is also needed. Bladder cancer victims are older and commonly have other medical problems, such as lung and heart disease. An internist can help evaluate surgical risks. There is no reason to go to a major university hospital or cancer center for the treatment of this disease; good urologists, internists, and radiation oncologists are available in most large communities.

Before surgery is performed, three factors must be considered. First, is your general health good enough to tolerate extensive surgery? Second, is there any evidence that surgery will not be curative? (To decide this the surgeon will perform a number of tests, which have already been mentioned.) Third, can the person tolerate and care for the substitute bladder that the surgeon will construct?

Surgery   For people in good general health who need surgery, the usual procedure is total removal of the bladder along with the draining lymph nodes, the prostate (in males), and some of the urethra. This operation is termed a radical cystectomy. The surgeon must take the ureters (the tubes that connect the kidneys to the bladder) and implant them into an artificial bladder.

The Artificial Bladder.   Three types of artificial bladders are currently used: the ileal loop, the rectal bladder, and the ureterocutaneous bladder. An ileal loop is a section of the small intestine that is removed from the intestinal stream and isolated. The ureters are connected to this and a tube is then connected to a bag that the patient wears on his abdomen or his leg. A rectal bladder involves placing the ureters into the rectum so the patient urinates through the rectum; however, a colostomy must be performed so that the fecal stream is diverted into a bag (as discussed in chapter 13, "Cancers of the Gastrointestinal Tract"). The other option is to connect the ureters directly to an outside appliance (ureterocutaneous bladder). The surgery is complicated and the person must make a major adjustment to live successfully afterward. With all the available options, either urine or stool must be collected in a bag strapped to the body. Thus, psychological adjustments similar to those of a colostomy patient are necessary (see chapter 13).

The American Cancer Society in conjunction with the United Ostomy Association has twenty thousand volunteer members who have ostomies and who are available to help you adjust. A volunteer will visit you if you ask your doctor to call the American Cancer Society after surgery. He or she will be able to answer your questions and is proof that a person can live and function after this type of radical surgery. Few people adjust to such a change in their body image without help. In our experience, people who have undergone the same operation are the most help.

Radiation   Radiation therapy can be used instead of surgery to try to cure bladder cancer. The cure rate or survival rate with high-dose radical radiation is very similiar to that obtained with surgery. The side effects include irritation and sometimes permanent damage to the bladder and bowel within the radiated area. Therefore, pain on urination, urinary frequency, and diarrhea are common problems. These symptoms are usually temporary and can be controlled by medication. However, there are also late side effects of radiation. These occur many months after the radiation has been completed and include a contracted and small bladder, ulceration and hemorrhage from the bladder, and radiation damage to the bowel (which can cause bleeding and obstruction). Therefore, radiation, like surgery, has many side effects, but it may spare the person the problem of an artificial bladder.

Combination Therapy: Surgery and Radiation   Some people with advanced bladder cancer are now treated with both radiation and surgery. The aim of this is to use each type of therapy in the manner that works best. Radiation controls the metastases to the nearby lymph nodes better than surgery. Surgery is better at removing the bulk of the cancer in the bladder. When radiation and surgery are used together, less radiation is needed and less extensive surgery is done. However, an artificial bladder is necessary. It is possible that the combination of surgery and radiation will cure more than either radical surgery or radiation or will cure the same number with fewer side effects.

Chemotherapy   The treatment of bladder cancer that has metastasized to other organs is not very encouraging. Usually, once metastases appear, bladder cancer tends to progress quite rapidly and survival is generally short. Chemotherapy is relatively ineffective, but has improved since the introduction of a drug called cis-platinum. Approximately 40 percent of patients will improve but usually only for a short period of time. Some people do respond well, feel better, and live longer with chemotherapy. High-dose combination or experimental chemotherapy might help, but the odds are heavily against anyone who tries such toxic chemotherapy at the present time. Therefore, we recommend no chemotherapy or low-dose chemotherapy. However, for those people who cannot accept the ineffectiveness of standard therapy, experimental drug programs are available.

The case of J.L. illustrates many of the difficulties that arise while living with this cancer.

J.L., a fifty-five-year-old sheep farmer, one evening felt crushing chest pain and collapsed. He was rushed to a local hospital, where he almost died from a massive heart attack. He had smoked two packs of cigarettes daily since he was fifteen years old. A routine urinalysis during his hospitalization revealed a small amount of blood in his urine. His doctor decided not to do any further tests while J.L. was recovering from his heart attack, but to perform them after several months. J.L. was discharged from the hospital in three weeks and was back at work on his ranch within six weeks.

When he saw his doctor three months later, another urinalysis was performed that again showed small amounts of blood. His doctor ordered an intravenous pyelogram, which was normal. He then made an appointment for J.L. with a urologist. However, J.L. was feeling well and was tired of seeing doctors, so he did not keep the appointment.

Six months passed and then J.L. began to have painful urination with bright red blood and blood clots. He went to his doctor, who immediately sent him to the urologist. He was hospitalized and the following morning underwent a cystoscopy. The urologist found two large and one small bladder tumors near the bottom of the bladder partially obstructing the urine flow. He was able to remove all three tumors with the cystoscope. The pathologist examined the tumors and found that they were well differentiated (not very malignant) and did not invade the muscle tissue. J.L.'s bleeding stopped and he was discharged from the hospital.

J.L. was told that the cancers were superficial and that most likely this relatively simple treatment had removed all the cancers. However, the urologist also told him that once bladder cancer develops, the chances are high that more will develop. Therefore, cystoscopies should be performed several times a year on a regular basis for the rest of his life. At first J.L. was frightened and planned to keep his appointments. However, as the first checkup approached, he decided that he was feeling well and did not need another cystoscopy. Two years went by without symptoms and without further medical care.

The tumors returned insidiously. First, J.L. had difficulty and pain when he urinated. This progressed until one morning he was unable to pass any urine although his bladder was full and painful. His wife drove him to a local emergency room, where he was catheterized (a rubber tube was placed through his penis into his bladder) and two quarts of urine were emptied from his bladder. He was seen by his former urologist, who cystoscoped him the following day. Unfortunately, a large cancer obstructing the passage of urine was found and a biopsy showed that it penetrated the bladder wall. An intravenous kidney x-ray showed damage to the kidneys from the pressure exerted by the urine and also evidence that the tumor had spread to the posterior abdomen.

Exploratory surgery was performed three days later. J.L.'s entire bladder was removed and the ureters were transplanted into a loop of bowel, an ileal loop, which was then left to drain into a bag worn on the abdomen. Examination of the bladder by the pathologist showed that the tumor had penetrated entirely through the bladder and had also involved several nearby lymph nodes. J.L. was next sent to a radiation oncologist for extensive radiation of his lower abdomen. Despite this very aggressive treatment the cancer spread to his bones and lung. J.L. died six months after his surgery from shortness of breath.

What happened to J.L. was indeed unfortunate but it happens all too often. J.L. did not return to his urologist for his regular cystoscopies. Rather, he waited for the bladder cancer to recur. He gave his cancer the chance to grow, invade deeply, and spread, and therefore become incurable. In contrast to the case of M.H., who saw his urologist regularly, had regular cystoscopies, and is alive, J.L. died of bladder cancer unnecessarily. Had the cancer been removed through cystoscopy early, many years of normal life could have been assured. Be sure that you take the time to have cystoscopy performed several times a year if you have had one bladder cancer.

CANCER OF THE PROSTATE

Cancer of the prostate is the most common cancer in men over the age of fifty. Fortunately, it is relatively uncommon in younger males. It only becomes common as men grow older and has a peak incidence at about seventy. Each year, approximately 60,000 cases are diagnosed and 20,000 Americans die from this disease.

When prostates are examined microscopically in men who have died from other conditions, unsuspected cancer is found in 15 to 50 percent of all men over the age of fifty. In these men, cancer of the prostate was of no consequence. It can be a very slow growing and therefore silent cancer. However, it cannot be ignored. While many men harbor asymptomatic cancer of the prostate that is discovered only at autopsy after death occurs from other causes, many others will have progressive disease and die from it unless it is treated.

Diagnosis

Cancer of the prostate can be discovered when it is still asymptomatic. Physicians often discover a lump in the prostate during a routine physical examination in older men, and it turns out to be cancer about half the time. Also, examination of the tissue removed during surgery done to relieve the obstruction of urine flow from benign prostatic hypertrophy, a very common problem in elderly men, can show deposits of prostate cancer. When symptoms do develop, the most common ones are due to enlargement of the prostate. This often causes difficulty starting urination, a small urine stream, or bleeding from the penis. Some people also go to a doctor with bone pain from metastatic cancer of the prostate. This cancer frequently spreads to bone, and may do so before causing any problems with urination.

The Rectal Examination   A rectal examination should be part of every physical examination for men over fifty. This will not only detect prostate cancer, which the physician feels as a hard lump in the prostate, but some rectal cancers as well. Asymptomatic prostate cancer has a better chance of being cured. Localized cancer can be cured with either surgery or radiation. Yearly rectal examinations after the age of fifty can detect cancer of the prostate before it causes symptoms. About half of nodules in the prostate that physicians feel in a rectal examination prove to be cancer. Therefore, once a prostatic nodule is discovered, the patient should be sent to a urologist for diagnosis and treatment.

A urologist will determine if cancer is present by obtaining a biopsy. He or she will usually do this by inserting a needle, either through the skin between scrotum and the rectum or through the rectum itself, to obtain tissue from the suspicious areas in the prostate.

Evaluating the Extent of the Disease

Once cancer is found, several tests should be performed to determine if it is localized. These should include x-rays of the bones and a bone scan, since prostate cancer usually spreads to the bones. A blood test called an acid phosphatase may be abnormal if the cancer has spread. An intravenous pyelogram checks for spread to the region around the prostate and bladder and a chest x-ray looks for spread to the lungs.

Treatment

Cancer of the prostate is a relatively chronic disease that usually occurs in elderly men who have other ailments such as diseases of the heart and lungs. Often their medical care become somewhat fragmented, with a urologist caring for their prostate cancer and an internist or general practitioner performing the remainder of their medical care. It is important that the doctors and the patient all communicate with one another. There is little to be gained by attempting aggressive treatment at a cancer center. What is required for adequate treatment of prostate cancer is the availability of a well-trained, board-certified urologist and a radiation oncologist. Radiation therapy may be used at several points in the disease: for initial treatment, for treatment of bone pain that has not responded to drugs such as stilbesterol (a female hormone), and occasionally in very low doses to relieve breast tenderness caused by stilbesterol.

If both the urologist's careful examination and the laboratory tests indicate that the cancer is still localized to the area of the prostate, then the aim of treatment should be to eradicate the cancer and hope for a cure. In contrast, if the tests indicate that the cancer has spread, the aim of treatment changes from cure to controlling symptoms.

Treatment for Cure

If the prostate cancer is still localized to the area of the prostate, there are two potentially curative therapeutic approaches—surgery or radiation.

Surgery   The curative operation for prostatic cancer is called a radical prostatectomy. The prostate gland, seminal vesicles, and part of the bladder are removed. This treatment is reserved for prostatic cancer that is still localized in men who do not have other diseases that are likely to end their life before the cancer spreads. About one prostatic cancer patient in ten has this radical surgery and about half are cured. Almost all become impotent and about 10 percent are unable to control their urine. Even in older men, impotence is a devastating development. Fortunately, several devices have been developed that can be implanted in the penis and allow the patient to have sexual intercourse again.

Radiation   Radiation to the prostate and draining lymph nodes is another approach that yields about the same cure rate as surgery. A big advantage is that potency is preserved in most patients and there are no problems with controlling urine flow. Complications of radiation include inflammation of the rectum during radiation, which can cause troublesome diarrhea and bleeding. Inflammation of the bladder can cause irritation on urination and bleeding in the urine.

If you have localized and therefore potentially curable cancer of the prostate, take your time to consider both options (surgery and radiation). Talk to both your urologist and a radiation oncologist personally to get both sides of the story. Find out about the effectiveness, cost, and side effects of each treatment. You need not make a decision overnight.

Metastatic Prostate Cancer

In most men with prostate cancer, the disease has spread and is, therefore, incurable. However, all is not lost. Metastatic cancer of the prostate does not signal impending suffering or death. The disease may remain stable or progress very slowly, which is why treatment is indicated only for metastases that cause problems such as bone pain. Prostatic cancer often is a very slowly progressing disease, one a man can live with, often for years.

If metastases are present but the patient feels well, the standard approach is merely to wait and see what happens. For example, H.R., a seventy-eight-year-old retired bus driver, found out he had cancer of the prostate when his doctor felt a nodule in his prostate on rectal examination during his yearly physical examination. He was sent to a urologist, who performed a biopsy that showed cancer of the prostate. X-rays of his hip and back bones showed changes characteristic of metastases of the prostate cancer to these bones. He had not had any pain in his bones and they weren't even tender when the urologist banged them gently with his hand. The urologist told H.R. about the metastases and that he might feel well and not need treatment for a long time. He wanted to wait and give treatment only when the cancer progressed and caused symptoms. He reassured H.R. that effective treatment was available. He felt well and had no bone pain for three years. Then his hips and back began to hurt. During these three years he was seen by the urologist on a regular basis and checked by examination and tests for advancing disease that might warrant treatment. When the pain did develop in his back and hips, H.R. had complete relief two weeks after starting stilbesterol, given in pills. He felt well for two years and had no further pain from his cancer. He died of a heart attack shortly after his eighty-fourth birthday.

Treatment of Metastases

Once problems from metastases do occur, up to 80 percent of patients will improve when placed on stilbesterol. An alternative treatment in men who cannot tolerate stilbesterol is surgical castration. Response to castration is similar to that with estrogens, because castration may aggravate heart disease.

Radiation   Radiation can relieve bone pain, a common problem with prostate cancer. It has few side effects and can be used in low doses given just to the areas that hurt.

Chemotherapy   Chemotherapy for prostate cancer is not very effective. Only about 10 percent of people improve. Because of the low response rate and the age of the typical patient (who may often have other medical problems), most oncologists either recommend no chemotherapy or low doses of relatively nontoxic drugs. Chemotherapy is only used in men who fail to respond to estrogens or castration.

The following case highlights some important aspects of the treatment of metastatic prostate cancer.

L.R., an eighty-five-year-old man, went to the emergency room of his local hospital because of some nagging low back pain. He had been working in his yard that day and after digging up six rose bushes had stabbing pain going down his left leg. He had been in excellent health and had not seen a doctor in sixty-two years. The emergency room physician took an x-ray of his lower back, and his bones were found to be riddled with unsuspected cancer. He was admitted to the hospital and a bone biopsy was performed. It showed extensive replacement of the bone with cancer, most likely from the prostate. Indeed, his acid phosphatase, a blood enzyme that is elevated almost exclusively in prostatic cancer, was 600 times greater than normal.

L.R. was examined by a urologist, who did not feel any surgery was indicated since the patient's prostate was not very large, although it contained a probably cancerous nodule. It was causing him no problem. Since he had pain in one area of the back, he was treated with radiation over a two-week period, with complete relief of pain.

Two years later his condition is absolutely unchanged. He is still planting roses, and despite his extensive cancer has had no further problems whatsoever. The only change in his routine is that he visits his urologist every few months to detect significant progression of the cancer so that hormones can be started if they are needed.

If a person with metastatic prostate cancer lives to be very old, he will probably die from the disease, but the course can be very, very slow. Both H.R.'s and L.R.'s case histories show that people can live normal lives despite widespread prostate cancer. Pain, the major problem, can almost always be relieved with either stilbesterol or radiation. Death, as often as not, occurs from other ailments associated with advanced age. We also wish to stress that for the rare man in his fifties or sixties with localized prostatic cancer, aggressive surgery and radiation should be used to attempt to cure.

Cancer of the Testes

Although cancer of the testes represents only about 1 percent of all cancer in men, it is the most common cancer in the eighteen to thirty age group. The only confirmed risk factor for this cancer is an undescended testicle.

The Undescended Testicle

The risk of developing testicular cancer is increased fiftyfold in men with an undescended testicle. Therefore, an undescended testicle should not be left in the abdomen. As it is hidden, if cancer develops there, it won't be diagnosed until it has become far advanced. The undescended testicle should be surgically brought into the scrotum or removed by a urologist. Any male whose testicle has been brought down into the scrotum surgically should be fully informed of the increased risk of testicular cancer and instructed and encouraged to examine his testicle every few months for early detection of cancerous lumps.

We feel that undescended testicles should be surgically removed and an artificial testicle placed in the scrotum. Many urologists don't agree, but we have now seen two young men die from testicular cancer that developed in undescended testes that were surgically brought into the scrotum. The undescended testicle is usually unable to produce viable sperm, and unless both testes are undescended, we see no reason to run the risk of cancer.

Diagnosis

There are really no early symptoms of testicular cancer. Usually the man goes to see a physician because of a painless enlargement of a testicle. This may be discovered by the person himself or by his spouse or sexual partner. Occasionally, symptoms of advanced cancer are present before enlargement of the testicle is noticed. It is not unusual for men to delay seeking help due to embarrassment or anxiety about the enlarged testicle. Testicular cancers also frequently produce hormones that cause breast enlargement and loss of libido, or sexual potency. Any man with enlargement of one testicle or the breasts should see his family doctor immediately. If his doctor suspects cancer, he should then be sent to a board-certified urologist.

If after examination the urologist feels that cancer is likely, he will undoubtedly operate as soon as possible. The first operation for testicular cancer is called a radical orchiectomy. This procedure involves removing the single enlarged testicle along with all the structures around it. It does not affect the other testicle and thus will not affect the ability to have intercourse or father children.

A pathologist will then examine the testicle to determine what type of cancer is present. The most important distinction to make is between seminoma and nonseminomatous tumors, which are far more malignant. The latter include embryonal cancers, teratocarcinomas, and chorio-carcinomas. If a nonseminomatous testicular cancer contains two or three of these types of cancer it is called a mixed cancer. These two basic sub-types of testicular cancer (seminomas and nonseminomatous tumors) will be discussed separately. The staging evaluation, treatment, and prognosis for each differ considerably.

Who Should Treat Testicular Cancer? A Team of Cancer Specialists!

Unlike the previous cancers discussed in this chapter, it is imperative that cancer of the testes be treated with a team approach. A urologist, a radiation oncologist, and a medical oncologist should examine the patient and then decide together with the patient the best treatment for his cancer. Testicular cancers are highly malignant and usually will be fatal in less than a year if not controlled. For the best results this cancer must be carefully staged. Then surgery, radiation, and chemotherapy, all effective forms of treatment, must be used to the best advantage. The exact treatment needed will depend upon the type of cancer and the stage, or extent of disease.

It Pays to Go to a Cancer Center or Large Medical Center   With cancer of the testes, you need a team composed of well-trained and experienced cancer physicians. Because this is a rare disease, most urologists do not do enough testicular cancer surgery to be truly expert at treating it. Also, not all medical oncologists are experienced enough with the high-dose, highly toxic combination chemotherapy necessary to cure this cancer. Therefore, we recommend that you ask to be sent to a major medical or cancer center. There a urologist specializing in cancer therapy who is experienced in the surgical treatment of testicular cancer will be available, as well as medical oncologists who are experienced and comfortable with very toxic, high-dose combination chemotherapy. In addition, larger hospitals or medical centers have experienced nurses who are invaluable in helping you through the difficult times and making life more tolerable while you take these very toxic treatments.

Testicular cancer is potentially curable and affects young people. Therefore, it is important that every effort be made to insure that the patient receives the best possible treatment. For many people not living near major medical centers, this may mean months of treatment far away from home. However, this could be a small price to pay for a cure. In summary, there is little doubt that treatment by a team of experts gives a man with testicular cancer a better chance for cure than can be achieved by any single physician or team of physicians without extensive experience in the evaluation and treatment of this disease.

NONSEMINOMATOUS TESTICULAR CANCER

Evaluating the Extent of the Disease

Men with a nonseminomatous cancer need a number of tests to determine whether the cancer has spread. These include a chest x-ray and tomograms of the lungs (a series of x-rays that will detect metastases that are not seen on the usual chest x-ray), a liver and a bone scan, and a lymphangiogram (to find out whether the lymph nodes in the abdomen are involved with the cancer). Several blood tests are done, including a human chorionic gonadotropin (HCG) and alpha fetal protein determinations, which measure hormones that can be made by these cancers. If the levels of these substances in the blood are elevated, these tests can allow the doctor to follow the progress of treatment and determine whether or not the cancer is still present after surgery. The oncologist can also tell whether the cancer is responding to chemotherapy by following the levels of either HCG or alpha fetal protein. These are termed *tumor markers*.

Treatment

Surgery   If the chest x-ray and tomograms and scans are normal and do not show spread beyond the lymph nodes in the abdomen, the next step is to perform an operation called a radical lymphadenectomy. The aim of this surgery is to evaluate the extent of the disease and to remove as much of the cancer as possible. The surgeon should be a board-certified urologist. He or she will remove all the draining lymph nodes on one side of the abdomen up to the level of the kidneys and some of the lymph nodes on the opposite side. Occasionally, extensive surgery is done on both sides of the abdomen. This is a long major operation; it can take up to eight hours. About 50 percent of men who have extensive pelvic surgery to remove the lymph glands from both sides of the lower abdomen become sterile. Although they can have normal erections and orgasms, they no longer ejaculate because the nerves that control ejaculation were cut during surgery. Unfortunately, this extensive surgery may be necessary to save your life. We recommend that you discuss the operation with your urologist beforehand. Only if he removes lymph glands from both sides of the pelvis will this complication occur. You must decide, with your doctor's help, if you are willing to accept this complication.

The decision whether further treatment is needed and whether radiation or chemotherapy should be used depends on the results of the lymphadenectomy. If none of the lymph nodes removed at surgery is cancerous, no further treatment is needed, and the chances for cure are 80–90 percent. If cancer is present in the abdominal lymph nodes, further treatment, either radiation or chemotherapy, is needed.

Radiation   Radiation has a role in the initial treatment of the nonseminomatous testicular cancers. Men who undergo radical lymphadenectomy and who are found to have only a small amount of disease in their abdomen may be given radiation after they recover from surgery. Approximately 75 percent are cured. Typically, radiation therapy is given to men who have only a few lymph glands (five of fifty, for example) with cancer. None of the nodes should be more than two inches in diameter and no tumor masses should have been left behind during surgery.

The decision to use radiation must be carefully considered in each case. Radiation will damage the bone marrow (where blood cells are made) and thus decrease the amount of chemotherapy that can be given if the cancer does recur. This may decrease the chance for cure later. We cannot emphasize too strongly that an experienced team of specialists who deal with many patients with testicular cancer is needed.

R.B. noted a lump in his right testicle and went to see his family doctor after three months. His doctor felt the hard testicle and immediately sent him to a urologist. The urologist removed the testicle two days after he first examined R.B. R.B. had a mixed nonseminomatous tumor composed of embryonal cell carcinoma and teratocarcinoma.

A series of tests that included the ones mentioned earlier in the chapter showed no evidence of metastases. One week after his orchiectomy, R.B. underwent a radical lymphadenectomy, which revealed that only three of fifty lymph nodes contained cancer. All were fairly small, measuring less than one inch in diameter.

After R.B. recovered from surgery, his urologist reviewed his situation with him. He first assured R.B. that he had discussed his case at the hospital tumor board. Many other doctors, including two radiation oncologists and three medical oncologists, attended the tumor board. Everyone at the tumor board felt that radiation therapy was best for R.B. It offered him a good chance for cure without many side effects.

R.B. underwent radiation over a five-week period of time. He experienced some nausea and diarrhea and lost ten pounds. Three months later he was back to normal. It is now six years since the cancer was found. R.B. still feels fine and is cured.

This case illustrates the place of radiation therapy in the initial treatment for nonseminomatous testicular cancer. R.B. had a small amount of disease in his abdomen. Therefore, radiation was chosen to eradicate any remaining tumor cells present in the abdominal lymph nodes not removed at surgery. Although the surgeon removed fifty lymph nodes during the radical lymphadenectomy, no doubt some were left behind.

If we change the case somewhat, we can illustrate how a different decision might have been made. If at surgery, thirty-five of the fifty nodes contained cancer and many of them were three to four centimeters in size, no doubt the urologist and the specialists at the tumor board would have decided that chemotherapy was the treatment of choice. Radiation therapy only treats cancer within the radiated area. Extensive abdominal cancer probably means that microscopic cancer is present in the lungs, liver, or bones. Therefore, the more cancer that is found at the time of lymphadenectomy, the less likely it is that radiation will treat all the cancer and cure the patient. If R.B. had had many, large, involved lymph nodes, he would have received intensive chemotherapy. Although this is much more toxic, it would have been necessary to give him a chance to be cured.

Chemotherapy Remarkable advances have been made in chemotherapy for nonseminomatous testicular cancer. Even with advanced metastatic disease, cure can be expected with aggressive chemotherapy in more than 50 percent of men. Chemotherapy is definitely indicated if the cancer has spread to the lungs, bones, or liver. It is also used if extensive cancer is found in the abdomen at the time of radical lymphadenectomy. Chemotherapy is currently being tested instead of radiation for patients who have lesser or limited amounts of cancer found in the abdomen at the time of radical lymphadenectomy.

The chemotherapy for testicular cancer involves a combination of three or more drugs given in high doses for periods of one to two years. The most commonly used drugs are vinblastine, cis-platinum, and bleomycin, though there are other drugs that are also very effective against this cancer. To cure half of the men with widespread testicular cancer, the drugs must be given in high doses. The side effects with this type of chemotherapy are considerable. People feel extreme nausea, lose weight, and generally feel rotten. Other side effects include temporary hair loss, muscle pain, extreme fatigue, and serious but treatable infections from the low white blood counts due to the therapy. Hospitalization is needed to give the drugs and to treat some of the side effects. The man may, in fact, spend much of several months in the hospital.

It is obvious that this type of chemotherapy can only be given successfully if the patient understands and is willing to fight for a cure. His physician must be both understanding and willing to use his every resource to help his patient. He must cajole, encourage, and even threaten his patient to try to keep him taking the very toxic treatment regimen. Without this treatment, death is certain. With it, cure is possible.

The following two case histories illustrate some very important points about chemotherapy for nonseminomatous testicular cancer.

C.R., a twenty-four-year-old Ph.D. student in comparative religion, was very depressed. His girlfriend had left him three months earlier, and he had lost interest in school and in life. He noticed a painless lump in his left testicle but waited six months as it continued to enlarge before he went to the student health service.

The physician in the student health service immediately referred him to a urologist, who admitted him for surgery as soon as he had examined him. The urologist was sure that C.R. had testicular cancer. A chest x-ray obtained before surgery showed multiple small tumors in his lungs. This could only be metastatic cancer that had spread from his testicle. The urologist nevertheless removed the involved testicle to find out what type of testicular cancer C.R. had.

C.R. had embryonal cell cancer of the testes. Because the cancer had spread to his lungs and was therefore beyond the reach of surgery or radiation, C.R. was referred to a nearby university-run Veterans Administration Hospital since he had little money and his insurance would not have paid for most of the high cost of treatment. The medical oncologist explained the situation to C.R. He had a very malignant tumor that would kill him unless very toxic chemotherapy could control it. C.R. had a chance for cure, but it would be a very difficult fight.

C.R. agreed to take chemotherapy and the oncologist started him on a program of chemotherapy with a combination of drugs every three weeks. Every third Sunday for four months, C.R. was admitted to the hospital. He received five days of treatment each time. He dreaded the treatments after his first, which had made him extremely nauseated. He vomited for five days without letup with the first course. He was so ill with his first treatment that from then on he felt ill just entering the hospital for his next treatment. This is not unusual for patients who become very nauseated and vomit with chemotherapy. Merely the thought of more chemotherapy may be upsetting enough to cause nausea and vomiting.

He was taken care of by different interns and residents or doctors in training. But at C.R.'s insistence he was always admitted to the same floor of the hospital and, therefore, had the same nurses. He became close to several of them. He also had one medical oncologist who directed his care.

After three courses of drug treatment, his chest x-ray became completely normal, and his alpha fetal protein, which had been elevated before the start of therapy, became normal. His medical oncologist was greatly encouraged, and told C.R. that he had a good chance for cure. He spent many hours encouraging C.R. to continue treatment.

However, after four months of treatment, C.R. simply disappeared for six weeks. During this time he fought an emotional battle with himself, trying to determine whether he could stand more treatment. He wanted to take a chance and live life as it was. He was really torn between stopping treatment completely to enjoy whatever time he had left without the agonizing and the indescribable nausea and vomiting from the treatment or continuing treatment to try for cure of his disease.

Fortunately, and partially because he had a close relationship with his medical oncologist and the nurses on the ward, C.R. chose to come back and continue treatment, and did so eighteen additional months. He received several additional courses of high-dose chemotherapy and for the remainder of the treatment got lower but still toxic doses of chemotherapy. He has now been off all treatment for two years and his cancer has not recurred. He is almost certainly cured. Since this is a fast-growing cancer, if it is going to recur it will usually do so rather rapidly. C.R. finished his Ph.D. and at last word was feeling well and traveling in Europe.

C.R.'s case illustrates the difficulty that people have taking the course of chemotherapy necessary for cure of testicular cancer. Almost all patients become extremely ill from the treatments. Even if the tumor melts away and the chance for cure is high, it is still difficult to convince some people to continue with chemotherapy. Fortunately, C.R. had a close relationship with his oncologist and several nurses in the hospital. These people helped him to finish the therapy and his cancer was cured.

If you have testicular cancer and must take chemotherapy, you need a medical oncologist who is not only an expert in treating testicular cancer but also a physician you trust and can confide in. Chances are slim that you will continue and finish your course of treatment if you do not have a close relationship with your medical oncologist. Therefore, you should not hesitate to ask to see a second oncologist. You need a doctor who suits you.

C.F., a thirty-two-year-old school teacher, married and the father of three children ages three, six, and eight, had an undescended testicle as a child. At age four he had an operation and the testicle was brought down and placed in his scrotum. He went to his family doctor when he noticed painful enlargement of both his breasts. His doctor found a painless lump in the undescended testicle. C.F. was immediately sent to a urologist, who performed an orchiectomy two days later. The pathologic diagnosis was pure choriocarcinoma, the kind of testicular cancer with the worst prognosis. Chest x-rays, a liver scan, and a bone scan all were normal. However, the human chorionic gonadotropin titer was very, very high and lymphangiogram showed a massive amount of cancer in the abdominal lymph nodes.

The urologist next performed a radical lymphadenectomy. This confirmed that many large lymph nodes contained cancer. Some of the cancer could not be removed at surgery.

Because a large amount of tumor was found at surgery, and because of the very high HCG titer, C.F. was referred to a medical oncologist after he recovered from surgery. The medical oncologist explained to him that he had advanced choriocarcinoma and that choriocarcinoma was the worst of all the testicular cancers. He would need to receive a very toxic course of combination chemotherapy. C.F. wanted to try anything that might give him a chance to live. He wanted to see his children grow up. He decided to take experimental combination chemotherapy. He became very interested in his own care and read about his disease and the drugs; he even read the package inserts that list all possible complications of the drugs he was to take. C.F. was, in fact, a perfect patient. He was cooperative, informed about his cancer, and a full partner in his treatment.

For three months he took high-dose therapy. He got severe nausea, vomiting, and weakness with each treatment, but seemed to be responding very well. His HCG fell from over 50,000 to 200. The masses in his abdomen got smaller. However, despite continued high-dose chemotherapy his HCG titer began to rise.

When this happened both C.F. and his oncologist knew that a cure was no longer possible. Their objectives changed from cure to control of symptoms. It was now important to allow C.F. as much time as possible with his family. Chemotherapy was stopped and was only started again several months later when he developed symptoms from metastases in his lungs and liver. He died at home, eleven months after the onset of his illness, with progressive choriocarcinoma in his liver and lungs.

C.F.'s case shows that despite the striking advances in chemotherapy for testicular cancer, half the victims are not cured. The medical oncologist and C.F. both tried for a cure. When a cure became an impossible goal, they wisely decided to stop the toxic chemotherapy, allowing C.F. to spend as much time as possible with his family and his friends.

We cannot stress too strongly the difficulties in taking toxic chemotherapy for several years. We have not illustrated this with any case histories, but we have both had patients responding well to chemotherapy who quit and died of a possibly curable cancer. It is essential that the patient not only have faith in the medical capabilities of his medical oncologist but also have a close working relationship with the physician as a person. This is needed to get through the one to two years of high-dose chemotherapy. One of the major causes of death in patients with testicular cancer is failure to continue chemotherapy. In fact, that happens as often as death from failure to respond to chemotherapy.

Finally, we must emphasize again that optimal treatment for nonseminomatous testicular cancer can only be obtained if a team of experts, including a board-certified urologist, radiation oncologist, and medical oncologist, all of whom have experience in treating this cancer, work together to plan and deliver treatment. With this cancer good treatment can save your life.

SEMINOMA

When the pathologist finds that a testicular cancer is a seminoma, the patient can breathe easier. The chances for cure are excellent and the therapy is less toxic than with nonseminomatous testicular cancers. Adequate therapy can be given by a radiation oncologist.

Staging

The staging evaluation for seminomas is almost the same as for non-seminomatous testicular cancers. People should have a chest x-ray and chest tomograms, a liver scan, and a bone scan. Blood is collected for HCG and alpha fetal protein levels. A lymphangiogram is done to evaluate the status of the lymph nodes in the abdomen. However, in contrast to nonseminomatous testicular cancers, a radical lymphadenectomy is not needed. In fact, no more surgery is needed to evaluate the extent of this disease. With the tests mentioned above, treatment decisions can be made that offer the patient a high chance for cure.

Treatment

Radiation   We strongly recommend being evaluated and treated by a board-certified radiation oncologist. Because seminomas are very radio-sensitive, radiation is the standard treatment. Seminomas can almost always be cured with relatively low doses of radiation. Even if the lymphangiogram does not show involvement of the abdominal nodes, radiation to the abdomen is given. With this treatment more than 90 percent of men are cured. There are only mild side effects, such as nausea and diarrhea. Thus, most men with seminoma do not need any chemotherapy.

If the lymphangiogram indicates that there is cancer in the abdominal lymph nodes, the standard treatment is to radiate the abdomen and also the lymph nodes in the chest and left side of the neck. More radiation is used because there is greater chance that the cancer has spread to these lymph nodes. Radiation cures more than 80 percent of men with seminoma even with an abnormal lymphangiogram.

If a seminoma recurs in organs such as the lungs or bones, or if it is widespread when first diagnosed, radiation can still be used as treatment. These tumors are radiosensitive, and therefore low doses of radiation can even be given to the lungs. Men have been followed for years after radiation for widespread seminoma and some have done well.

Chemotherapy   Most patients with widespread disease cannot be cured with radiation. They are treated with chemotherapy. Although not many men with seminoma have received chemotherapy, the disease seems to respond well. At present most men with advanced seminoma who need chemotherapy are treated with the same toxic, high-dose combinations as nonseminomatous testicular cancers.

SUMMARY

Kidney Cancer

1. Cancer of the kidney should be evaluated and treated by a board-certified urologist.
2. Surgical removal of the kidney is the standard treatment and cures one-third of people with this cancer.
3. Chemotherapy is relatively ineffective against cancer of the kidney.
4. Hormones and radiation are used to treat metastases.
5. Patients with metastatic kidney cancer should not give up hope, since the course can be very unpredictable. The cancer may grow very slowly, stop growing, or, rarely, even disappear without treatment.

Bladder Cancer

1. Blood in the urine may signal bladder cancer. Even if it goes away, see your doctor and make sure bladder cancer or kidney cancer or other disease is not present.
2. If you have blood in your urine, a urologist will use a cystoscope to look inside your bladder to be sure that cancer is not present. Superficial or early bladder cancers can be removed at cystoscopy with an 80 percent chance for cure.
3. In contrast, advanced bladder cancer that has deeply invaded the bladder wall must be treated aggressively with radical surgery and/or radiation. The chance for cure is less.
4. Any person who has had one bladder cancer is prone to develop further bladder cancers and should have cystoscopy on a regular basis. Aniline dye workers also have an increased incidence of bladder cancer and should be regularly checked.

Prostate Cancer

1. All men over the age of fifty should have a yearly rectal examination. Asymptomatic prostate and rectal cancer can be discovered by a rectal examination.
2. If it is still localized, prostate cancer can be cured with surgery or radiation therapy.
3. Men with metastatic prostate cancer can live for years. The disease progresses slowly and responds to hormonal treatment.

Testicular Cancer

1. Cancer of the testicle is a very malignant cancer and it usually occurs in younger men.

2. An undescended testicle is at high risk for developing testicular cancer. Therefore, if your child has an undescended testicle it should either be brought down into the scrotum or removed surgically. We recommend removal, although this is a controversial topic.

3. The treatment of nonseminomatous testicular cancer is complex. In contrast to the other cancers discussed in this chapter, it should only be done by a team of experts that includes a urologist, a radiation oncologist, and a medical oncologist with experience in the treatment of testicular cancers.

4. In contrast to renal cell, bladder, and prostate cancer, which can be usually treated in most communities, we think it pays to go to a large medical or cancer center to receive the best treatment for nonseminomatous testicular cancer.

5. The nonseminomatous testicular cancers are treated with surgery, radiation, and chemotherapy. The method of treatment depends upon how far the cancer has spread. Decisions are complex, and the appropriate choice of treatment may determine whether a young man with this cancer lives or dies.

6. Men with seminomas are more fortunate. They have a good chance for cure and usually need only radiation therapy. This is less toxic than the high-dose combination chemotherapy used to treat nonseminomatous testicular cancer.

16

Skin Cancers

The skin is by far the most common site of cancer. Over 100,000 people have skin cancers diagnosed and treated each year in the United States. Luckily, the skin is our most visible organ, so cancer there can be diagnosed and treated early. Less than 5,000 Americans die of the more common types of skin cancer each year. Most of these deaths are preventable and are due to delay in diagnosis. In this chapter we will discuss the three major types of skin cancer: basal cell and squamous cell cancers of the skin, which are somewhat similar, and malignant melanoma, which is a highly malignant and much less common tumor.

Basal Cell and Squamous Cell Cancers of the Skin

Both basal cell and squamous cell cancers of the skin tend to grow slowly and spread to other parts of the body late in their course. Compared to many other cancers, they remain localized and are curable for long periods of time. However, if they are ignored they will eventually become incurable. Delay in seeking attention for skin cancer will also increase the amount of normal tissue destroyed by the cancer and increase the amount of normal tissue that must be removed for adequate treatment. These cancers commonly arise on sun-exposed areas such as the face and hands. The disfigurement that results from removal of large tumors can be considerable, while small tumors can be removed with minimal cosmetic effect. In summary, early skin cancer is almost 100 percent curable by simple treatment that leaves minimal scarring.

Who Should Treat Basal and Squamous Cell Cancers?

Treatment for basal cell and squamous cell skin cancers should be directed by a dermatologist. This is a doctor who has had at least three years of training in diagnosing and treating skin diseases. After this training an examination is given to test the doctor's knowledge in skin diseases. A certificate stating that your doctor is a board-certified dermatologist insures that he or she has had adequate training and has passed this examination.

Another physician who is often involved in treating skin cancer, particularly large cancers that involve the face, is a plastic surgeon. This surgeon has had training in general surgery and additional training in the surgical specialty of plastic surgery. He or she is an expert at performing surgery with the best possible cosmetic results. Thus, if you have a cancer that necessitates removal of part of your face, the plastic surgeon will plan the treatment so your appearance will be as close to normal as possible.

While early or small basal cell and squamous skin cancers are adequately treated by a board-certified dermatologist, larger ones deserve a team approach for the best results. Some skin cancers are treated with radiation, which should be performed by a board-certified radiation oncologist.

Causes

We know more about what causes skin cancer than we do about most other types of cancer. In fact, a type of skin cancer was the first cancer associated with environmental factors. In 1775, Percival Pott described a type of skin cancer that arose in the scrotums of chimney sweeps in England and related it to exposure to chimney soot. Later, in the 1800s, skin cancer was associated with arsenic exposure. Many studies have also related skin cancer with intense exposure to the sun, showing that chronic exposure to intense sunlight is the most important contributing factor in the development of skin cancer. The incidence of skin cancer increases as one approaches the equator and also with increasing altitude. Both of these factors correlate with the amount of ultraviolet radiation, the dangerous rays in sunlight that cause sunburn as well as cancer.

Another important factor is genetic and relates to how your skin reacts to ultraviolet sunlight. The less pigmentation in your skin, or the lighter you are, the more likely you are to develop skin cancer with exposure to intense sunlight. Thus, blacks are relatively protected compared to fair-skinned Scandinavians, Scots, and Irish. The importance of skin pigmentation is highlighted by the very high incidence of skin cancer in blacks who have a rare genetic defect called albinism, which results in a white appearance due to a lack of skin pigmentation.

Another factor associated with the development of skin cancer is exposure to radiation. In the 1930s and 1940s, many people were treated with radiation for acne, or pimples. Twenty to thirty years later many of these people developed multiple skin cancers. If you have been exposed to radiation, you should be checked regularly for the development of skin cancer. You should also avoid excessive exposure to sunlight. As with other cancers, exposure to more than one carcinogen probably has more than an additive effect.

How to Protect Your Skin against Sunlight

You can protect yourself from exposure to ultraviolet light by using suntan lotions containing para-aminobenzoic acid, commonly abbreviated PABA. PABA effectively prevents the penetration of ultraviolet light into the skin. Suntan lotions that do not contain this ingredient or similar substances are ineffective. If you have had any skin cancers or are light or fair skinned, you should protect all sun-exposed areas of your skin using a PABA-containing sunscreen. This is very important if you are going to be exposed to intense sunlight, such as when skiing or swimming.

BASAL CELL CANCER OF THE SKIN

Diagnosis and Treatment

Basal cell cancers are the most common type of skin cancer. These cancers are related to sunlight exposure, and light-skinned people are the most susceptible. Most basal cell cancers occur in areas of the skin that are exposed to sunlight, such as the face, neck, and arms. Especially common sites include the nose, the forehead, and the cheeks.

Basal cell skin cancer usually begins as a small firm, somewhat waxy protrusion of the skin that may ulcerate in the center as it enlarges. The edges of the bump become elevated and may look somewhat waxy or pearly. Cancers that develop on the midportion of the body may have a flatter appearance and may be scaly. They usually have a crusted center with a raised pearly border. They can also appear somewhat pigmented, that is, they can be somewhat dark in appearance.

Fortunately, basal cancers grow slowly and never spread to distant areas of the body unless they are totally ignored for many years. Rather, these cancers tend to invade the normal tissues around them. It is important to diagnose them early, as the larger they are, the greater the cosmetic damage may be.

Basal cell cancer, like other cancers, is diagnosed by a biopsy. No staging procedures or tests to look for metastases are usually done. The usual type of biopsy that is performed is called a punch biopsy and can be done by any physician but is usually performed by a dermatologist. A sharp instrument called a punch cuts out a tiny segment of the skin.

Usually the area to be biopsied is locally anesthetized so you feel little pain. The size of the biopsy is usually tiny, about one-eighth inch in diameter.

If you are found to have one basal cell cancer, you should be carefully examined for other basal cell cancers, because anyone who develops one skin cancer is likely to develop others. A very careful examination of the skin becomes the most important part of your physical examination. You should be examined completely naked and closely observed by your physician in good light.

A.H., a fifty-four-year-old Swedish sailor, noticed a small nodule on his nose. For two and a half years this nodule slowly grew and became large enough to be quite noticeable. He usually avoided doctors, but he became worried about this growing lump. He saw a family physician, who immediately told him that he probably had a basal cell cancer. A.H. was sent to a dermatologist, who examined the lump on his nose and then examined him carefully for other skin cancers. The dermatologist was rather upset. He told A.H. that basal cell cancers could be treated easily when they are small, but that this cancer had grown to a large size and had invaded the nose extensively. He now needed extensive surgery with removal of most of his nose or extensive radiation to cure the cancer. With either treatment, he would need plastic surgery to reconstruct the nose. He saw a radiation oncologist and a plastic surgeon. Then all three doctors met and decided that surgery followed by a plastic reconstruction of his nose was the best approach. A.H. had the surgery and soon after had his nose rebuilt by the plastic surgeon.

It has been four years since this treatment was done, and the cancer has not recurred. However, A.H. has developed three additional small basal cell cancers on his face. All were treated in the dermatologist's office before they became troublesome.

This case illustrates several important points. A.H. was the typical kind of person to get skin cancer. He was a sailor with years of exposure to intense sunlight, was of Scandinavian descent, and was light skinned with blue eyes and blond hair. Also, basal cell cancers rarely spread, and they remain curable for long periods of time. When small they can be effectively treated in the physician's office with any of several simple procedures. A.H. delayed two and a half years and needed rather extensive treatment to cure his cancer.

Basal cell cancers can be treated by several methods, any of which can cure the cancer and, depending on its size, leave minimal scars. Most dermatologists use either electrosurgery, traditional surgery, cryosurgery (using liquid nitrogen), or radiation therapy. The goal of treatment is to destroy the cancer and leave the normal tissue intact. The type of treatment you will be given for basal cell cancer depends upon the size, the location, and the preference of your dermatologist. Some of the details of these treatments are explained later in this chapter.

SQUAMOUS CELL CANCER OF THE SKIN

Squamous cell cancer, the second most common type of skin cancer, is somewhat more malignant than basal cell cancer. It develops in sun-exposed areas and is related to arsenic and radiation exposure. It can also develop in burn scars and from precancerous skin lesions called solar, actinic, or senile keratoses. Squamous cell, like basal cell, cancer tends to occur most frequently on the face and neck and is more common in light-skinned, fair-haired individuals.

Some squamous cell cancers have a much higher rate of metastases than basal cell cancers. These include ones that arise in the mouth or on the lips or ears, or those that arise in skin not damaged by sunlight, that is, in burn scars. If they are ignored, they can spread to nearby lymph nodes and from there to distant organs and can cause death. Most of the 5,000 Americans who die yearly from skin cancer die from squamous cell cancer of the skin that they ignored. When squamous cell cancers are small, more than 90 percent can be cured. If the cancer has spread to nearby lymph nodes, only 50 percent can be cured.

Diagnosis

The diagnosis of squamous cell cancer of the skin is made by a punch biopsy. Staging for this cancer is simple: careful examination of the skin and nearby lymph nodes is adequate. If the cancer is large, your physician will probably take a chest x-ray to make sure the disease has not spread to the lungs.

Squamous cell cancer may appear different from basal cell cancer. At first, it looks like a hard, scaly lesion. As it enlarges, the center breaks down and ulcerates and becomes covered by a scab. In general, any sore on your skin that does not heal should be evaluated by a physician. Your physician should biopsy the sore to determine whether or not it is cancerous. A simple biopsy will cure the cancer if it is tiny. However, if the cancer is larger, and most are, a small amount of the cancer is removed for the initial diagnosis and then a decision will be made on what is the best treatment.

Treatment

The treatment for both basal cell and squamous cell cancers is similar. The object is to remove the cancer completely but leave as much normal tissue as possible and thus minimize cosmetic side effects. Current treatments include electrosurgery, excisional surgery, chemosurgery, cryosurgery, and radiation. Any of these treatments can be curative in better than 90 percent of cases if the cancers are small. If the cancer is large, or if it is in an area that is difficult to treat, such as the eyelid, a team approach is to your advantage. Best results can be obtained if the dermatologist works with a radiation therapist, a plastic surgeon, and sometimes even an ophthalmologist. The utilization of a team of experts offers you the best chance for good treatment with the best cosmetic results.

Electrosurgery　Electrosurgery involves the use of an electric needle that burns the cancerous tissue. This is most often used with a technique called curettage in which the tissue is scooped out. The area of the cancer is first anesthetized with a local anesthetic much like what a dentist will apply before doing dental work. Then a curette is used to remove some of the cancer, after which the underlying cancer is destroyed by the intense heat of the electric needle. The curetting and burning is continued until all the cancer is removed as well as some of the surrounding normal tissue. It should be done by an experienced dermatologist, since inexperienced physicians often do not remove enough tissue and the cancer recurs in the same area. Adequate treatment usually involves at least three curettings and three applications of the electric needle at one time. A scab forms after this procedure and falls off in four to six weeks, usually leaving a small scar. This is very satisfactory treatment for small squamous and basal cell cancers (less than a centimeter in size). It can be done simply in the dermatologist's office and leaves a good cosmetic effect.

Excision Surgery　Another alternative with excellent results involves surgically removing all the cancer and some normal surrounding tissue. After removal of the cancer, the wound edges are brought together with sutures. Larger lesions may require more extensive procedures, such as skin grafting, to fill the defect. Surgical excision is often the treatment of choice for skin cancers that border on mucous membranes such as the lips, anus, vulva, and penis.

Chemosurgery　This approach involves surgery that is monitored very exactly so that enough tissue is removed for cure but not too much. It is frequently used for large lesions or for ones in areas difficult to treat with other techniques or especially for ones in which it's difficult to determine precisely the edges of the cancer. Zinc chloride is applied to the cancer and kills the cancerous cells after several hours. At this time, a section of the tumor is removed and looked at under the microscope to see if the whole cancer and enough normal tissue was removed. If examination under the microscope shows that not enough tissue was taken out, more zinc chloride is applied, and after several hours another section of tissue is removed and looked at under the microscope. This is repeated until all the cancer is removed and enough of a normal margin is removed to insure local control. A newer modification of this technique involves the excision of dried pieces of tissue under local anesthesia for microscopic examination, rather than zinc chloride fixation. This is an excellent approach, since it yields excellent cure rates for difficult lesions. It requires a specially trained surgeon, usually a dermatologist.

Cryosurgery   Cryosurgery involves using liquid nitrogen to freeze the cancer. It should be used for very, very small skin cancers and for precancerous lesions. It is not one of the established, time-tested treatments for moderate-sized or large skin cancers.

Radiation   One can give enough radiation to eradicate skin cancers completely. But this takes up to four weeks and therefore is much more time consuming and more costly than the alternative forms of treatment. However, it is an effective form of treatment and may be the treatment of choice where disfigurement will result from extensive surgery. It is especially useful in elderly or debilitated people who may not be candidates for extensive surgery for a large skin cancer.

Chemotherapy   Chemotherapy for skin cancer that has spread and cannot be cured is relatively ineffective, though it does offer temporary improvement for some people. We recommend either no chemotherapy or low doses of nontoxic chemotherapy. We believe that high-dose toxic chemotherapy is much more likely to hurt than help.

PRECANCEROUS SKIN LESIONS

Precancerous skin lesions are lesions that, if left untreated, may become cancerous. Therefore, if you have one or, more likely, many precancerous skin lesions, you must watch them very carefully yourself and see a dermatologist on a regular basis. In this way the dermatologist can treat any cancers that develop. An alternative is to treat these premalignant lesions before they become malignant and prevent cancer from developing. The following is a descriptive list of the more common precancerous skin lesions.

Actinic, Solar, or Senile Keratoses

These are premalignant lesions of the skin related to chronic exposure to ultraviolet light or intense sunlight. Approximately 5 million to 20 million Americans have solar keratoses. Their incidence, as expected, is directly related to chronic intense exposure to sunlight and to the lightness of the person's skin. They occur mostly on the face, neck, and hands. Initially they resemble red to brown or gray discrete lesions that are usually covered with a firmly attached dry scale. As they progress, they become more scaly or even horny. Most will remain premalignant but some develop into squamous cell cancer. Signs of possible malignant transformation include increasing size, increasing thickness, increasing redness, ulceration, bleeding, or oozing.

Arsenic Keratoses

Arsenic keratoses result from chronic exposure to arsenic. People can be exposed to arsenic at work in smelting foundries, from some insecticides, from drinking water (which contains arsenic), and from a variety of other sources. These look different from solar keratoses. They are hard, yellow, scaly lesions that tend to occur on the palms and soles. Like solar keratoses, they may develop into squamous cell cancer.

Radiation Dermatitis

Radiation exposure, mainly in the form of therapeutic radiation used by doctors in the past to treat acne and other skin conditions, predisposes the area irradiated to skin cancer. Irradiated areas of the skin tend to become mottled and pigmented, atrophic (thin skinned), scarred, and telangiectasic (developing many small vessels). Cancer can develop as early as one year and as late as sixty years after radiation exposure. If you've been irradiated to any area of skin, you have to watch the area or have it watched regularly by a dermatologist for the rest of your life. Squamous cell cancer arising from an area of radiation tends to be aggressive, that is, it spreads quickly. It is very important, therefore, to notice and have it treated as soon as possible.

Burn Scars

Scars from serious burns or from other causes may develop into cancer and should be watched.

Albinism

Albinism results from an inherited disorder that causes the absence of pigment formation. Albinos are very light skinned and therefore are very prone to develop skin cancer. In addition, they tend to have multiple solar keratoses.

Treatment of Precancerous Skin Lesions

With any of the premalignant or precancerous skin lesions, two alternative approaches are possible. One is to watch the lesions or have them watched closely by a dermatologist and to treat at the earliest sign of any change that suggests cancer. The other is to treat these precancerous lesions immediately and avoid cancer. More often than in the past, preventive treatment is being resorted to, especially for solar keratoses. An effective method of treatment for these lesions (if there aren't too many) involves freezing with liquid nitrogen. However, many patients have hundreds of these lesions. For such individuals, a very effective treatment is to use topical chemotherapy. A drug used intravenously to treat many different types of cancer, 5-Fluorouracil (5-FU), can be used topically or applied just to the skin to treat these precancerous lesions. The drug, which comes in various concentrations and as either a cream or solution, is applied once or twice a day, first by the dermatologist and then by the patient himself after he has been taught how to apply it properly. Treatment continues until there is an intense local reaction around and involving the solar keratoses, indicating that destruction of the keratoses is occurring. Within one to two weeks of the reaction, the solar keratoses are destroyed and the local reaction slowly subsides. The end result is excellent, with normal skin growing in the area of previous keratoses.

Finally, immunotherapy, which involves the topical application of a chemical agent against which the body reacts immunologically, can also be used to treat solar keratoses. The chemical is applied to the solar keratoses, and when the body reacts to the chemical, it destroys the premalignant lesion.

Topical chemotherapy or immunotherapy requires an experienced dermatologist and should not be administered by an untrained physician.

MALIGNANT MELANOMA

Fortunately, malignant melanoma is much less common than the other types of skin cancers. Unlike basal and squamous cell cancer, malignant melanoma is a very malignant cancer, and it kills many of its victims. It can occur at any age, but most commonly occurs between the ages of twenty to fifty. Malignant melanoma is more common in whites than in blacks. When it does occur in blacks, it usually arises on the more lightly pigmented parts of skin, such as the palms of the hands. Although exposure to sunlight definitely has some relationship to this disease, the connection is by no means as clear-cut as with the other skin cancers. Melanomas may start in sites that are never exposed to sun, such as inside the mouth, on the bottom of the feet, on the retina of the eye, or even inside the bowel.

This cancer arises from the pigmented cells in the skin called melanocytes. Many malignant melanomas develop in moles or birthmarks. The average white person has about thirty to forty pigmented moles on his skin. However, the chance of any pigmented mole developing into malignant melanoma is very small, approximately 1 in 1 million. Therefore, it makes very little sense to remove all pigmented moles from everyone. If a mole gets chronically irritated by rubbing it, etc., and gets sore, red, or itchy it's probably wise to have it examined and possibly removed. Also, if you have a mole that appears to be changing, growing, changing color in any way, bleeding, or itching, you should see a doctor without delay. If a mole changes, and especially if it becomes blacker, develops tiny satellite moles, or starts to get larger, it is highly suspicious for malignant melanoma and should be checked by a doctor.

Most melanomas are black but some can actually be red brown, or blue or even have white areas in them. Malignant melanomas are very malignant. They spread widely throughout the body and, unless removed before they have spread, they cannot be cured.

Diagnosis and Treatment

If you and your doctor suspect that you have a malignant melanoma, you should immediately be referred to either a general surgeon or a dermatologist for an excisional biopsy. The diagnosis and treatment of malignant melanoma is surgical. The tumor is resistant to radiation therapy. If the lesion is a malignant melanoma, the patient should be sent to a general surgeon for surgery. The suspected melanoma should be completely removed, along with a margin of normal tissue. Even for a small melanoma, a fairly large area of normal tissue (two to three inches) around the cancer should be removed. A skin graft is often needed to cover the surgically created wound.

The most important prognostic factor in melanoma is how deeply the cancer has penetrated into the skin. If it only involves the surface of the skin, the chances for cure are 80 to 90 percent. By contrast, if the tumor has penetrated into the layer of fat under the skin, the chance for cure falls to 10–15 percent.

Surgery is the only effective treatment for malignant melanoma, and it can only be effective or curative if the cancer has not spread. In addition to examining the melanoma, your physician should examine the nearby lymph nodes very carefully. Melanoma spreads through the blood and the lymph system to nearby lymph nodes. Malignant melanoma tends to metastasize widely. The tests that are usually obtained include a chest x-ray and liver, bone and brain scans. If the melanoma has spread to any of these organs, cure is currently impossible.

Should the Nearby Lymph Glands Be Removed?   There is still serious debate about how much surgery should be done to treat melanoma. Surgeons agree that the least amount of surgery should be a wide excision of the cancer. They also agree that enlarged lymph nodes in the region of the melanoma should be removed if there is no spread to other organs such as the lung or liver. However, there is much controversy about whether or not nearby lymph nodes that are not enlarged should be removed. For example, if a melanoma arises in the thigh or the foot, some surgeons will remove the melanoma and normal-sized lymph glands in the groin. Other cancer surgeons will not remove those lymph nodes if they appear normal on examination. In general, most surgeons feel that, if a melanoma is deeply penetrating the skin, the nearby lymph nodes should be removed because there is a good chance these nodes have small deposits of cancer even though they are not enlarged. If there are microscopic deposits of melanoma cells in these lymph nodes and it has not spread to other parts of the body, the disease can be cured by removing them.

For many melanomas, removal of the nearby normal-sized lymph nodes as part of the initial treatment is not possible. These melanomas are situated where they can spread to several lymph nodes areas, i.e., a melanoma in the middle of the back can spread to the nodes under either armpit or in the groin. Removing the nodes in all areas is obviously not worth the surgical risks.

Lymph node dissections should be performed by experienced cancer surgeons. Although they provide good treatment for other skin cancers, dermatologists are not trained to do the types of surgery necessary to cure malignant melanoma. After a melanoma is diagnosed, you should be referred to a surgical oncologist or at least to a surgeon who has extensive experience in treating the cancer.

Radiation Melanoma is very resistant to radiation; therefore, radiation plays a small role in the treatment of this disease. However, it is used to treat some local problems such as painful bone metastases. Unfortunately, radiation is less effective at controlling problems from melanomas than from most other cancers.

Chemotherapy Chemotherapy is somewhat effective against this disease. About 15 percent of people with metastases will improve temporarily with chemotherapy. The standard treatment is a drug called DTIC, usually given intravenously for five consecutive days each month. The side effects are loss of appetite, nausea, and vomiting that can be severe even if the patient takes pills to prevent or decrease nausea and vomiting. High-dose combination chemotherapy is more toxic and isn't more effective against this cancer. Therefore, we recommend either no chemotherapy or DTIC. Otherwise you are much more likely to be hurt than helped.

Immunotherapy There has been much information both in the lay press and the medical press about the use of immunotherapy in this disease. Immunotherapy involves bolstering the body's defenses so it can attack cancer cells and kill them. A weakened tuberculosis bacterium known as BCG has been extensively tried in clinical trials. Thus far the results of these trials are at best inconclusive. At present there is no proven benefit from taking BCG for melanoma. Other drugs that may boost the body's immune defenses (such as levamisole) are also currently under study. At the present time, there is no firm evidence that immunotherapy of any kind is of benefit in this disease.

We do not recommend traveling to a cancer center for experimental chemotherapy or immunotherapy, as trials to date have not shown these methods to be of benefit in this disease. Adequate treatment is available where there are experienced, board-certified general surgeons and medical oncologists.

Melanoma is a strange cancer. Patients with widespread disease may have a spontaneous disappearance of all their disease that can last for many years. Other patients who appear to be cured by the initial surgery relapse many years later. The unpredictability of this type of cancer makes it a fairly difficult disease for both physicians and their patients.

D.S., a twenty-five-year-old schoolteacher of Norwegian ancestry, was in excellent health. She was married, had one small child, and had no family history suggesting a predisposition to cancer. For several weeks she had noticed that the back of her bra strap occasionally was somewhat bloody. She asked her husband to check her back, and he found that she had a 1/2 cm blackish crusted mole in the midportion of her back. Neither she nor her husband was worried by this; however, she did see her family physician, who referred her to a dermatologist.

The dermatologist performed a small punch biopsy and asked her to return in four days. When she returned, he explained that she had a type of highly malignant skin cancer called a malignant melanoma and that the biopsy showed deep penetration into the skin. Also, he wanted to send her to a surgeon for further surgery. The area around the cancer as well as the cancer should be cut out. D.S. still did not realize that a small skin cancer such as this could be so serious.

She saw a surgeon two days later. He examined her carefully, especially for enlarged lymph nodes under the armpits and in the groin. The examination was normal. He then explained the need for further surgery to D.S. and her husband. He arranged for her admission to the hospital. Under general anesthesia, he performed a wide excision of the cancer. He removed the rest of the melanoma and several inches of surrounding normal tissue. A skin graft was taken from an area on her thigh and used to cover the wound. Lymph nodes were not removed because the melanoma was situated where it could spread to several different areas. D.S. had malignant melanoma that had penetrated into the underlying fat. Her chances for cure were not good.

When her surgeon visited the next morning, he told her that although he had removed as much of the cancer as possible, there was a still a high probability that it had spread to other areas of the body and that she might require further treatment. He ordered a bone scan, a liver scan, and a brain scan, all of which were negative. Her chest x-ray was also normal. She was extremely upset and asked if anything further could be done. Her surgeon felt she needed the hope of experimental treatment.

D.S. lived in a city with a university medical center, to which she was referred for possible experimental treatment. After careful examination and review of her records and tests, she was offered a chance to participate at an experimental study testing the effectiveness of immunotherapy with BCG. It was explained to her that this type of treatment was yet unproved but might be beneficial. She was desperate. She was young and knew that her chances of being cured with just the surgery were poor.

D.S. chose to try the experimental immunotherapy. She received BCG by what is called scarification. The bacteria are placed on the skin and a series of scratch marks are drawn on the skin with a fine needle. The bacteria can penetrate the skin and set up a local infection. This leads to some scarring and some local irritation. The bacteria, however, are usually not capable of causing serious infection in man. She received treatment every month for two years. During the entire time she felt well and had regular checkups every three months that included a chest x-ray, a liver scan, and a bone scan.

Then she began to develop headaches on the left side of her head that were especially severe in the morning. She called the doctor who was giving her the BCG and told him about the new symptoms. He ordered a brain scan, which showed two metastases in the brain. She was treated with a drug called Decadron to decrease the swelling in the brain and she started on a course of radiation to her brain. She developed increasing symptoms with weakness, severe headaches, and progressive paralysis of her right side. Within eight weeks she lapsed into coma, and she died shortly thereafter.

Although D.S. had no evidence of metastases after surgery, she undoubtedly had microscopic disease in her brain and possibly elsewhere in her body. We cannot tell whether or not her immunotherapy helped prolong her life. However, it is highly doubtful it would have had any effect on the brain metastases. It is also not uncommon for brain metastases in this disease not to respond well to radiation. Melanoma is a highly radiation-insensitive tumor. Therefore, radiation therapy plays only a small role in the treatment of this disease. Chemotherapy isn't effective either to treat brain metastases.

S.R., a fifty-five-year-old bank vice-president, had a mole on his arm that he noticed was increasing in size. It had also changed color and was somewhat blacker than it had been previously, and there were several tiny black areas around it. At the time of his yearly physical examination, he showed the mole to his internist. The internist was almost certain by the appearance of the mole that it was a malignant melanoma and immediately referred him to a surgical oncologist.

S.R. was hospitalized and underwent what is called an excisional biopsy, where a wide area around the tumor was removed along with the entire tumor. He too required a skin graft. Unlike D.S., his tumor did not penetrate the skin; it was confined to the upper layer.

His surgeon told him he had melanoma but the chance for cure was good. He also discussed with him the possibility of surgically removing the nearby lymph glands in his armpit. However, he believed it wasn't necessary as the melanoma wasn't penetrating the skin deeply. He felt no further treatment was required.

It is now two years after his initial operation, the tumor has not re-curred, and S.R. is still enjoying excellent health. He is probably cured, but it is possible that sometime within the next several years the cancer may return, in the lymph nodes that were not removed, in other areas of his skin, or in his liver, lungs, or brain.

Many melanomas are caught early enough that the cancer has not pene-trated deeply into the skin. Surgery can remove all the cancer, and the person is cured. If the melanoma has penetrated through the skin into the fat, chances for cure are small, as the cancer has probably spread to other organs such as the liver, lungs, or bone. Radiation is quite ineffective, and chemotherapy offers only temporary improvement for some people. Immunotherapy is still unproven and experimental.

SUMMARY

1. If you have very light skin or if you have been exposed to many years of intense sunlight or to skin irradiation, you are more prone to develop skin cancers. If you develop one skin cancer, you are likely to develop more. You can protect yourself from the dangers of intense sun-light by using suntan lotion with PABA in it.

2. If you have nonhealing sores on your skin or lesions that are enlarg-ing or changing in color, you should see your doctor immediately. Any change in a pigmented mole, either enlargement, change in color, bleed-ing, or the development of pigmented areas around the mole, may indi-cate a malignancy. The doctor best able to evaluate these potential can-cers is a board-certified dermatologist.

3. Basal cell and squamous cell skin cancers are the most curable of all cancers. They can be cured by many different methods. However, if you let a skin cancer grow big enough that it spreads, it can kill you.

4. Melanoma, a cancer that arises in pigmented cells such as are found in moles and birthmarks, is a very malignant tumor and must be caught early if you are to be cured.

5. Malignant melanomas need to be treated by either a general sur-geon, a plastic surgeon, or a surgical oncologist, as they require major surgery for removal. Dermatologists should not treat this type of skin cancer by themselves. They will biopsy the mole and should refer you to a general surgeon if the biopsy shows cancer.

6. Radiation is relatively ineffective against melanoma, but it is some-times used to treat troublesome metastases.

7. Chemotherapy for melanoma offers temporary improvement for some patients. At present, we advise a drug called DTIC.

8. Immunotherapy for melanoma is unproven as yet and is still experi-mental.

17

Brain Tumors

The central nervous system is composed of the brain and the spinal cord. Tumors of the central nervous system are not rare. Approximately 20,000 Americans develop tumors of the brain or spinal cord each year and about 9,000 die from them. Tumors arising in the central nervous system may be malignant or benign. The malignant tumors are either primary in the brain or, more commonly, start elsewhere and metastasize to the brain. Tumors such as breast cancer, lung cancer, and malignant melanoma commonly spread to the brain. These different types of brain tumors will be discussed in this chapter because the symptoms, the evaluation, and the treatment for these different tumors are similar.

Malignant brain tumors grow and invade the surrounding normal brain tissue. Unlike most other cancers, they rarely spread beyond the central nervous system to other parts of the body. Benign brain tumors do not invade the surrounding brain tissue. However, even these "nonmalignant" tumors are dangerous if not treated.

There is little room for growth within the central nervous system. The brain is tightly enclosed in the skull and the spinal cord is surrounded by the parts of the vertebral bodies that make up the spinal canal. Neither place allows room for expansion. In fact, in most normal people there is room for only 100 grams, or one-fifth of a pound, of tumor in the brain before increasing pressure causes severe symptoms and death. Therefore, anything that causes expansion of the brain or spinal cord, even if it is benign and only pushes on the surrounding brain tissue, will produce increased pressure. This pressure is responsible for most brain damage from tumors, and, if unchecked, will eventually cause death. Perhaps the use of the word *benign* to describe a brain tumor is misleading. No brain tumors are really benign. All are dangerous. The benign tumors differ from malignant ones in that they tend to grow much more slowly and can often be either controlled or cured by surgery or radiation.

Prognosis

The prognosis with brain tumors varies considerably with the type of tumor and its location. Tumors on the surface of the brain are easier to treat than tumors deep within the brain. Deeper tumors, even if benign, cannot always be completely removed without much damage to the normal brain tissue. Many parts of the brain are critical to normal functioning.

Benign tumors such as meningiomas tend to occur on the surface of the brain and don't invade the normal surrounding tissue. Therefore, they can often be cured by surgery. In contrast, malignant tumors tend to occur deep within the brain and invade normal tissue. Many cannot be completely removed.

Treatment

The primary treatment for brain tumors is surgical. If a malignant brain tumor cannot be completely removed by the neurosurgeon, radiation therapy is given after surgery. Radiation therapy by itself is seldom curative. The amount of radiation necessary to cure a brain tumor is often more than normal brain tissue can tolerate. Therefore, if a malignant brain tumor cannot be removed, it is usually incurable. Many tumors cannot be completely removed by the surgeon because that would destroy too much normal brain tissue.

Chemotherapy is not very effective against brain tumors. It helps some temporarily. The usefulness of chemotherapy in combination with surgery and radiation is currently being evaluated. At present, research centers are also investigating methods of increasing the sensitivity of brain tumors to radiation. However, thus far the results of such studies are not very encouraging.

Who Should Treat You? The Neurosurgeon   The physician who should treat you if you have a tumor of the brain or spinal cord is a neurosurgeon. This is a surgeon who has had four to six years of specialized training in the evaluation of and surgery for tumors and other diseases of the central nervous system. He or she also knows about the need for radiation and possibly chemotherapy after the surgery has been completed. A physician who has received this specialized training and passed a test evaluating his or her knowledge becomes a board-certified neurosurgeon.

A board-certified neurosurgeon is available in most middle-sized and all larger communities. Therefore, adequate treatment for brain tumors is available in most communities. It does not pay to travel to a cancer center far away from home unless you are referred by your neurosurgeon. There are few promising experimental approaches to the treatment of brain tumors at the present time.

Medulloblastoma: The Need for a Team Approach   The one exception to the advice in the previous paragraph is with a tumor called a medulloblastoma. This tumor occurs solely in children. It is highly malignant but can be cured with aggressive treatment. Like many other childhood cancers, a combined approach employing surgery, radiation, and often chemotherapy is used to cure this otherwise rapidly fatal cancer. Therefore, children with this tumor should be referred to a major childhood cancer center or children's hospital for the best treatment.

Symptoms of Brain Tumors

Brain tumors produce symptoms in two ways: they damage or irritate the specific area of the brain in which they grow, and they also cause more generalized symptoms by increasing the pressure inside the skull.

The symptoms due to damage of normal tissue in the area of the tumor are called "localizing" signs. The specific symptoms depend upon where the tumor is located. For example, if a tumor is growing in the area of the brain that moves your arm or leg, you may develop arm or leg weakness; if a tumor is growing in the cerebellum, the part of the brain that coordinates movement, you may develop poor coordination; if a tumor is affecting the part of the brain that controls vision, you may develop partial blindness.

Seizures   Another local sign of a brain tumor is the onset of epilepsy or seizures. Brain tumors cause seizures by irritating the area of the brain around the tumor. People who develop seizures for the first time in adulthood should be evaluated for the possibility of a brain tumor. A person may be completely well between seizures and yet have a tumor. Almost one-third of adults who develop seizures have a brain tumor. The tumor may be a benign meningioma. As with other tumors, early diagnosis is important. The larger the tumor grows, the more of the normal brain it damages. Newly diagnosed epilepsy in an adult should not merely be treated with drugs. All adult epileptics should have at least one thorough evaluation for small brain tumors. The tests needed include an electroencephalogram, skull x-rays, and a CAT scan or a brain scan. These tests are described later in this chapter.

Symptoms from Increased Intracranial Pressure

Brain tumors may produce generalized symptoms due to increased pressure within the brain. Rapidly growing tumors do this more often than do slow-growing tumors. Symptoms of increased pressure include headaches, nausea and vomiting, and decreases in mental functioning. A person may become forgetful or undergo a personality change.

Headaches   Headaches are a very common symptom and are rarely due to brain tumors. Therefore, you need not fear that you have a brain tumor merely because you have headaches. But if you have severe headaches you should see your family doctor. If he, or she, finds no hint of localized brain damage or of increased pressure in the brain, nothing further need be done. However, if your headaches are persistent and severe, your family doctor may send you to a neurologist or you should request a referral to one.

Neurologists are diagnosticians, not surgeons. They have taken three or more years of specialized training in the evaluation and treatment of diseases of the nervous system. The neurologist will carefully examine you for evidence of nervous system damage. If he, or she, finds nothing else wrong with you even though you have headaches, you can be almost sure you do not have a brain tumor and do not need further testing. Thus, although severe headaches are common with brain tumors, millions of people have headaches and do not have brain tumors. Even severe headaches should not make you overly worried about brain tumors.

The Evaluation for a Suspected Brain Tumor

People with signs of localized brain damage, with epilepsy starting in adulthood, or with signs of increased intracranial pressure should be sent to a board-certified neurosurgeon or board-certified neurologist. Both neurosurgeons and neurologists are qualified to evaluate these symptoms. However, only a neurosurgeon can operate on a brain tumor.

The neurosurgeon or neurologist will first perform a careful history and physical examination. Then, if he feels a tumor or other disease may be present, he will obtain a series of tests. First he will usually order x-rays of the skull. These are abnormal in 30 percent of people with brain tumors. Skull x-rays may show calcium if the brain tumor is a craniopharyngioma or a meningioma. They may also show changes from increased intracranial pressure and whether or not one side of the brain has become enlarged. Although skull x-rays are seldom conclusive, they can be helpful and are necessary to eliminate head trauma as a cause of the symptoms. The remainder of the evaluation for brain tumors includes four tests: an electroencephalogram, a brain scan, a CAT scan, and an arteriogram.

The Electroencephalogram (EEG)   The electroencephalogram (EEG) is a recording of brain waves. For this test, wires are taped on a person's scalp and brain waves are recorded. The test is difficult to interpret and must be read by a board-certified neurologist or neurosurgeon. It may show abnormal brain waves over the area of a tumor (the EEG is abnormal in approximately three-quarters of people with brain tumors). It is a simple and safe test. Even if it shows an abnormality, further tests must be done before surgery to define more accurately the exact location and extent of the tumor.

The Brain Scan   A brain scan is performed by injecting a small dose of radioactive material into an arm vein. This material accumulates uniformly in the normal areas of the brain. Tumors often have a richer blood supply than normal and accumulate more radioactivity than the surrounding normal brain. A camera is used to take pictures of the radioactivity in the brain. In about 80 percent of people with brain tumors, the brain scan is abnormal and shows increased radioactivity over the tumor. A brain scan shows the location of the tumor much more accurately than an EEG. If a brain scan is normal and a tumor is still suspected, the next test that should be done is a CAT scan.

The CAT Scan   Computerized axial tomography, or CAT scanning, is a major advance in x-ray technology that has recently become widely available. Many x-rays are taken, and a computer integrates them and can give very detailed pictures of the brain. This test is totally without risk or discomfort. It is more sensitive than a brain scan and may show tumors or other problems when a brain scan is normal. If an EEG, a brain scan, and a CAT scan are normal, the chances that symptoms are due to a tumor become very small.

The Arteriogram (Cerebral Angiogram)   If these tests show that a tumor is probably present, an angiogram is usually done. Unlike the previous tests, this must be done in the hospital. Cerebral angiograms are done by injecting an iodine-containing material into one or more of the four major arteries that supply the brain: the left and right carotids and the left and right vertebrals. The carotid arteries supply most of the upper portions of the brain. The vertebral arteries supply the lower and back part of the brain.

To perform cerebral angiography, a catheter is placed into an artery in the neck or the leg under local anesthesia. Using x-ray control, the neurosurgeon positions the catheter into the artery that goes to the area of the brain involved by the tumor. Then the dye is rapidly injected and many x-rays are taken quickly. Angiography shows not only the exact site of the tumor but also its blood supply. This helps the neurosurgeon plan the operation. Unlike the previous tests, however, there are some rare side effects from this procedure. The main one is bleeding from the site where the artery is punctured. However, this small risk is more than balanced by the valuable information obtained.

Is the Brain Tumor a Metastasis?

Before the neurosurgeon proceeds to operate on a presumed primary brain tumor, he or she must be sure that the tumor has not originated in another part of the body and spread to the brain. If the CAT scan, brain scan, or angiogram shows multiple tumors, metastases are likely. Primary brain tumors are almost always single. If a person has a history of a "cured" cancer, such as breast or lung cancer, even if only a single tumor is found, it is also likely to be metastic. However, even if there is no history of cancer and tests indicate a solitary brain tumor, a thorough cancer examination should be done. Before brain surgery, the neurosurgeon should obtain a chest x-ray to check for lung cancer and, for women, do a breast examination and probably also obtain mammography to check for breast cancer. He, or she, should carefully examine the skin for malignant melanoma, check a urine sample for microscopic blood from a kidney cancer, and test several stool samples for blood from colon cancer. Cancers from these areas frequently spread to the brain. It is not too unusual for breast or lung cancer to present first with symptoms from brain metastases. But if these tests are all normal and if there is only a single abnormal area in the brain, most likely it is due to a primary brain tumor.

Surgery for Diagnosis and Treatment   The next step for the person with suspected primary brain tumor is surgery. (More details about the actual surgery are included in the section on gliomas. This is similar to brain surgery for other brain tumors.) Neurosurgery for brain tumors should be done only by a board-certified neurosurgeon in a hospital large enough to have certain specialized facilities, including a neurosurgical intensive care unit and full rehabilitation facilities. The first several days after surgery are a critical time. Brain swelling from the surgery can develop quickly, and life-threatening infections of the nervous system can occur. Nurses specially trained in neurosurgical postoperative care should be watching people after brain surgery. Even if your community hospital has a neurosurgeon, it may not have the intensive care facilities or the rehabilitation facilities necessary for someone who has had brain tumor surgery. Therefore, your neurosurgeon may refer you to a large hospital.

We will discuss some of the more common types of brain tumors: gliomas, nongliomas, benign tumors, and metastatic tumors. In this chapter, we concentrate mainly upon tumors that originate in the central nervous system, despite the fact that most brain tumors are metastases from cancers that originate in other parts of the body.

Malignant Brain Tumors

GLIOMAS

Gliomas are the most common type of malignant brain tumor. About half of all brain tumors in adults are gliomas. They occur most often between the ages of thirty and sixty. Two factors affect how well a person with a glioma fares. The first is the location of the tumor in the brain, which determines how accessible it is to the surgeon. For example, if a glioma arises in an area such as the cerebellum, the surgeon can remove the whole tumor without removing too much normal brain tissue. However, most gliomas occur deep in the brain and cannot be entirely removed. The other important factor is the pathologic grade of the tumor, that is, how malignant the tumor looks under the microscope. A grade 1 glioma contains cells that act somewhat malignant but look almost normal. If the tumor appears more malignant it is given a higher grade, up to 4. Generally, the higher the grade of the tumor, the faster the tumor grows, and, therefore, the worse the prognosis.

The most common type of glioma is an astrocytoma. Grades 1 and 2 grow slowly, and people can survive for years and some are cured. However, people with grades 3 and 4 astrocytomas rarely live more than one year. Grade 4 is sometimes also called glioblastoma multiforme. This is the most malignant brain tumor in adults.

Treatment

Steroids A drug called dexamethosone, or Decadron, is often given by mouth as soon as the diagnosis of a brain tumor is made if the brain is under increased pressure. This drug will usually decrease the brain swelling and relieve symptoms such as headaches. Steroids don't shrink the tumor itself but rather decrease the inflammation of the surrounding brain. They are used to decrease brain swelling temporarily before surgery. They are also used if brain swelling occurs during radiation therapy.

Surgery Surgery is the first and main form of treatment for gliomas as well as for most other brain tumors. Most gliomas and most other malignant brain tumors are not cured by surgery because they cannot be completely removed without damaging too much of the brain. Although it is beyond the scope of this book to give a detailed explanation of what brain surgery is like, perhaps a brief description will be helpful.

Under general anesthesia, the part of the skull over the tumor is cut with a saw and lifted up so that the brain can be seen. The neurosurgeon then locates and removes as much of the tumor as possible. Some normal brain tissue surrounding and covering the brain tumor also must be removed. After the surgeon has finished, the skull is closed and the wound heals like any other bone fracture.

Brain damage from surgery. The type and degree of brain damage after surgery depend upon the location of the tumor, the damage to the surrounding brain caused by the tumor before surgery, and the amount of normal brain tissue that had to be removed at the time of surgery. Destruction of brain tissue by the tumor and surgery almost always cause some brain damage.

The brain is divided into a dominant hemisphere and a nondominant hemisphere. In right-handed individuals, the left hemisphere is dominant; conversely, the right hemisphere is dominant in left-handed people. If a brain tumor occurs in the dominant hemisphere, both the tumor and the surgery produce greater abnormalities than if it is on the nondominant side. However, in younger individuals, even fairly marked damage present immediately after surgery may improve. It is important that neither the brain tumor victim nor his family assume that brain damage present immediately after surgery will be permanent. Some of the apparent damage is due to brain swelling from the surgery. It resolves in a matter of days. The brain also has a remarkable ability to transfer function from one area to another. Therefore, the remaining normal brain tissue may take over some of the duties of the damaged tissue, and the patient may improve over a period of weeks to months. Rehabilitation therapy is important in helping this transfer of function.

Prognosis. The prognosis with gliomas depends on the degree of malignancy. Only rarely are gliomas completely removed by surgery. Usually the tumor invades deep parts of the brain and cannot be removed without producing too much brain damage. The neurosurgeon tries to take out as much of the tumor as possible to relieve pressure on the brain. After surgery, people usually feel better; the symptoms of increased pressure such as headache disappear and some local defects such as arm or leg weakness may improve.

Unless the tumor is completely removed, it grows again. The higher the grade of the tumor, the faster it tends to come back. Grades 1 and 2 astrocytomas grow slowly, sometimes taking many years. The more malignant grades 3 and 4 tumors tend to come back rapidly, usually in months. Some astrocytomas can be completely removed and cured. For example, occasionally children develop a low-grade astrocytoma of the cerebellum, a surgically accessible part of the brain. Many of these tumors can be cured.

Radiation Following surgery for most gliomas, patients are referred for radiation therapy. Radiation therapy is used to buy additional time. It slows down the regrowth of the tumor. Unfortunately, this effect is usually somewhat short lived. Few people with grades 3 or 4 tumors live more than two years even with surgery and radiation. In the rare situation where the surgeon cannot remove any of the tumor because it is too deep in the brain, radiation is used as the primary treatment. This is not as good as a combination of surgery and radiation.

The side effects of brain radiation are temporary hair loss and mild sores in the mouth. The dosage of radiation must be carefully gauged because the brain has limited radiation tolerance. If too much is given, brain damage can occur from six months to a year later. If not enough is given, the tumor will not be controlled. Sometimes it is difficult to distinguish between brain damage due to radiation and that from a recurrence of the tumor. CAT scans are useful in making this distinction. In modern radiation facilities, the dosage is carefully controlled by computers, and radiation damage to the brain rarely occurs. Radiation should be given by a board-certified radiation oncologist with modern facilities.

Chemotherapy Chemotherapy for brain tumors is currently under investigation. Most anticancer drugs are not useful for the treatment of brain tumors, because they do not enter the brain and spinal cord. However, a group of drugs called nitrosoureas readily enters the brain. Two drugs within this group, BCNU and CCNU, have been used experimentally in combination with surgery and radiation to treat malignant gliomas. Studies have shown modestly increased survival when CCNU was used after surgery and radiation. However, further clinical trials are needed to determine the value of these drugs in therapy for brain tumors. Their beneficial effect is temporary and they do have side effects, including nausea and vomiting, that may last from several hours to several days. Nitrosoureas also suppress bone marrow function and may lead to life-threatening complications such as bleeding and infection.

Other experimental approaches to the treatment of malignant brain tumors include the use of drugs that increase the tumor response to radiation without increasing the radiation toxicity of normal brain tissue. These studies are just getting underway. You may want to ask your neurosurgeon and radiation oncologist about these drugs, which are called "radio-sensitizers."

In summary, people with low-grade (1 and 2) astrocytomas can live for years with their tumors. Some are cured by surgery. Surgery alone or with radiation helps people to live symptom free for years. On the other hand, people with the more malignant (grades 3–4) astrocytomas rarely survive for more than two years. Relief of symptoms for some months can usually be obtained with surgery and radiation. The tumors do regrow quickly and are usually rapidly fatal. Occasionally, even a high-grade glioma can be completely removed if it is accessible to the surgeon, and thus is cured.

R.T., a single mother of two children, ages four and six, was on welfare. On a visit to her home, her welfare case worker found her acting bizarrely. She had become increasingly suspicious and thought he was out to get her. She was not taking care of her children, and they were underfed and dirty. Her apartment was filthy. Previously, although she had many problems, she had been a scrupulous housekeeper and had taken excellent care of her children. The case worker was worried about the children and visited her weekly for the next two weeks. Each time, she was more withdrawn and increasingly bizarre. On the second visit she said he was the devil, and she tried to kill him with a kitchen knife. He called the police. The children were taken to the children's shelter and R.T. was taken to a large city hospital for psychiatric evaluation.

R.T. seemed well physically but was suspicious, withdrawn, and hallucinating. She said she had talked to God. God had told her to kill the social worker because he was an agent of the devil. The psychiatry resident examined her and did not detect any neurologic abnormalities. Therefore, R.T. was placed under observation in the city psychiatric hospital for three days and then transferred to the state psychiatric hospital. She remained there for the next month but did not improve with drugs that usually help paranoid schizophrenics.

One morning six weeks later, she did not wake up. She was rushed back to the city hospital, where evaluation showed that she had a marked increase in intracranial pressure. The pressure had severely compressed a vital area of her brain. The damage was permanent. She died three days later. At autopsy, a large glioblastoma (grade 4) was found in the right frontal lobe of her brain.

A common but often unrecognized symptom of brain tumors can be a change in personality. R.T. was examined but no abnormalities were found that gave a hint that her personality change was from a brain tumor. The tumor was located in a so-called "silent" area of the brain. The only symptom it produced was her personality change. Had it been diagnosed earlier, at best only several months of useful life might have been salvaged. The message from R.T.'s case is that anyone who has a marked change in personality should not automatically be assumed to be just mentally ill. Personality changes such as forgetfulness, paranoid delusions, exhibitionism, or inappropriate anger can result from frontal lobe brain tumors. Before a person is labeled as psychotic and committed to a state hospital, a thorough examination by a neurologist should be performed. If any abnormalities are found that suggest brain damage, further tests should be done. Unlike R.T., a person might have a personality change from a highly treatable or even a curable tumor.

A.K., a forty-two-year-old married arc welder with four children, developed weakness in his left arm. He assumed he had hurt his arm and continued to work. As time went on, the weakness progressed and involved his left leg and even the muscles on the left side of his face. After he developed difficulty walking, he saw his family physician. A.K.'s doctor found weakness of his left arm and leg and immediately sent A.K. to a neurologist. The neurologist found the same neurologic abnormalities and ordered an electroencephalogram, a brain scan, and skull x-rays. The skull x-rays were normal but the EEG and the brain scan both showed a tumor in the right side of the brain.

A.K. was admitted to a large hospital in his community and examined by a neurosurgeon. His tests were reviewed and the neurosurgeon did a carotid angiogram the following day. The angiogram showed the exact location of the tumor in the right side of his brain. The results of these tests and the proposed surgery were discussed with A.K. and his wife the next day. He was told that he probably had a brain tumor. Surgery was necessary to find out what kind of tumor it was and to try to remove it. The neurosurgeon told him he would try to remove as much of the tumor as possible.

A.K. and his wife were extremely frightened. They asked questions about what he would be like after he awoke from surgery. Would he be crippled? Would be be able to think normally? Would he ever be able to go back to work? The surgeon explained that although surgery was dangerous, he might wake up with less weakness than he had before surgery. He also told A.K. that it was very unlikely that he would have a personality change or difficulty talking or understanding. This was because the tumor was in the nondominant half of his brain. A.K. was right-handed, and therefore the dominant part of his brain was the left side.

At surgery the following day, a large grade 2 astrocytoma was found involving the area of the brain called the motor cortex. The motor cortex controls the motion of the opposite side of the body, i.e., right-sided tumors cause left-sided weakness. Unfortunately, the tumor extended deeply into the brain and could not be completely removed. The bulk of the tumor was removed. A.K. felt better after surgery. He still had some weakness of his left arm and leg, but his leg was stronger than before and he walked normally. Even though the tumor was not completely removed, it was a low-grade tumor and could take years to regrow.

Several days after surgery, the neurosurgeon met with A.K. and his wife. He told them that A.K. had a malignant brain tumor that could not be completely removed. He recommended radiation as soon as A.K. recovered from his operation. Radiation would not cure him but probably would give him more time by slowing the regrowth of the tumor. A.K. and his wife asked questions about radiation and found out that the side effects were not bad: he would lose his hair temporarily and might have some soreness in his mouth.

A.K. decided to take radiation. The possible benefits greatly outweighed the side effects. He was sent to a radiation oncologist in the same hospital, who planned a course of radiation to the whole brain. For these treatments, A.K. had to go to radiation therapy five days a week for treatments that lasted only about one-half hour. During the radiation he felt well enough to drive himself to and from the hospital.

A.K. planned to go back to work after the course of treatment was completed. He enjoyed his family and his job. Even though he had a brain tumor, there was nothing in his life he wanted to change. He and his family tried to maintain as much normalcy as possible.

After he started radiation, A.K. and his wife decided to tell their children about his illness. They had already talked about these matters between themselves for several weeks. The children were told that he had cancer in his brain and that he was receiving treatment. A.K. also told the children he did not expect to be cured but that he would live for many years. The whole family was extremely upset and cried that night and for several days afterward. However, this open conversation allowed the whole family to share A.K.'s illness with him. He did not feel as alone as do many people who are unable to share their problems. Surprisingly, the children were reassured. They had been afraid that their father was going to die any day.

A.K. received radiation with few side effects. He felt well and returned to work. His only reminder of the brain cancer was some mild weakness of his left leg and arm. Four years later the increasing weakness began again in his left arm and leg. He began to get headaches, which were most severe in the morning. He went back to his neurosurgeon, who found that A.K. was weaker and had signs of increased intracranial pressure. A CAT scan showed that his tumor was back. A.K. underwent surgery, and the neurosurgeon again removed most of the tumor. He recovered quickly from surgery and felt well for two additional years.

Then he began to develop headaches. These were worst in the morning and soon became almost intolerable. His neurosurgeon again obtained a CAT scan, which showed the tumor enlarging again. He told A.K. that further surgery was not possible and that more radiation could not be given without destroying normal brain tissue. Chemotherapy might, however, buy a short period of time. A.K. decided to take chemotherapy because he wanted as much time as possible with his wife and children. He was placed on dexamethasone (Decadron), which relieved the increased pressure in his brain and relieved his headaches. He also received a dose of BCNU intravenously. He was nauseated for several hours. Over the next six months, however, he became increasingly weak and soon was unable to walk. Luckily he was conscious and in full control of his mental facilities and therefore able to communicate with his family during this time.

A.K. and his family decided that he should die at home if at all possible. His wife helped him get around. The American Cancer Society loaned them without charge a hospital-type bed, a wheelchair, and other devices to help care for him at home. He lapsed into coma and died at home. His family felt good that they were able to share his last moments.

This case typifies the course of people with low-grade astrocytomas. Often surgery and radiation can offer relief of symptoms for years, but the tumor will eventually recur. Treatment gave A.K. six good years.

This case also illustrates how well some families deal with the crisis presented by a progressive and eventually fatal cancer. A.K., his wife, and his children all came to terms with his illness while he was still alive. They communicated their feelings and therefore were able to become closer. A.K. was self-sufficient for six years. When the tumor progressed and the fatal outcome was certain, the family decided that it was best for A.K. to die at home. They were helped by services provided by the American Cancer Society and by the support offered by their neurosurgeon. A.K. and his family felt good about their ability to have some control over his illness and his death.

A.K. and his family resisted the temptation of going to a cancer center far from home for experimental treatment. The neurosurgeon explained to them that there were no promising experimental approaches for the treatment of this brain tumor. If A.K. and his wife had traveled to a cancer center, he might have lived for two or three months longer if experimental treatment had worked, but much of the additional time would have been spent away from his family and friends.

Adequate treatment for most brain tumors can be offered if a board-certified neurosurgeon, a board-certified radiation oncologist, and rehabilitation facilities are available. These specialists are generally available in most moderate-sized and large communities. Since brain tumors are usually fatal, it is best that the person spend his good time with family and friends instead of in a distant cancer center undergoing experimental treatment that is unlikely to help.

MEDULLOBLASTOMA

A tumor related to gliomas called medulloblastoma occurs only in young children. Medulloblastomas account for 30 percent of brain tumors in children. The disease usually arises in the cerebellum, the area of the brain that coordinates motion. A frequent symptom is lack of coordination. Medulloblastomas not only are fast growing, but unlike other brain tumors they spread by seeding cells into the spinal fluid and so metastasize to other parts of the brain and spinal cord. They often produce symptoms of increased intracranial pressure such as headaches. Although this is an extremely malignant tumor, it is very radioresponsive and can be cured.

Medulloblastoma Can Be Cured

Children with medulloblastomas should be sent to a major children's cancer center or to a large children's hospital. Only these centers have the treatment facilities and psychological support systems that children and their families need. (See chapter 23, "Cancer in Children.")

The treatment for medulloblastoma involves a combination of surgery for diagnosis and to remove as much of the tumor as possible, followed by radiation and chemotherapy. The value of chemotherapy is currently under study. After surgery, high-dose radiation is usually given to the whole brain and the spinal cord. Without radiation, medulloblastomas are rapidly fatal. With aggressive therapy, children are cured. Chemotherapy is given both intravenously and into the cerebral spinal fluid. The latter procedure is performed by inserting a needle into the spinal cord in the lower portion of the back (a lumbar puncture). With modern treatment, between 50 and 70 percent of children with this very malignant tumor are alive five years after diagnosis.

There are long-term side effects from radiation to the spinal cord in children. Radiation interferes with normal bone growth. Therefore, children who receive radiation as infants will be short. They may also develop curvatures of the spine if they are not carefully watched for this complication. Perhaps chemotherapy will allow the dosage of radiation to be lowered in the future. The lower the dosage, the more normal growth becomes.

Benign Brain Tumors

Almost one-half of brain tumors are benign. Meningiomas, acoustic neuromas, pituitary tumors, and craniopharyngiomas are common non-malignant brain tumors. In contrast to the malignant tumors, benign tumors grow slowly and do not invade the normal surrounding brain tissue. However, although these tumors look benign under the microscope, they are still dangerous. Because the brain is encased in a rigid bony structure and therefore cannot tolerate any increase in size, even a benign tumor will cause problems. If left untreated, a benign brain tumor can kill.

MENINGIOMAS

Meningiomas are benign, slowly growing tumors. They usually occur near or on the surface of the brain. Thus, they can often be completely removed surgically. Even if they can't be completely removed, surgery can provide years of symptom relief. The symptoms of meningiomas, which depend upon the location of the tumor, develop slowly. Seizures and localized brain malfunctioning are most common. Common symptoms also include a change in thinking ability or a personality change that could lead to admission to a psychiatric hospital.

The prognosis with meningiomas is excellent if they are treated. The evaluation is the same as for malignant tumors and is most easily made by a brain scan or a CAT scan. Meningiomas can be either entirely removed or at least mostly removed by a neurosurgeon. If they are not completely removed they grow back, and a second operation is needed. However, symptoms are controlled for long periods of time. Surgery can usually be done without damaging normal brain tissue.

ACOUSTIC NEUROMAS

Acoustic neuromas are benign tumors that arise in the nerve going to the ear. The usual symptoms from this tumor are ringing in the ear, decreased hearing, and decreased coordination due to damage to the cerebellum. These tumors, like meningiomas, are usually curable, although the surgery is very delicate. Some small tumors are treated by otolaryngologists. Larger tumors are treated by neurosurgeons.

PITUITARY TUMORS

The pituitary gland is a small gland at the base of the brain that secretes hormones that control the secretion of many other hormones. It regulates the thyroid, the adrenal gland, and sexual hormone production. Several benign tumors arise in this area. The usual symptoms of pituitary tumors are from hormonal imbalance. Either too little or too much pituitary hormone production occurs. If the tumor is large, partial blindness occurs, since the tumor can press on the optic or visual nerve. Pituitary tumors are benign and can be controlled or cured.

Treatment

Treatment options for pituitary tumors include surgical removal of the tumor, cryosurgery—that is, destroying the tumor by freezing it—radiation, or a combination of surgery and radiation.

Radiation   Radiation for the treatment of pituitary tumors must be performed in centers that have very specialized equipment. The proper treatment has few side effects. The pituitary is a very small gland; high doses of radiation are delivered to only the gland and nearby surrounding area, so most of the brain escapes radiation. It pays to go to a larger center so that you can receive expert radiation for a pituitary tumor. Small community hospitals rarely have the equipment necessary to give this type of specialized treatment.

Treatment, whether it be surgery and radiation or radiation alone, usually controls pituitary tumors. Headaches and other symptoms such as decreased vision will improve. However, the tumor may have already destroyed the pituitary gland. Therefore, even a person with a cured pituitary tumor may need replacement hormones the rest of his or her life. They should have their hormone status checked: thyroid, adrenal, and sexual hormone function can be below normal. The hormonal evaluation may require referral to another specialist called an endocrinologist. This is an internist who specializes in hormonal problems. He or she will decide after a series of blood tests whether you need hormones. If you do, he, or she, will prescribe them and see you on a regular basis to check your hormonal status.

METASTATIC TUMORS OF THE BRAIN

Perhaps the most common type of brain tumor is one that originates in another organ and spreads to the brain. Breast and lung cancers account for a majority of brain metastases, but malignant melanoma, kidney cancer, and gastrointestinal cancer also can spread to the brain. The symptoms from brain metastases are similar to those of primary brain tumors: headaches and signs of local brain dysfunction such as arm or leg weakness and seizures. The development of severe headaches or of a focal defect such as arm weakness in a patient who has cancer in another part of the body is always a cause for concern. If you or someone in your family has a cancer and develops headaches or other neurological problems, you should immediately call your physician. He or she will quickly perform tests to see if a metastatic tumor is present.

It is important to diagnose and treat metastases to the brain as soon as possible. The results with therapy are best when there is minimal brain damage from these metastases. The evaluation of metastatic brain tumors is the same as that for primary brain tumors. Usually a brain scan is obtained first. If this does not show metastases, a CAT scan is done. If these tests show tumors in the brain in someone with known cancer elsewhere, no further tests are needed. The person can be sent to a radiation oncologist for radiation therapy without surgery. If more than one abnormality is seen on the brain or CAT scan, even if you have no known cancer, the tumors are also likely to be metastatic.

Treatment

Radiation   The treatment of metastatic brain tumors is usually radiation given over two to three weeks. Before radiation is started, dexamethasone (Decadron), a steroid hormone, is usually given to decrease brain swelling. This often dramatically relieves the symptoms. Radiation of metastatic brain tumors can control them for months or even years. Frequently people die from metastases to other organs such as the liver rather than from a regrowth of metastatic brain cancer. Malignant melanoma is an exception. This cancer does not respond well to radiation. If possible it is treated surgically.

Surgery   Surgery is sometimes used to treat metastatic brain tumors. It should only be used for single metastases in patients who are otherwise well and who are expected to live several years. Sometimes these people can live for years and occasionally are cured. However, surgery is not generally used to treat metastases because there are many of them and because survival is already limited by the cancer elsewhere in the body.

P.S., a Catholic nun and school principal, had a mastectomy for breast cancer. She felt well and continued as principal of her school for two and a half years. Then she gradually began to develop aches and pains in many of her bones. She went back to her surgeon, who found that several of her bones were tender to pressure and suspected bone metastases. He ordered a bone scan, which showed many abnormal areas due to metastases. Three previous bone scans had been normal. He told P.S. that although she had metastases to bone her cancer was progressing slowly and she had a good chance of responding to hormones. She was placed on estrogens, and over the next month her pain improved and then disappeared completely.

She felt well for about one year and then developed increasingly severe headaches. The headaches awakened her in the morning and were localized to the left side of her head. She thought they might be due to tension and therefore she medicated herself with a tranquilizer and aspirin. However, over the next several weeks, the headaches increased in intensity and became totally unbearable. Unfortunately, her surgeon had died and she had no other physician.

P.S. went to a family physician recommended by one of her friends. He did not know much about breast cancer, and was not aware that it often spread to the brain. Therefore, he did not do a thorough neurologic examination and did not examine her eyes thoroughly. An examination of her eyes would have shown signs of increased pressure. He prescribed codeine and told her that her headaches were most likely migraine. The codeine temporarily helped, but after another week she developed weakness on the left side of her body.

She returned to the family physician, who realized his mistake, hospitalized her, and asked a neurologist to see her. She had greatly increased pressure inside her head and definite muscle weakness in her left arm and left leg. He ordered a brain scan, which showed three separate abnormalities that were suspicious for tumors.

The neurologist started P.S. on Decadron to decrease the pressure in her brain and had a radiation oncologist see her that same day. Radiation started that evening, and within twenty-four hours her headaches had improved. After a two-week course of radiation, her headaches were gone and her weakness had improved considerably. But because of the delay in treatment, she still had some weakness in her leg and arm. However, within one month she was back at work.

She felt well for two more years but then again developed headaches, weakness, and difficulty remembering simple things. She would forget her telephone number, forget where she had placed her pencils, and often repeat things several times. She was under the care of a medical oncologist, who was giving her estrogen to control her bone metastases. When he saw her with these symptoms, he suspected a recurrence of the brain tumors and sent her to the neurologist who had seen her previously. A brain scan showed that the three tumors were larger than before.

The medical oncologist, neurologist, and radiation oncologist reviewed her problems. They decided that P.S. could not receive more radiation since she had received as much as her brain could tolerate. Further radiation would damage her brain. She was again started on Decadron, which improved her symptoms temporarily. However, within the next few weeks she became weaker and eventually lapsed into coma. She was hospitalized and then transferred to a nursing home. She died one month later in coma.

This case illustrates several important points about metastatic brain tumors. In a patient like P.S., with cancer elsewhere that can spread to the brain, any neurologic symptoms require tests to see if brain metastases are present. If the brain scan or CAT scan is abnormal, surgery is not necessary. Metastatic brain tumors are treated with Decadron to decrease swelling quickly and with radiation to the brain. The radiation usually controls the tumors. Brain radiation controlled P.S.'s brain cancer for two years. Although she died of recurrent brain cancer, many patients with breast cancer and other cancers with brain metastases die from the cancer elsewhere while the brain cancer is still well controlled by radiation. P.S. was lucky to respond so well to radiation. It is important to be treated as soon as possible. Two-thirds of the people with metastatic brain tumors respond well to radiation. How much people recover depends on how much damage has already occurred to the brain. For example, slight weakness of the arm or leg will almost always get better after radiation; however, if the leg and arm are severely weak, a good response is less likely.

A.T., a sixty-year-old retired construction worker, had slowly progressive but incurable lung cancer. Six months after this diagnosis was made, he developed headaches. His doctor suspected brain metastases and obtained a CAT scan, which showed two tumors. These were also certainly metastases from the lung cancer. He told A.T. that his cancer had spread to his brain but that radiation could probably control it.

A.T. was sent to a radiation oncologist, who explained the radiation treatment he would be given and the side effects. A.T. received Decadron tablets to decrease his brain swelling and then started four weeks of radiation. He felt well during the treatment. His headaches disappeared shortly after he started Decadron.

After the radiation was completed, he felt fairly normal and spent his time fishing and playing golf. One year after receiving radiation to his head, his appetite decreased and he developed pain in the right side of his abdomen. His physician found an enlarged liver. A liver scan showed spread to the liver. The surgeon talked with A.T. about metastases to his liver. He told him that chemotherapy was not very effective for his type of lung cancer, but that if he wanted treatment, he would send him to a medical oncologist. The oncologist was not enthusiastic. He said that chemotherapy offered only temporary benefit and more often than not harmed more people with its toxic side effects than it helped.

A.T. decided that he would not take chemotherapy. Instead he would take pain medications to control his symptoms. He lived four more months and had good pain relief with a "pain cocktail" that he took every six hours. The cocktail contained methadone, a narcotic, and a mild tranquilizer. A.T. died from his liver metastases at home and was quite comfortable until the end.

A.T.'s brain metastases responded well to radiation. Unfortunately, there was no good treatment for his lung cancer and he died of metastases to his liver. It is not unusual for radiation to control brain metastases long enough that the person dies of metastases elsewhere.

SUMMARY

1. The brain is enclosed in a rigid case (the skull), and any expanding growth is dangerous. Therefore, if they are not treated, both benign and malignant brain tumors damage the brain and can kill.

2. A brain tumor should be evaluated by either a board-certified neurosurgeon or a board-certified neurologist. However, only the neurosurgeon can operate on a brain tumor.

3. Adequate care for adults with brain tumors is available in most large communities. A board-certified neurosurgeon, a board-certified radiation oncologist, a neurosurgical intensive care unit, and a rehabilitation medicine department are needed.

4. People who develop seizures for the first time in adulthood need to be evaluated for the possibility of brain tumors. Approximately one adult in three who develop seizures has a tumor.

5. Benign brain tumors such as meningiomas or acoustic neuromas can be cured or controlled for long periods of time with surgery. Other benign brain tumors, such as pituitary tumors, are usually controlled by surgery and/or radiation.

6. Malignant brain tumors usually are not curable. High-grade tumors are usually rapidly fatal, but people can live for years with low-grade tumors.

7. The treatment for malignant tumors is surgery, often followed by radiation. Unfortunately, tumors can rarely be completely removed. Radiation can only rarely prevent regrowth of the cancer.

8. The place of chemotherapy in the treatment of malignant brain tumors is still being evaluated. Some people improve temporarily with it.

9. Medulloblastoma, a very malignant brain tumor in children, should be treated at a large cancer center that treats many children. It is curable with a combination of surgery and radiation, and often chemotherapy.

10. If you have cancer and develop headaches or other signs of brain dysfunction such as weakness in an arm or leg, you should go to your doctor immediately for evaluation and treatment. Certain cancers

commonly metastasize, or spread, to the brain. These include cancers of the breast, lung, kidney, and intestinal tract, and malignant melanoma.

11. Metastatic brain tumors are usually treated with radiation. They generally respond well and can be controlled for long periods of time. Surgical removal of metastic brain tumors is rarely done, but is indicated if there is a single metastasis, especially in a person who otherwise appears to be cured of cancer.

18

Cancers of the Blood Cells
and Lymph Glands

The cancers discussed in this chapter arise from the bone marrow and from lymphoid tissue. The bone marrow is the spongy tissue filling the center of the bones, a site of blood cell production. Blood cells perform four important functions: red blood cells carry oxygen to the tissues of the body; platelets are important in preventing and controlling bleeding; granulocytes, or "polys," help control infection by engulfing and killing bacteria; and lymphocytes also help fight infection by producing antibodies and may protect the body against some cancers. The cancers that start in the bone marrow are the acute and chronic leukemias and multiple myeloma. They are characterized by the uncontrolled growth of blood cells.

The major lymphoid organs of the body are the lymph nodes and the spleen. Lymphocytes are manufactured, reside, and function there and circulate in the peripheral blood. Cancers that arise from the lymph nodes and spleen are called malignant lymphomas. The two major categories are Hodgkin's disease and non-Hodgkin's lymphoma.

Each year, approximately 50,000 Americans develop, and 35,000 die from, leukemias and lymphomas. These cancers occur in young people more often than many other more common cancers. Therefore, although they account for only 8 percent of all cancer deaths, almost 50 percent of cancer deaths before the age of thirty are due to these cancers. They have a greater impact than their incidence would suggest.

Cancers arising from the bone marrow and lymphoid tissues are discussed separately, since their prognosis, need for and response to treatment, and need for specialized care vary. The cancers included in this chapter are Hodgkin's disease, non-Hodgkin's lymphoma, acute myelocytic or acute nonlymphocytic leukemia, chronic myelocytic leukemia, chronic lymphocytic leukemia, and multiple myeloma. Acute lymphocytic leukemia is primarily a disease of childhood and is discussed in chapter 23, "Cancer in Children."

Malignant Lymphomas

The malignant lymphomas are cancers that arise from the lymph nodes, the spleen, or lymph glands such as the tonsils. These cancers are divided into two major subtypes, Hodgkin's disease and non-Hodgkin's lymphoma. Though they share characteristics, they differ in important ways and will be discussed separately.

HODGKIN'S DISEASE

Since 1832, when Thomas Hodgkin described seven people who died with the disease that bears his name, there has been striking progress in both the understanding of and the ability to treat this malignant disease of lymph nodes. Hodgkin's disease usually attacks people between the ages of fifteen and thirty-four and over the age of fifty. Each year, approximately 8,000 Americans develop and 3,000 die from it. The treatment of Hodgkin's disease is one of the major success stories in cancer therapy. Most people with this disease are now cured. Twenty years ago, it was invariably fatal.

Diagnosis

Although Hodgkin's disease can start anywhere, it usually starts as a painless swelling of lymph nodes, often the lymph nodes in the neck. Someone with early Hodgkin's disease may feel entirely well or may feel tired or have fevers, drenching sweats at night, weight loss, or severe itching.

Lymph nodes enlarge in response to infections. For example, the lymph nodes in the neck will enlarge if you have infected teeth, tonsilitis, or an ear infection. You should not go to your doctor every time you notice swollen lymph glands in your neck. Most lymph node enlargements are due to infections and not to cancer. In young adults, infectious mononucleosis is a common cause of neck node enlargement. However, persistently enlarged lymph glands, especially if not tender, merit a visit to your doctor. Lymph nodes enlarged from nonmalignant conditions are usually single, not larger than one to two inches in diameter, somewhat soft, and often tender. Lymph nodes are more likely to be malignant if they are hard or rubbery, not tender, or matted together or if they involve more than one area, for instance, both the neck and the axilla (armpit). If the doctor thinks your lymph nodes are suspicious for malignant lymphoma or another cancer, he or she should refer you to a general surgeon for a biopsy.

The Lymph Node Biopsy   A persistently enlarged lymph node may contain Hodgkin's disease, non-Hodgkin's lymphoma, or another cancer, and therefore should be biopsied. The biopsy should be done by a board-certified general surgeon. This is a fairly simple procedure and can usually be done with local anesthesia. Depending upon the location of the suspicious lymph node, the biopsy is done either in the surgeon's office or in a hospital. The surgeon should remove an entire lymph node. This makes it easier for the pathologist to make the diagnosis. It may be difficult for the pathologist to tell what is wrong even with a large lymph node to study. In this situation the slides are sent to another pathologist, who specializes in disorders of lymph nodes.

The Four Subtypes of Hodgkin's Disease   If Hodgkin's disease is present, the pathologist must decide its "subtype," or classification. The four subtypes, called lymphocyte predominant, nodular sclerosis, mixed cellularity, and lymphocyte depleted Hodgkin's disease, are guides to therapy and how well someone is likely to do. People with lymphocyte predominant and nodular sclerosing Hodgkin's disease have a better chance of being cured than those with mixed cellularity and lymphocyte depleted Hodgkin's disease. Some decisions about staging and treatment depend on the subtype of Hodgkin's disease.

Staging: How Far Has Hodgkin's Disease Spread?

Hodgkin's disease starts in one area of the lymph system—the lymph glands of one side of the neck or the groin, for instance—and then metastasizes, or spreads, through the system to other organs of the body, such as the liver, bone, bone marrow, and lungs. It is very important to find out how far Hodgkin's disease has spread.

There are two very effective forms of treatment for Hodgkin's disease: radiation and chemotherapy. Radiation can only cure Hodgkin's disease if the cancer is within the lymph glands and spleen. Chemotherapy reaches all areas of the body and is used to treat widespread Hodgkin's disease. It is important to pick the correct treatment the first time. Hodgkin's disease is more likely to be cured on the first try than if it relapses. Therefore, if your physician knows exactly how far Hodgkin's disease has spread, he or she can choose the right treatment the first time.

The tests needed to assess spread in Hodgkin's disease are more extensive than those for many other cancers, since so much depends on them. The tests are:

—A chest x-ray to see if the lymph nodes in the chest or the lungs are involved.

—A liver-spleen scan to determine if the liver or spleen is enlarged and therefore possibly involved with Hodgkin's disease.

—A lymphangiogram to determine if the lymph nodes in the abdomen are involved with Hodgkin's disease. (This is done by injecting a radiopaque dye into small lymphatics, or vessels, in the feet. The dye then spreads into the lymph nodes along the spine deep inside the abdomen and can be seen on x-ray. If they are involved by Hodgkin's disease, they appear enlarged and "foamy.")

—One or more bone marrow biopsies to see if the disease has spread to the bone marrow.

—An exploratory laparotomy if the other tests are not conclusive regarding abdominal spread of Hodgkin's disease.

The exploratory laparotomy is the best method of determining whether Hodgkin's disease has spread to the abdomen. It should be done by a board-certified general surgeon, preferably one who has done many such operations to stage or evaluate Hodgkin's disease. Although an exploratory laparotomy is major surgery, it is safe and worthwhile.

After opening the abdomen, the surgeon will carefully look and feel for areas of Hodgkin's disease. For example, he checks for enlarged lymph nodes and removes any that are enlarged or any that looked abnormal on the lymphangiogram. He also removes the entire spleen, takes several biopsies of the liver, and usually takes a large bone marrow biopsy. These specimens will all be examined under a microscope to see if Hodgkin's disease is present.

The spleen is removed to see if it has Hodgkin's disease and to decrease radiation damage to the left kidney. The spleen is a lymphoid organ and routinely must be treated with radiation unless it is removed. Removal of the spleen appears to have minimal long-term side effects in adults. However, the organ does play a role in fighting infection, and a person without a spleen is somewhat more susceptible to severe bacterial infections.

The Four Stages of Hodgkin's Disease   After the "staging" tests have been completed, the person with Hodgkin's disease will have his disease classified into one of four stages. Stage 1 disease is limited to one lymph node area (for example, the left side of the neck or the right armpit). Stage 2 disease is limited to several lymph node areas either above or below the diaphragm (the muscular wall separating the lungs from the abdomen). For example, Hodgkin's disease involving the left side of the neck, the left armpit, and the nodes around the heart (mediastinal lymph nodes) is stage 2 disease.

In stage 3, there is disease on both sides of the diaphragm but limited to the lymph nodes and the spleen. For example, involvement of the neck, armpit, and spleen is stage 3 disease. Stage 4 disease has spread beyond the lymph nodes and spleen to other organs such as the lungs, the liver, or the bones.

Each of these four stages of Hodgkin's disease is given an additional classification, A or B. People with weight loss, fever, or night sweats are said to have B disease; those without the symptoms have A disease. People without symptoms tend to do better and usually require less treatment than those with B symptoms. For example, a person with Hodgkin's disease localized to the left side of the neck without any symptoms is classified as having 1-A disease. The same person with disease localized to the neck but with night sweats would be classified as having 1-B disease. There is a relationship between the extent of the disease and the presence or absence of symptoms. People with early stages (1 and 2) of Hodgkin's disease tend not to have symptoms, and those with more extensive disease (stages 3 and 4) tend to have symptoms.

Treatment

Radiation, chemotherapy, or a combination of both are used to treat Hodgkin's disease. The treatment depends upon the disease stage and whether or not symptoms are present. Radiation is used alone for early stages of Hodgkin's disease and cures the large majority of patients. However, radiation is a local form of treatment; it must be directed to specific areas of the body. If the disease has spread beyond the area radiated, it will recur.

Chemotherapy is used to treat extensive or widespread disease since it reaches all parts of the body. It is effective treatment for Hodgkin's disease: most people with advanced disease improve and live longer with chemotherapy. In fact, almost one-half of people treated with chemotherapy are cured.

Stages 1 and 2-A Hodgkin's disease are treated with radiation therapy, and about 90 percent of people are cured. Stages 1, 2-B, and 3-A Hodgkin's disease are treated with either extensive radiation or radiation and chemotherapy. About 50 percent are cured with radiation alone. Clinical trials strongly suggest that the combination of radiation and chemotherapy cures more people. However, doctors will need more time to evaluate fully the benefits of combined treatment. Stages 3-B, 4-A, and 4-B disease are treated with chemotherapy. Approximately 40 percent of people with advanced Hodgkin's disease are cured.

In summary, Hodgkin's disease is curable by either radiation or chemotherapy. Early or localized disease without B symptoms is treated with radiation. Advanced disease is treated with chemotherapy. Intermediate-stage disease is usually treated with a combination of radiation and chemotherapy, but radiation alone is still an acceptable alternative.

Surgery Surgery has no place in the treatment of Hodgkin's disease except for the initial lymph node biopsy and, if necessary, an exploratory laparotomy.

Radiation High doses of radiation therapy are needed to eradicate Hodgkin's disease reliably. The standard treatment is to irradiate not only the areas involved but neighboring lymphoid areas as well. This is called extended field radiation. Its aim is to treat the known areas of involvement as well as other areas that are likely to contain microscopic nests of tumor cells. The treatment is usually given in two stages. First, lymph node areas above the diaphragm are radiated over four to six weeks. This is called mantle radiation. After several weeks of rest, the areas of the spleen and the upper abdominal lymph nodes are radiated. If abdominal lymph nodes are also involved (stage 3-A), all abdominal (upper abdominal and pelvic) nodes are radiated. This is called an inverted Y radiation field. The treatment, therefore, takes several months to complete, and it often takes several months after completion of radiation for a person to feel normal again.

The side effects of radiation vary considerably, ranging from very mild to severe. The common short-term side effects include fatigue or tiredness, loss of appetite, nausea and vomiting, and irritation or reddening of the skin over the areas radiated. Irritation of the lungs can cause coughing, inflammation of the esophagus can cause difficulty swallowing. Bowel irritation with diarrhea and loss of appetite can occur during the radiation of the abdominal lymph nodes. These side effects are temporary, and most patients have only some of them. Most people feel tired during radiation but can continue many normal activities, such as housework, schooling, or a job. During radiation, the blood counts are checked regularly because radiation depresses the blood count.

Serious long-term side effects of radiation for Hodgkin's disease are rare if the treatment is done well. We recommend that radiation be given by a board-certified radiation oncologist associated with a large medical center. Since the dosage needed to cure Hodgkin's disease is close to the tolerance level of normal tissues such as the heart, lungs, and spinal cord, if the radiation is not given by an expert, either the disease may not be cured or serious side effects can occur. These side effects include damage to the heart resulting in inflammation to the lining (pericarditis) or to the heart muscle. The lungs can be permanently scarred, causing shortness of breath.

For women who may want to have children in the future, a simple operation that moves the ovaries out of the radiation field can preserve fertility. If this is not done, radiation results in sterility. Males are not rendered sterile because the testes are not in the field and can be shielded from radiation.

Chemotherapy High-dose combination chemotherapy is used to treat widespread Hodgkin's disease. Fortunately, many drugs are effective against this disease. When used in combination, they are even more effective. About 80 percent of people with widespread Hodgkin's disease go into complete remission with high-dose combination chemotherapy.

This means that all evidence of disease disappears; it does not mean that the disease is cured. Microscopic deposits of tumor may still remain. However, half of the people who go into complete remission are, in fact, cured. Therefore, high-dose combination chemotherapy can control the disease for four out of five people and cure the disease in almost one-half.

The standard chemotherapy for Hodgkin's disease is a combination of four drugs called MOPP. These drugs are given for two weeks every month for six or more months. Two drugs are given intravenously twice each month and two drugs are taken in pill form for two weeks out of each month. The side effects are considerable, but almost all people can be treated in the physician's office or in a clinic. Common side effects of MOPP are a loss of appetite, nausea and vomiting, fatigue, hair loss, and depression of the bone marrow functioning, which can cause infections or require platelet transfusions. Usually the nausea and vomiting occur only on the two days of intravenous therapy each month. Although most people on chemotherapy do not feel normal, they can function fairly well. Most are able to continue working.

Most men treated with MOPP will become sterile, some temporarily but many permanently. If a man who wants to father children needs chemotherapy for Hodgkin's disease, sperm can be stored frozen and used up to several years later for artificial insemination.

Combination Radiation and Chemotherapy For 1-B, 2-B, and 3-A Hodgkin's disease, the combination of high-dose radiation and combination chemotherapy is being compared with radiation as the initial therapy. The combination of both seems to cure more people than radiation alone. However, doctors still aren't sure it is better treatment. People who are treated with radiation alone and who aren't cured are treated with combination chemotherapy when the disease recurs. The chemotherapy can often control the disease and cures some people. Several more years of testing are needed to see which approach is best for these stages of Hodgkin's disease. Ask your medical oncologist or radiation oncologist about the latest information.

Both radiation and chemotherapy have similar side effects, and treatment must be coordinated to obtain the maximum benefit with the fewest side effects. Radiation and chemotherapy are given in sequence. The chemotherapy is given for four to six months either before or after the radiation. Generally, side effects are somewhat worse when both radiation and chemotherapy are given. The long-term side effects, which include a higher risk of developing second cancers, may outweigh the benefits of an increased cure rate.

Who Should Treat Hodgkin's Disease? The staging, evaluation, and treatment of Hodgkin's disease is complex. This is one of the most curable cancers with good treatment. However, if not treated correctly, the chance for cure can be lost. It is important to stage the disease properly and then give accurate radiation, combination chemotherapy, or both. Optimal treatment demands at the very least a team of two specialists, a board-certified radiation oncologist and a board-certified medical oncologist or hematologist.

Although adequate treatment of Hodgkin's disease can be obtained in most moderate-sized communities that have a board-certified radiation oncologist and a board-certified medical oncologist, we recommend that you go to a large medical center to ensure that you receive the best treatment. At larger centers, there are usually several radiation oncologists and several medical oncologists, including some who specialize in treating Hodgkin's disease. Your case will be reviewed at a tumor board, a conference where many specialists are present. This minimizes the chance for error.

S.W., a twenty-six-year-old lawyer, went to his family doctor two months after he noticed a painless lump on the right side of his neck. Otherwise he felt entirely well. His physician found several large lymph nodes in his neck. He sent S.W. to a general surgeon, who removed one of the large lymph glands in his office under local anesthesia. The gland showed Hodgkin's disease, lymphocyte predominant type.

The surgeon told S.W. that he had Hodgkin's disease. Fortunately, there was effective treatment for Hodgkin's disease and he had the easiest type to cure. S.W. lived in a large city and was therefore sent by the surgeon to a radiation oncologist at a university hospital. The radiation oncologist examined S.W. He had no B symptoms, such as sweats, fevers, or weight loss, and the disease was apparently limited to lymph nodes in the neck. The radiation oncologist talked at length with S.W. about his disease and the need for further testing to see if it had spread to other areas of his body. He also spoke about radiation and the high potential for cure. He told S.W. that most probably he had early or localized Hodgkin's disease and would receive radiation after a series of tests were completed.

S.W. felt a little better. The shock of finding out that he was a victim of cancer, that he might not live out his expected lifetime, still dominated his thinking. He was mildly depressed. The radiation oncologist seemed very optimistic about his prospects for cure. S.W. still wondered whether the radiation doctor was merely reassuring him. He decided that he would go to a medical library and find out for himself while undergoing the tests he needed.

Over the next several days S.W. had a series of tests including a blood count, a chest x-ray, a bone marrow biopsy, and a liver-spleen scan. They were all normal. However, his lymphangiogram showed some suspicious lymph nodes in his abdomen.

He met again with the radiation oncologist, who explained to S.W. that he had to undergo an exploratory laparotomy to see whether the lymph nodes in his abdomen were indeed involved in Hodgkin's disease.

Although the lymphangiogram showed suspicious lymph nodes, it was not a conclusive test. He assured S.W. that his case had also been reviewed by other specialists at a tumor board. All had agreed that a laparotomy was needed.

S.W. was admitted to the hospital and underwent an exploratory laparotomy. The surgeon found nothing suspicious in the abdomen. He removed several lymph nodes and the spleen and took three liver biopsies and a large bone marrow biopsy. All of the biopsies were negative. S.W. indeed had early, localized Hodgkin's disease, stage 1-A.

Several days after the surgery, the radiation oncologist explained to S.W. that he would be treated with radiation therapy and had a better than 90 percent chance for cure. S.W. started radiation therapy two weeks later. He received four weeks of five-day-per-week radiation to the lymph nodes of his neck, armpits, and chest. During this time he felt tired and lost his appetite and sense of taste. He was given three weeks of rest and then four weeks of radiation to his upper abdomen, which made him feel worse than the chest radiation. He lost about six pounds, felt very tired, and vomited several times. However, two months after he finished with the radiation, he felt entirely well again.

S.W. was examined by the radiation oncologist every two months for two years. Then he was given some good news: he was probably cured. Hodgkin's disease usually recurs within two years after radiation therapy. Seven years later, S.W. is still alive and well without any evidence of Hodgkin's disease and is almost certainly cured.

S.W.'s story illustrates several important features of Hodgkin's disease. He had enlarged lymph nodes in the neck as his only symptom. This is the most common presentation for Hodgkin's disease. S.W. received excellent treatment. His family physician sent him to a general surgeon for a lymph node biopsy. The surgeon then referred him to a large medical center, where he received expert care. He was carefully evaluated and then received radiation therapy. He had the benefits both of a close relationship with his radiation oncologist and of the expertise of other radiation oncologists and medical oncologists who consulted on his case at the tumor board. Like most people with early Hodgkin's disease, S.W. was cured with two months of radiation.

If S.W. had lived in a small town, we would hope that, rather than receiving the treatment there, he would have been referred to a large medical center where specialists with experience and training in the treatment of Hodgkin's disease are available. If you have Hodgkin's disease, it pays you to travel even a long distance. Several months of dislocation are worth the years of normal life that are obtained with accurate staging and excellent treatment.

B.W. was less lucky than S.W. He had B symptoms and advanced Hodgkin's disease when the diagnosis was first made.

B.W. was a fifty-three-year-old carpenter who went to his doctor because he felt tired and had lost his appetite. He told his doctor that he had drenching sweats at night and sometimes needed to change his pajamas twice. He had gone from 160 to 140 pounds. His family physician thought that B.W. looked ill. He found enlarged lymph nodes under his left armpit and an enlarged spleen. He told B.W. that he might have a lymphoma and that the lymph node in his left armpit must be biopsied. He sent B.W. to a board-certified general surgeon, who removed a large lymph node from under the armpit under local anesthesia in the hospital. The lymph node showed mixed cellularity Hodgkin's disease. B.W. was sent to a medical oncologist at a large clinic nearby.

The medical oncologist examined B.W. and reviewed the biopsy. He told B.W. that he had Hodgkin's disease and that although it was probably advanced, several tests were needed before treatment could be started. A blood count, a chest x-ray, and a bone marrow biopsy were normal. A liver-spleen scan showed an enlarged spleen, and a lymphangiogram showed very abnormal lymph nodes that were almost certainly involved in the disease.

The medical oncologist reviewed B.W.'s case at his clinic's weekly tumor board. All the specialists agreed that B.W. had at least stage 3-B Hodgkin's disease and should receive only chemotherapy. They thought a laparotomy was not needed since chances were slim that it could change the treatment. The oncologist met with B.W. and explained the results of the tests and his decision to start with chemotherapy. He explained that chemotherapy had an excellent chance of controlling the disease and might even cure him. He also explained that chemotherapy had some bad side effects, such as nausea and vomiting, hair loss, and fatigue. He assured B.W. that these side effects did not mean the treatment was not helping him. The oncologist told B.W. that most people are able to continue work and other normal activities while taking chemotherapy.

B.W. started chemotherapy that day. He was treated with MOPP, given in two intravenous injections twice each month and pills for two weeks weeks each month. At first he was discouraged because, as the oncologist had explained, the drugs made him sick. With each injection, he developed nausea and vomiting that lasted about twenty-four hours. He felt weak and tired during the first two weeks of treatment. Then he noticed that the lymph nodes got smaller and the fevers and sweating went away. He began to feel stronger. Over the next five months he received five additional courses of treatment, and with each course he improved. Although he did not feel completely well, he felt better.

After six months of treatment, the medical oncologist repeated the staging tests and told B.W. that he had a complete remission. This did not mean B.W. was cured, although a cure was a possibility. He wanted to follow B.W. carefully.

Over the next fifteen months, B.W. felt entirely well. Then he again developed fever and night sweats. The oncologist found enlarged nodes under his armpit. B.W. was depressed. A cure was no longer a possibility. Hodgkin's disease had come back. The oncologist prescribed MOPP again.

B.W. received six more courses over six months, and again had a complete remission. However, this remission only lasted seven months.

When the disease came back a second time, B.W. was sicker than before. He had severe night sweats and high fevers with chills, and he felt awful. His oncologist explained that a different combination of drugs might help him. B.W. was again started on chemotherapy, and the drugs again controlled the disease. The sweats and fevers went away and the lymph nodes decreased in size. B.W. went into his third complete remission. This time he did not feel as well as he had during his two previous remissions.

After the six cycles were completed, treatment was stopped. Within three months he was sick again. The medical oncologist told B.W. that he would only try to control the symptoms of the disease. Further high-dose therapy could no longer help him.

B.W. was upset but still felt fortunate. It had been four years since the diagnosis was made. He had expected to die within a few months, as many of his friends with other cancers had. Instead, he had lived four years and felt well much of the time. The time had been well spent with his wife, his children, and his grandchildren.

Over the next several months, Hodgkin's disease inexorably progressed. B.W. died at home from an infection.

This case also illustrates some very important points about advanced Hodgkin's disease. Treatment is quite effective. MOPP or other combinations of drugs can usually control the disease completely. About half the patients who obtain a complete remission are cured. B.W. was not cured but he had four good years. The therapy has side effects but most people can continue many of their normal activities while receiving it. It does not require hospitalization and is almost always given in the doctor's office or clinic. Despite the side effects, chemotherapy makes a person with Hodgkin's disease feel better because it controls the symptoms of the disease.

Hodgkin's disease should be evaluated and treated by a team of specialists that includes a radiation oncologist and a medical oncologist. It pays to travel to a major center to receive optimal treatment. Radiation and chemotherapy are both effective forms of treatment and can cure this disease. Radiation is indicated for early Hodgkin's disease. A combination of radiation and chemotherapy is often used to treat intermediate stages of Hodgkin's disease. Chemotherapy is used for late stages of the disease. Almost all people with this disease benefit from treatment; in fact, most are cured.

NON-HODGKIN'S LYMPHOMAS

Non-Hodgkin's lymphoma tends to occur in older people than does Hodgkin's disease. It is most common in persons over fifty and afflicts more men than women. Approximately 14,000 Americans develop this cancer and 11,000 die from it each year. Non-Hodgkin's lymphoma, like Hodgkin's disease, is a cancer of the lymphoid system, the lymph nodes, and the spleen. However, there are significant differences between these two kinds of malignant lymphoma.

Diagnosis

The diagnosis of non-Hodgkin's lymphoma is made exactly as with Hodgkin's disease—by a biopsy of an enlarged lymph node or of other organs if the cancer starts elsewhere.

The first symptoms of non-Hodgkin's lymphoma are more variable than those of Hodgkin's disease. People may notice enlarged lymph glands in any area—the neck, the armpit, or the groin. The first symptom could be a swollen abdomen due to a large liver or spleen. Almost one time in three, the disease starts outside the lymph system. It may arise in the stomach or bowel, causing obstruction or bleeding. It can start in a bone, causing pain, or in the skin. Lymphoma of the skin, called lymphoma cutis, starts as either an itching rash or as lumps in the skin with no other symptoms. In contrast, it is rare for Hodgkin's disease to start outside of the lymphoid system.

The Four Subtypes of Non-Hodgkin's Lymphoma   As with Hodgkin's disease, the pathologist subclassifies non-Hodgkin's lymphoma into four histologic subtypes according to what cells are seen under the microscope: well-differentiated lymphocytic lymphoma, poorly differentiated lymphocytic lymphoma, mixed lymphoma, and histiocytic lymphoma. Each of these four is further classified as diffuse or nodular. The histologic type and whether a lymphoma is diffuse or nodular is of great prognostic importance. Well-differentiated lymphocytic lymphomas and the nodular types of the others tend to progress slowly. Before the era of modern treatment, many people with these types lived for many years. In contrast, the diffuse varieties of poorly differentiated lymphocytic lymphomas, mixed lymphomas, and histiocytic lymphomas progress rapidly; twenty years ago the average length of survival was less than one year. Because people with modular lymphomas and well-differentiated lymphocytic lymphomas can live for years even without treatment, they are treated differently from people with the more aggressive diffuse lymphomas.

Staging

Non-Hodgkin's lymphomas, like Hodgkin's disease, need careful evaluations to determine the extent of the disease. Radiation and chemotherapy are both effective treatments: radiation can successfully treat localized non-Hodgkin's lymphoma; chemotherapy is used to treat widespread disease. Non-Hodgkin's lymphomas are staged or evaluated somewhat differently from Hodgkin's disease. A blood count and a chest x-ray are obtained as with Hodgkin's disease. However, the next tests usually done are two bone marrow biopsies. These are done by inserting a needle under local anesthesia into the bone. A core of bone containing bone marrow is then removed. Some pain cannot be blocked by the local anesthesia, but it occurs only when the marrow cavity is entered. Bone marrow biopsies are safe and only take five to ten minutes. Non-Hodgkin's lymphoma involves the bone marrow much more often than Hodgkin's disease: approximately 30–40 percent of people with non-Hodgkin's lymphoma have bone marrow involvement. If the bone marrow biopsies are positive, the disease is stage 4, and no further tests are needed. In contrast, only 1–2 percent of people with newly diagnosed Hodgkin's disease have marrow involvement.

If the bone marrow biopsies are normal, a liver-spleen scan and lymphangiogram are done next. In most cases, the lymphangiogram shows lymphoma. This means that a person has stage 3 disease. An exploratory laparotomy is not usually done to evaluate the stage of the disease further in non-Hodgkin's lymphoma. Some cancer centers are studying its value, but its usefulness is not established at the present time.

After staging tests have been completed, a person with non-Hodgkin's lymphoma has his or her disease classified into four stages according to the extent of the disease. Non-Hodgkin's lymphoma tends to be more widespread at the time of diagnosis than Hodgkin's disease. Only 15–20 percent of people have stage 1 or 2 disease, compared to almost half of the people with Hodgkin's disease.

The Four Stages of Non-Hodgkin's Lymphoma   Stage 1 disease is limited to one lymph node or to a single localized non–lymph node area such as the stomach. Stage 2 disease is limited to lymph node areas on one side of the diaphragm or to a non–lymph node area and neighboring lymph nodes. For example, if the stomach and the lymph nodes in the area of the stomach were involved, the disease would be stage 2.

Stage 3 disease involves lymph node organs above and below the diaphragm. Disease that has spread outside the lymph system and beyond the one extranodal area (such as the stomach) is classified as stage 4. For example, if the lymphoma involves the liver, the bone marrow, the lungs, or the skin, it is stage 4.

Although B symptoms can be present in non-Hodgkin's lymphoma as well as in Hodgkin's disease, their importance is less clear. However, most lymphoma victims with B symptoms do have widespread and aggressive diseases and are treated with chemotherapy. Only rarely do patients with nodular lymphomas have B symptoms.

Treatment

As with Hodgkin's disease, the treatment for non-Hodgkin's lymphoma is radiation, chemotherapy, or a combination of both. Radiation is used to treat localized (stage 1 or 2) disease, and chemotherapy is used for widespread disease (stages 3 and 4). Since most people with non-Hodgkin's lymphoma have stage 3 or stage 4 disease when they first see a doctor, only a few people are treated with radiation; more receive chemotherapy as the first treatment. Radiation can cure localized non-Hodgkin's lymphoma. Chemotherapy can often control widespread disease. However, in contrast to Hodgkin's disease, where 40 percent of people are cured with chemotherapy, responses are most often temporary in non-Hodgkin's lymphoma. A few patients are cured, but usually the disease recurs. Therefore, chemotherapy is less effective against non-Hodgkin's disease.

The diffuse, aggressive lymphomas and the more benign nodular lymphomas are treated quite differently and are discussed separately. Survival with aggressive non-Hodgkin's lymphomas depends almost entirely upon controlling the disease by effective treatment. On the other hand, people can live for years with the less aggressive or more benign forms of lymphoma, even without effective treatment.

Treatment for Aggressive Diffuse Lymphomas   The aggressive lymphomas include the diffuse, poorly differentiated lymphocytic lymphomas, the diffuse mixed lymphomas, and histiocytic lymphomas. These diseases need intensive treatment. The average survival without effective control of the disease by therapy is under two years. If totally untreated, many patients would die within a few months.

Treatment for localized disease (stages 1–2).   Radiation is the standard treatment for stage 1 or 2 non-Hodgkin's lymphomas. It can reliably kill all lymphoma cells in a localized area and cure the disease. Usually radiation is given to the area or areas of obvious lymphoma and to neighboring lymph node areas, much as with Hodgkin's disease. About 75 percent of people with stage 1 and 50 percent of people with stage 2 non-Hodgkin's lymphoma are cured. Those who are not cured and go on to develop recurrent lymphomas do so because there were microscopic deposits of cancer beyond the areas radiated.

Studies are in progress at present to test the advantage of adding chemotherapy to radiation for stages 1 and 2 lymphoma. The aim of chemotherapy is to treat the microscopic deposits of tumor cells that have spread beyond the areas that are radiated, and thus possibly increase the cure rate. Although it is too soon to tell whether this approach is effective, the early results are promising.

Treatment for extensive disease (stages 3–4).   About 80 percent of people with non-Hodgkin's lymphoma have stage 3 or 4 disease and receive chemotherapy as their first treatment. There are many drugs that are effective against non-Hodgkin's lymphomas, and they are more effective when used in combination. With high-dose combination chemotherapy, about 50–60 percent of people with aggressive non-Hodgkin's lymphoma go into complete remission. These people feel better and live longer. Most of the patients who do not get a complete remission will get a partial remission; their tumor shrinks by at least 50 percent and they also feel better. Thus, chemotherapy benefits most people with aggressive lymphoma.

Several combinations of drugs are used, but the standard and most popular treatment in the United States at present is called CHOP. This is a four-drug combination that is given over several days each month for six or more cycles. Three of the drugs are given intravenously on the first day of each cycle and then a pill (prednisone) is given for five days. The intravenous drugs are cyclophosphamide (Cytoxan), hydroxydaunarubicin (Adriamycin) and vincristine (Oncovin). This treatment almost always can be given in a doctor's office.

Side effects from high-dose combination chemotherapy vary considerably from person to person. The more common side effects are loss of appetite, nausea, and vomiting from the intravenous medication; this usually lasts less than one day. Almost everyone loses most or all of his or her hair. Low blood counts one to two weeks after treatment can be dangerous and can lead to bleeding or infection. The dosage of the drugs is adjusted so that this complication is rare. Bleeding can occur with low platelet counts and infection with low granulocyte counts. Platelet transfusions or hospitalization for infection are occasionally necessary. Although most people suffer some side effects, they are able to continue many of their activities. Even with the side effects, some people feel better while taking chemotherapy because their cancer symptoms disappear. They feel stronger and, if they had pain, become pain free.

Chemotherapy is usually given for a finite period of time. For example, CHOP is given for six cycles and then treatment is stopped if the lymphoma has gone into remission. The patient is watched carefully. Some medical oncologists follow combination therapy with low-dose "maintenance therapy." Others do not. In most cases, the lymphoma recurs. Treatment is less effective for each recurrence; that is, the chance for complete remission decreases and the remissions are shorter. The picture is not all gloomy. Some people with aggressive lymphoma who go into a complete remission are cured. In fact, with diffuse histiocytic lymphoma, formerly the worst lymphoma, there is a good chance for cure if complete remission is obtained. However, few people with diffuse poorly differentiated lymphocytic lymphoma or diffuse mixed lymphoma are cured with chemotherapy.

L.H., a fifty-nine-year-old schoolteacher, went to her doctor because of vomiting after meals. She noticed that she usually vomited up undigested food. Her doctor found a dilated stomach on examination. X-rays of the stomach showed a mass where the stomach emptied into the small bowel (the pylorus). He suspected cancer and therefore sent her to a general surgeon. The surgeon examined her, reviewed the x-rays, and admitted L.H. to the hospital. He explained that she needed an operation to see what was wrong.

The surgeon operated the next day and found a large mass at the lower end of the stomach. He took a biopsy and waited for the pathologist's report. Tissue can be frozen and then looked at under a microscope in a matter of minutes during surgery. In twenty minutes he had an answer: L.H. had non-Hodgkin's lymphoma, probably histiocytic type. The surgeon realized that it was important to determine the extent of the disease. Therefore, he carefully looked around the abdomen, especially for large lymph nodes and nodules in the liver or spleen. He removed several nearby lymph nodes, removed the spleen, and did several liver biopsies and a bone marrow biopsy. Microscopic examination showed that all these tissues were normal. L.H. had stage 1 non-Hodgkin's lymphoma.

The surgeon told L.H. that she had a lymphoma. However, it seemed to be localized to the stomach itself. Chances were good that radiation could effectively control or cure it.

She was sent by the surgeon to see a radiation oncologist at a university hospital. He questioned and examined her and reviewed all her tests. Then he talked with her about her disease. L.H. had diffuse histiocytic lymphoma, one of the worst types of non-Hodgkin's lymphomas. Fortunately, the very thorough evaluation during surgery showed that it was limited to the stomach. Radiation was the treatment of choice for localized lymphoma. In fact, the oncologist was very optimistic about her chances for cure with just localized radiation therapy.

After recovering from surgery, L.H. returned to the radiation oncologist. He explained that the radiation would be carefully planned and that it would take only twenty minutes a day. She would receive radiation five days a week for four to five weeks to the area of the stomach and the neraby lymph nodes, even though they were not obviously involved with lymphoma. The treatment had some side effects. She might lose her appetite, become nauseated, or have diarrhea. The skin overlying the radiated area would become irritated and red. These side effects were temporary, and she would feel completely well in several months. He also told her that her case had been presented at the weekly tumor board conference and that other radiation oncologists and medical oncologists had agreed that radiation was the correct treatment and that her chance for cure was good.

Over the next four weeks L.H. underwent radiation. She lost her appetite and had some nausea and vomited once. She lost eight pounds. However, two months after the treatment was completed, she felt completely well. It is now seven years since L.H. was found to have lymphoma, and the disease has not recurred. She is cured.

This case illustrates several important points. Non-Hodgkin's lymphoma can start outside of lymph nodes: in the bones, the gastrointestinal tract, the skin, or almost anywhere. L.H. received excellent treatment. Her family doctor sent her to an experienced surgeon. When he found that she had lymphoma, he did a careful evaluation of the abdomen. This helped the radiation oncologists and medical oncologists decide upon the correct treatment plan. She had the advantage of a close relationship with one radiation oncologist and the advice of other specialists who attended the tumor board conference. While most non-Hodgkin's lymphomas have spread too widely to be controlled or cured with radiation, localized disease can be cured. L.H. felt weak and nauseated during radiation treatment but felt well again soon afterward. Despite not feeling well, she was able to continue teaching while receiving therapy.

N.W., a thirty-one-year-old housewife, went to her family doctor because she felt tired, had lost fifteen pounds, and was sweaty at night. He found enlarged lymph nodes under her left armpit and in her right groin. He also found that her liver and spleen were enlarged. Her blood counts were abnormal: she was anemic and her platelets were low. He suspected a malignant lymphoma and sent her to a board-certified general surgeon to obtain a lymph node biopsy.

The surgeon placed her in the hospital and removed a large lymph node under her left armpit using local anesthesia. It showed diffuse, poorly differentiated lymphocytic lymphoma. The next day the surgeon told her that she had a bad type of malignant lymphoma and that he was referring her to a medical oncologist for treatment since she needed chemotherapy. She had at least stage 3 disease.

The medical oncologist examined N.W. carefully. He then told her that she had an advanced aggressive lymphoma. Without treatment she would probably not live many months. She needed high-dose chemotherapy. Although this had side effects, it would probably make her feel better and prolong her life. She asked whether chemotherapy would cure her. The medical oncologist had to tell her that very few people with her type of lymphoma could be cured with chemotherapy.

N.W. asked the medical oncologist for some time to think about treatment. In a matter of days, she had been transformed from a healthy young woman who had years of life to look forward to, into a person with a highly malignant cancer who might die in a matter of weeks or months. She was also faced with high-dose toxic chemotherapy. She talked to her husband, her mother, and two close friends. After two weeks she was still very frightened and could not decide what to do. She was depressed and anxious. Although she knew she needed therapy, she could not face the thought of having "poisons" injected into her body. Her family physician talked with her husband, and they suggested that she see a psychiatrist. Her physician felt that unless she could talk about some of her fears, she would not do well with therapy. She agreed and paid several visits to a psychiatrist who was experienced in dealing with cancer patients. The psychiatrist was able to help N.W. face her disease more realistically. She also placed her on antidepressive drugs. N.W. was still depressed and anxious but was now able to make decisions.

N.W. believed in and liked her medical oncologist. He was well trained, straightforward, and seemed warm and sincere. However, she didn't want to start chemotherapy until she had at least one other opinion. Her oncologist referred her to another oncologist at a large clinic. He reviewed her case, gave her a similar prognosis, and recommended the same treatment. She satisfied herself that there were no other options. If she wanted to feel better and live more than a few months, she needed chemotherapy. She went back to her medical oncologist.

Chemotherapy with CHOP was started, and N.W. had side effects. Despite the use of pills to decrease nausea, she became sick and vomited several times after the first intravenous injections and felt weak for several days. Then, to her surprise, she started to feel better. Her sweating decreased. She felt stronger, and she was hungry for the first time in months. She also noticed that her lumps were getting smaller. After the second course of chemotherapy, all the lumps disappeared and she started to feel almost normal again.

N.W. received six courses of chemotherapy over six months, and with each course felt better. At the end of her therapy, tests showed no lymphoma. All the lumps had disappeared, and her medical oncologist happily told her that she was in complete remission. He could find no enlarged lymph nodes. Her liver and spleen had shrunk to normal size and her bone marrow, which had been abnormal when he first saw her, was normal. The oncologist told her that he would have to watch her carefully and start treatment again if and when the lymphoma reappeared.

She felt well for eleven months. Then she started to feel tired and developed night sweats. The medical oncologist found that her lymph glands, her liver, and her spleen were enlarged. She was again started on combination chemotherapy. This time N.W. did not obtain a complete remission. The lymph nodes, liver, and spleen decreased in size but did not return to normal. She felt better with therapy but not as well as with the first course of treatment. After five cycles of chemotherapy, the lymphoma started to grow again. Despite changing treatment, the lymphoma continued to progress. She became more fatigued, continued to lose weight, and died of progressive lymphoma nine months after the tumor recurred.

N.W.'s course was quite typical for patients with extensive, aggressive lymphoma. She had symptoms from her lymphoma when she first saw her doctor. Chemotherapy gave her a complete but only temporary remission. Except for diffuse histiocytic lymphoma, the remission is usually only temporary. The lymphoma recurs, and chemotherapy is usually less effective the second and third times. Chemotherapy definitely helped N.W. She lived longer and felt well for a year and a half because of therapy. Unfortunately, it did not cure her disease. Clearly there is room for improvement in the treatment of widespread, aggressive lymphomas.

The Less Aggressive Nodular Lymphomas These lymphomas tend to grow slowly and rarely cause symptoms such as night sweats or fever. People therefore tend to feel well and live for years without treatment.

Well-differentiated lymphocytic lymphoma, nodular poorly differentiated lymphocytic lymphoma, nodular mixed lymphoma, and nodular histiocytic lymphoma are the more common types of nonaggressive lymphomas. The average survival before the era of modern radiation and chemotherapy was five to seven years with these lymphomas. Some people lived ten to twenty years with them. Therefore, aggressive treatment is not indicated for most people with these lymphomas.

Treatment for localized nodular lymphomas.   Stages 1 and 2 lymphomas are given radiation treatment similar to that described for Hodgkin's disease. Radiation is given to the areas that are involved with lymphoma and to nearby areas that might contain microscopic deposits of lymphoma. Unfortunately, only about 15 percent of people with nodular lymphomas have localized disease that can be cured by radiation.

Treatment for extensive nodular lymphomas.   The treatment of widespread, less aggressive lymphomas is either relatively low-dose nontoxic chemotherapy or a form of radiation called total body irradiation (see below).

Total Body Irradiation   Total body irradiation consists of low-dose radiation given to the entire body. It is a systemic form of treatment; it reaches all parts of the body. Radiation is given two to three times a week for several minutes. There is no loss of appetite, nausea, vomiting, or diarrhea, since the dosage is so low. The only troublesome side effect is depression of the blood counts, which are carefully checked by the radiation oncologist. Total body irradiation is as effective as chemotherapy for these lymphomas. About 60–70 percent of patients go into complete remission with this fairly simple form of treatment.

Chemotherapy   The chemotherapy for these lymphomas is either a single drug in moderate doses or a combination of drugs, also in fairly low doses. Recent studies have shown no advantage to high-dose combination chemotherapy when it was compared to daily oral low-dose therapy with drugs, like cyclophosphamide or chlorambucil, that rarely cause any side effects. About 70 percent of people with these lymphomas will go into complete remission with nontoxic chemotherapy. Chemotherapy is usually given for six to twelve months and then stopped if a person goes into complete remission; it is usually continued longer if the person doesn't go into a complete remission. For these lymphomas, it is thus quite effective. The disease can be controlled for many years with nontoxic doses of drugs.

T.H., a sixty-eight-year-old carpenter, noticed painless lumps on both sides of his neck while taking a shower. They didn't go away, and one week later he went to his family doctor. Although he felt entirely well, his physician found enlarged lymph nodes on both sides of his neck and in his armpits and a large spleen. A blood count and a chest x-ray were both normal. His doctor suspected that he had a malignant lymphoma and sent him to a general surgeon. The surgeon removed one of the large lymph nodes on the right side of his neck under local anesthesia in his office. It showed a nodular, poorly differentiated lymphocytic lymphoma. The surgeon told him that he had a lymphoma but that it was of a type that would probably allow him to live for years.

Nevertheless, T.H. was frightened. Friends of his with cancer had suffered and died. In fact, his closest friend had died of lung cancer only a year earlier. He wasn't sure that the surgeon was telling him the truth. Perhaps the surgeon just wanted to make him feel better. He was sure he too would die soon and painfully.

He was referred to a medical oncologist, who saw him, examined him carefully, and reviewed his record. He explained to T.H. that he had a lymphoma. Although it was a type of cancer, T.H. was fortunate to have one with which he could live a long time. His type of lymphoma grew slowly and only required simple, nontoxic therapy. Although he might have trouble soon, most likely he would live for many years. The oncologist explained that no further tests were needed since T.H. had lymphoma in both the lymph nodes in his neck and in his spleen. Therefore, his treatment would be chemotherapy and not radiation.

The medical oncologist placed T.H. on chlorambucil, a type of anti-cancer drug given daily in pill form. He took three pills every day and had no side effects. The oncologist carefully watched his blood counts. Chlorambucil depresses the marrow and can lead to anemia, low platelets, and low granulocytes. If any of these occur, the drug must be decreased or stopped for a while. Over several months all the lumps and his large spleen shrank to normal size. He continued on chlorambucil for about one year and then it was stopped. The oncologist told him that he had a complete remission; all evidence of lymphoma had disappeared. However, T.H. would need to restart treatment if and when his lymphoma returned.

For the next two years T.H. did well. His checkups each month were normal. Then he noticed that the size of the lymph nodes in his neck was increasing. The oncologist agreed that his nodes and spleen were enlarging. Because T.H. felt so well, the oncologist thought that it was safe to wait without chemotherapy and see what would happen.

For another year all was well. Although his lymph nodes were large, he felt perfectly normal. Then his liver and spleen became large enough to cause him some discomfort. The oncologist therefore started chlorambucil again, and after several months the disease disappeared. T.H. had a second complete remission, which lasted ten months.

The oncologist reviewed T.H.'s case at the hospital's weekly tumor board conference. Although T.H. probably would respond to chemotherapy again, the radiation and medical oncologists at the conference felt that total body irradiation might give a longer remission. T.H. was sent to a radiation oncologist, who explained the procedure. He received radiation for six weeks without any side effects and again had a complete remission.

The lymphoma did not return for two years. Then the lymph glands and spleen started to enlarge. For the first time T.H. felt sick from his lymphoma. He was tired and had sweating and fevers. He lost weight. The oncologist was worried because previously T.H. had always felt well despite his lymphoma. Chemotherapy was started again, but T.H. did not respond to chlorambucil. A combination of drugs was tried but he still did not respond. The lymph nodes did not disappear, and he felt worse.

The oncologist had to tell T.H. that his disease could not be controlled much longer. T.H. had realized that things were not going well. He told his oncologist that he was grateful for the many years of good life that he already had. He had spent the time with his family, friends, and grandchildren. He had done many of the things that he had planned to do during his retirement. He was no longer afraid to die. Several weeks later, almost seven years after his diagnosis, T.H. died from progressive lymphoma.

T.H.'s case illustrates a typical course of the nodular type of non-Hodgkin's lymphoma. These lymphomas grow slowly, and many people live for years with their disease. In contrast to that for aggressive lymphomas, treatment is nontoxic. T.H. received pills daily and then total body irradiation. Neither had side effects.

The Young Person with Less Aggressive Lymphoma   The survival rate with nonaggressive lymphomas is measured in years. Elderly people often die of other causes, such as heart attacks. However, if you are under age fifty and develop nonaggressive lymphoma, you will most likely die from it eventually. Although many medical and radiation oncologists give all people the same treatment regardless of age, many others treat young patients more aggressively. Their aim is to prolong life or to cure the person. The benefits of more aggressive combination chemotherapy and the use of chemotherapy and total body irradiation together are being studied. There is no evidence that more aggressive therapy prolongs life, but for the young person with this kind of lymphoma, more aggressive, experimental approaches make sense.

Who Should Treat You for Non-Hodgkin's Lymphoma?   The evaluation and treatment of non-Hodgkin's lymphoma are extremely complex. Aggressive and nonaggressive types should be treated with high-dose radiation to attempt to cure localized disease. With more extensive disease, the treatment diverges. High-dose chemotherapy is indicated for aggressive lymphomas, while fairly nontoxic low-dose chemotherapy or total body irradiation is used for less aggressive lymphomas.

As with Hodgkin's disease, a team of specialists is needed to evaluate you and plan and deliver treatment effectively. Your family physician or internist cannot offer you optimal treatment for this disease without some direction from cancer specialists. At the very least, a board-certified radiation oncologist and a medical oncologist or hematologist should plan and give treatment. If possible, you should be evaluated and treated at a large medical center or clinic where there are several such specialists present. At larger hospitals and medical centers, all cases are presented at tumor board conferences.

The Leukemias

The leukemias are a group of cancers that originate in the bone marrow. When the disease develops, the abnormal, or leukemia, cells accumulate in the bone marrow and crowd out the normal cells.

Each year approximately 22,000 people develop and 15,000 die from leukemia. The three common types that we discuss here are acute non-lymphocytic leukemia, chronic myelocytic leukemia, and chronic lymphocytic leukemia. These differ in their clinical course, their prognosis, and their need for and response to treatment, and therefore will be discussed separately.

ACUTE NONLYMPHOCYTIC LEUKEMIA

Acute nonlymphocytic leukemia, in which we include acute myeloge-nous leukemia, myelomonocytic leukemia, monocytic leukemia, pro-myelocytic leukemia, and erythroleukemia, is the most common form of acute leukemia in adults. It occurs with equal frequency in all ages, and is slightly more common in men than in women. People who have been exposed to radiation, anticancer drugs, and certain chemicals, such as benzene, are at increased risk for developing acute leukemia. People treated with radiation or chemotherapy for Hodgkin's disease develop the disease seven times as frequently as does the rest of the population. Likewise, survivors of the atomic bomb blast at Hiroshima and Nagasaki have a greatly increased incidence of acute leukemia.

Diagnosis

The symptoms of acute leukemia are most often due to a lack of cells normally produced in the bone marrow. The leukemic cells accumulate and crowd out the normal marrow cells. More than half of people with acute leukemia go to their doctor because they feel tired because of a low red blood cell count. Bruising of the skin or bleeding either from the gums or into the urine or stool is also common from a lack of platelets. Fever and infection from a lack of granulocytes can also be the first symptom. Less commonly the leukemia is diagnosed because of enlarged lymph glands or an enlarged liver or spleen.

The diagnosis of acute nonlymphocytic leukemia is not difficult to make. If a patient tells a doctor he or she is tired, the doctor will not often think of leukemia. Tiredness is most commonly caused by anxiety or depression. However, if the patient also has a severe infection, bruising, or bleeding, the diagnosis is usually made quickly. Leukemia is diagnosed when a blood count is obtained. With acute leukemia, the blood count is abnormal. Anemia, a low platelet count, and a decreased number of granulocytes are usually found and indicate a serious blood disease. The blood smear may show the blasts, or leukemic cells. That establishes the diagnosis.

If your physician suspects acute leukemia or another serious blood disease, he or she should immediately refer you to a board-certified hematologist or oncologist, who will review your case and do a bone marrow aspiration examination. This is done by inserting a needle, under local anesthesia, into one of the bones where blood is made, usually into the back of the hip bone. It is uncomfortable, since the anesthesia cannot completely control the pain. However, it is completely safe and takes only a few minutes. The diagnosis of acute leukemia can always be made with a bone marrow examination. Most of the marrow has been replaced with very immature, leukemic cells.

Treatment

Only ten or fifteen years ago, there was no effective treatment for acute leukemia. Now chemotherapy treatment can usually make patients feel better and prolong their lives. Although there is still much room for improvement, there has been great progress in the past decade.

Treatment should be started almost immediately with this disease. Life-threatening bleeding and infections are an ever-present threat because of the lack of platelets and granulocytes. The situation will not improve unless and until the leukemia is controlled by chemotherapy. Then the marrow can again produce the needed platelets, granulocytes, and red blood cells. Acute nonlymphocytic leukemia is treated with very high doses of toxic drugs. People become sicker before they improve. During this time they are totally dependent on the skills of their physicians and nurses and the capability of the blood bank to supply needed transfusions of platelets, red cells, and sometimes granulocytes. Thus, modern chemotherapy for acute leukemia benefits most people but is both complex and hazardous.

Who Should Treat You for Acute Myelocytic Leukemia?   Acute myelocytic leukemia is a life-threatening illness, and the treatment that is needed to control it is complicated and hazardous. High doses of drugs are used, which kill leukemic cells but which also further damage normal marrow cells. The treatment stops the production of platelets and granulocytes. Therefore, problems with bleeding and infection become worse before they become better.

Patients with acute leukemia need lots of help to survive the several-week period until the treatment has a chance to work. They must be watched carefully. They need red blood cell transfusions for anemia, platelet transfusions to prevent bleeding, and antibiotics to control infection. Complex decisions must be made on an hour-to-hour basis. These decisions can make the difference between life and death. Well-trained physicians must *always* be available.

Optimal treatment for acute leukemia can only be given by a board-certified medical oncologist or hematologist who treats many people with acute leukemia. Experienced nurses are also extremely important. Your doctor is not always in the hospital. If a fever develops at night, the nurse must understand that treatment with antibiotics needs to be started immediately. If he or she waits until the doctor comes the next morning, it can cost the patient's life. Finally, platelet transfusions must be readily available during the initial treatment. This means that the community in which you are treated must be large enough to have a large blood bank that has platelet transfusions available on short notice.

The best treatment for acute leukemia is available at large medical centers such as cancer centers and large university hospitals but may also be available at large community hospitals. If you live in or near a large city that has a cancer center or large university hospital, we recommend that you go there for treatment. If not, you must find out if treatment can be given in or near your community. You should ask your medical oncologist or hematologist whether he treats many patients with acute leukemia. If he treats only one or two a year, you probably should go to a more experienced doctor. It is also important to find out if the nurses where you are to be treated have experience caring for people with this disease.

Chemotherapy   The high-dose chemotherapy that has been developed in the past decade helps people with acute leukemia. There are several phases of treatment.

Induction.   Remission induction refers to the initial phase of treatment. The aim is to obtain a complete remission. With a complete remission, all evidence of leukemia is gone. The bone marrow and blood look normal. The marrow functions normally and produces adequate numbers of red cells, platelets, and granulocytes. When someone is in complete remission, he or she feels well.

Remission induction is a very hazardous and trying time. Three to six weeks of hospitalization are needed. People are usually very sick during this time. They are fatigued, feverish, and infected. They are often covered with bruises; they have sore mouths and nausea, and they lose ten to twenty pounds. They are sick from high-dose chemotherapy as well as from the disease. If the treatment is successful, they improve after several weeks, when the marrow starts to function again. When the blood counts become normal, a marrow examination is done. If it looks normal, a complete remission has been achieved. About four of five adults under fifty go into a complete remission with chemotherapy.

Consolidation.   After the leukemia goes into remission and a person has had several weeks to recover from induction therapy, the next phase of treatment, called consolidation, is started. Consolidation treatment consists of high-dose chemotherapy and requires another lengthy hospitalization. However, the hospitalization is shorter and people do not get as sick as they did with induction therapy. Lower doses of drugs are used and the person is in better condition.

Maintenance Therapy   After they have completed consolidation therapy, most patients are placed on low doses of chemotherapy given in a doctor's office or clinic. This is referred to as "maintenance" therapy. Although doctors think maintenance therapy prolongs remissions, they are not sure. Therefore, trials are in progress to compare how people do with and without maintenance therapy.

The majority of people with acute leukemia obtain complete remissions. However, in most cases this is temporary. The average remission lasts only about one to one and a half years. When the leukemia recurs, treatment can be given and some get a second and even a third remission. Each remission tends to be shorter than the one preceding it. The survival of a person with acute myelocytic leukemia depends upon obtaining a remission and staying in it.

Prognosis

Without treatment, survival with acute leukemia is short: most people die within a few months. High-dose combination chemotherapy allows up to 80 percent of young people and about 50 percent of people over the age of fifty to go into a complete remission. Older people have a lower chance of entering remission because they can't tolerate as much chemotherapy. Those people who obtain a remission feel well and live longer because of it. Those who do not, usually die quickly, often during their first hospitalization.

In almost all cases of complete remission, although the marrow and blood appear normal under a microscope, nests of leukemic cells still remain. The average remission lasts about one year, but some people have much longer remissions. About one remission in four is longer than two years, and there are an increasing number of people with acute leukemia who have been in remission more than five years and are off treatment. We do not know whether these people are cured or if their leukemia will recur. If you obtain a remission, there is hope that you may live for years.

E.H., a twenty-four-year-old college student, went to the university health clinic because of a sore throat, fever, and chills. The physician diagnosed acute tonsilitis and gave her penicillin. She improved but returned two weeks later, again with a sore throat and fever. Her physician suspected a more serious problem and therefore obtained a blood count. The red cells, platelets, and white cells were all decreased. He looked at the stained blood smear under a microscope and saw several very immature cells, which led him to suspect that E.H. had leukemia.

He sent her to a board-certified hematologist at a university hospital, who reviewed the blood counts and slides and did a bone marrow examination. This showed replacement of most of the marrow with leukemic "blast" cells. The hematologist told E.H. that she had acute leukemia and that she needed to be hospitalized immediately for intensive treatment. She was too upset to talk further and asked to talk to him later. She went home and talked to her fiancé and her parents. Her whole life was turned around. She was entering her senior year in college and she had planned a trip to Europe with her fiancé. Now her life was radically changed. She had a fatal disease and if she wanted any "normal time" she had to be hospitalized and given toxic therapy.

Her fiancé talked to the hematologist, who explained that there was no time to adjust to the situation. E.H. could develop a serious infection at any moment, and therapy should be started as soon as possible. With her family's support, she agreed to take therapy. She was admitted to the hospital and high-dose combination chemotherapy was started. She received several drugs intravenously and several by mouth. She had some nausea and vomiting. Over the next two weeks she felt sicker than she thought it possible to be and still be alive. She was extremely tired, she had a very sore mouth, no appetite, and continual fevers and chills. She spent almost the entire time in bed receiving continuous intravenous feedings and fluids. She also received red blood cells, platelets, and antibiotics. She lost fifteen pounds and all her hair.

She was very depressed and almost wished the end would come. She was sure the treatment wasn't working. Although the hematologist assured her that all people with leukemia get that sick, she didn't believe him. Then, during her third week of hospitalization, she started to feel a little better. Her doctor told her that there were signs of early improvement in her blood. Over the next two weeks, she continued to feel better and her blood counts became normal. The hematologist did a bone marrow examination. No leukemic cells were seen. He happily told her that she was in complete remission and could go home.

E.H. rested for two weeks at home and felt stronger each day. She then returned to her hematologist, who outlined the rest of the treatment program. He explained that another course of intensive treatment with hospitalization was needed. She questioned the need for more treatment since she felt so well and her blood and bone marrow appeared normal. He explained that she was in complete remission, but that she was not cured. Without continued treatment to suppress the leukemia, it would probably return quite soon.

E.H. agreed to another course of treatment and entered the hospital. She received the same drugs as before but in lower doses. She was not nearly so sick and spent several hours out of the hospital each day. The hospitalization lasted only two and a half weeks. Next she received "maintenance" therapy: each month for five days she took oral medications and gave herself injections under the direction of her hematologist.

All went well for twenty months. E.H. remained in remission and felt quite healthy. She had some tiredness when taking maintenance therapy but felt fine the rest of the month. She returned to school and graduated. She could not go on long trips, but she did go on several shorter vacations with her fiancé. After twenty months in remission, E.H. felt fatigued and developed fevers. A bone marrow examination showed recurrent leukemia.

She was admitted to the hospital again and received high-dose combination chemotherapy. After one month of hospitalization, in which she got as sick as she had on her first admission, she went into a second remission. The hematologist explained that this remission would probably be shorter, and indeed it only lasted six months.

When her leukemia came back for the second time her hematologist recommended low-dose chemotherapy. He did not want her to spend her remaining time in the hospital. Over the next three months she received drugs to suppress her leukemia. They did not help. She spent most of her time at home but was very tired. She needed blood transfusions and had several short hospitalizations to treat infections. She died three months after the second recurrence of a severe infection. She had just celebrated her twenty-sixth birthday.

This case highlights several points about leukemia. The treatment of acute leukemia is very hazardous. People feel worse before they get better. They are sick because their bone marrow does not function because of the leukemia. Chemotherapy damages the bone marrow further. Although E.H. felt as if she were dying and was so sick that she wanted to die, a week later she was in remission and feeling better.

The treatment for leukemia is complex. The doctor must be available and know when to give antibiotics, platelets, and red cells. E.H. was treated by an experienced hematologist in a big university hospital. The nurses on the ward were experienced in the care of patients with leukemia. E.H.'s twenty-month remission is fairly typical of acute leukemia. Acute leukemia usually recurs, despite continued treatment.

The Person over Age Fifty with Acute Leukemia

High-dose combination chemotherapy is very toxic. During the initial phase of treatment, the patient faces death from bleeding or infection until the bone marrow is cleared of leukemic cells and starts to function normally. Young people usually tolerate this very toxic therapy, and about 80 percent obtain a remission. However, as people get older they tolerate less stress. People over fifty often cannot survive the toxicity of high-dose combination chemotherapy. About half will die in the hospital of infections or other complications. Therefore, middle-aged or older people with acute leukemia are usually treated with lower doses of these drugs. Unfortunately, with lower-dose therapy the remission rate drops to 50 percent because the leukemic cells are not killed as well. There is no other recourse for middle-aged people, since with higher-dose therapy the remission rate is still about the same because so many people die in the hospital from treatment.

The treatment of acute leukemia in even older people, for example, over the age of seventy, should be even less intensive. They are usually treated with low nontoxic doses of drugs in the doctor's office or clinic, not in the hospital. The remission rate is low, but what time the person has left is spent at home, not sick from toxic chemotherapy in the hospital.

The treatment for acute leukemia has improved dramatically in the last decade but still is far from perfect. Young people often get a remission, feel better, and live longer with high-dose chemotherapy but leukemia almost always recurs. Older people can't tolerate as much therapy; therefore, fewer get remissions. Those who do also benefit greatly from treatment. The treatment for leukemia should be administered by a board-certified hematologist or oncologist experienced in treating leukemia. If your community does not have these resources, it pays to travel to a larger medical center where there are experienced hematologists or oncologists, nurses with experience in caring for people with leukemia, and a large blood bank to provide the blood products needed during the initial treatment.

The Chronic Leukemias

The chronic leukemias are so named because before anticancer drugs were developed patients with these diseases often lived for years. In contrast, survival with acute leukemia without treatment was very short. With chronic leukemia, the cancer cells grow in the bone marrow as they do in acute leukemia but the process is much slower. The symptoms are more subtle and develop more slowly. Fatigue, an enlarged abdomen because of an enlarged liver or spleen, enlarged lymph nodes, a tendency to bruise easily, and recurrent infections are common symptoms.

There are two main subtypes of chronic leukemia: chronic myelocytic leukemia and chronic lymphocytic leukemia. They will be discussed separately because they have little in common except that they both have prolonged courses compared to the acute leukemias.

CHRONIC MYELOCYTIC LEUKEMIA (CML)

Chronic myelocytic leukemia is slightly more common in males than in females and usually occurs after the age of twenty. People exposed to radiation or benzene are at increased risk of developing this disease. Chronic myelocytic leukemia is a cancer that involves marrow cells that normally mature and develop into red cells, granulocytes, and platelets. Fortunately, although the cells are cancerous, they function normally. Therefore, anemia, infection, and bleeding are not a problem at first.

Diagnosis

The diagnosis of chronic myelocytic leukemia (CML) is usually quite simple. People go to the doctor because they are tired, sweaty, and losing weight. Many have a fullness in their abdomen from a very large spleen. Occasionally CML is diagnosed in a well person during a routine blood count. The white cells in the blood are greatly increased and mostly mature. In CML, granulocytes do not respond to the usual regulatory mechanisms, and they overgrow. All forms of granulocytes, from the most mature to the most immature, normally only present in the bone marrow, are seen in the peripheral blood. In addition, there is a specific chromosomal abnormality in chronic myelocytic leukemia—the Philadelphia chromosome. A bone marrow examination with an analysis of chromosomes in the marrow cells is also usually performed.

Prognosis

People live for years with chronic myelocytic leukemia. Though cancerous, the cells develop into normally functioning red cells, platelets, and granulocytes. Therefore, people with this disease do not get anemic, bleed, or get infected. Symptoms can be controlled with low-dose chemotherapy.

Unfortunately, sooner or later chronic myelocytic leukemia transforms into acute leukemia, the so-called blast crisis. When this occurs, the situation is even worse than with acute leukemia. The marrow no longer makes platelets, granulocytes, or red cells. Blast crisis does not respond well to high-dose chemotherapy, and most people die within a matter of weeks to months once the crisis occurs. Survival in CML depends on how long the disease remains in its original chronic form. Some people develop blast crisis early and die within months; others live for ten or fifteen years. The average survival is three to four years.

Treatment

Chronic myelocytic leukemia is treated with low-dose, nontoxic chemotherapy, usually with a drug called Myleran. This is taken by mouth. There are usually no side effects other than a decrease in blood cell counts. If the blood counts drop too low, your doctor will stop the drug and wait for them to rise. With Myleran, the spleen will decrease in size and symptoms from the CML disappear. Then the treatment is stopped. In some cases treatment can be discontinued for months. In others, the disease rapidly recurs and more treatment is needed. Your doctor will decide whether Myleran is needed continuously or only occasionally to control the symptoms of the chronic phase of CML. Unfortunately, treatment does not prolong life. However, it does make people feel better.

Some cancer centers—for example, Sloan Kettering in New York City—are testing the effect of using high-dose combination chemotherapy early in CML to see if this will prolong life. Their initial results are promising but it is still too soon to know if this approach will be successful.

People with chronic myelocytic leukemia feel well as long as they are in the chronic phase of the disease. However, when the disease progresses to the accelerated blast crisis they become sick quickly. This occurs in almost all people with CML. Combination chemotherapy is usually tried, but blast crisis is more resistant to treatment than is acute leukemia. Chemotherapy is only rarely successful. There is no good treatment for blast crisis of this disease. For people under thirty with this disease, bone marrow transplantation should be considered (see chapter 24, "Experimental Treatment for Cancer").

Who Should Treat You for Chronic Myelocytic Leukemia?   If you have chronic myelocytic leukemia you should be treated by an experienced, board-certified hematologist or oncologist. These physicians know how and when to treat you and how to let you live with your disease. For most people, there is no advantage to traveling to a large medical or cancer center because there are few promising experimental treatments for this disease. The person with CML, however, may want to try experimental therapy like that offered at Sloan Kettering or to consider bone marrow transplantation before blast crisis occurs.

G.L., a forty-one-year-old taxi driver, went to his family doctor because for several months he had felt tired and had become full after eating only small amounts of food. His physician discovered an enlarged spleen that was pressing on his stomach. This explained his inability to eat normal amounts of food. A blood count showed that he had large numbers of immature cells and granulocytes in his peripheral blood. His family doctor suspected chronic myelocytic leukemia, told him about his suspicion, and asked him to see a board-certified hematologist.

The hematologist confirmed the diagnosis by looking at the stained blood smear. However, to be sure, he sent blood for a chromosomal analysis. This showed the Philadelphia chromosome, an abnormality that occurs only with this disease. The hematologist told G.L. that he had a chronic form of leukemia. Although problems could occur at any time, most likely he could live for years relatively normally. He told G.L. that he would need to take treatment in the form of pills. These would help his tiredness and shrink his spleen, allowing him to eat normally again. The hematologist told him he would probably die from his disease; it could happen in one year or in six years. Most people live about four years after their diagnosis.

G.L. was very upset but at least he had hope. There was a possibility of living for years with his disease. Over the next five and one-half years, he needed only occasional treatment with Myeleran to control the size of his spleen and make him feel better. He was able to live a normal life.

Then he became more tired. He developed fevers and started to lose weight. His blood showed blasts. He had developed blast crisis of his chronic myelocytic leukemia. The hematologist told him the bad news. He received chemotherapy in the clinic for four weeks but, like most people, he did not respond. Despite hospitalization and high doses of chemotherapy, he died of a severe infection six weeks after blast crisis occurred.

G.L.'s story illustrates some important features of chronic myelocytic leukemia. (a) The diagnosis is simple. (b) People can live with chronic myelocytic leukemia and feel normal for a long time. Fairly simple therapy can shrink the spleen and control fevers and fatigue. (c) The disease can transform to the acute, blast phase at any time. Unfortunately, treatment for blast crisis is not very effective, and death usually occurs in a matter of weeks or months.

CHRONIC LYMPHOCYTIC LEUKEMIA (CLL)

Chronic lymphocytic leukemia is more common in men than women and is a disease of middle-aged and elderly people. It is rarely seen before age thirty-five, and most commonly occurs after age fifty. In chronic lymphocytic leukemia there is an excessive growth of normal-looking lymphocytes. The lymphocyte has an important role in preventing infection. Therefore, as expected, one of the major problems with this disease is an increased susceptibility to infections. Bacteria are all around us and normally we live in harmony with them. However, with chronic lymphocytic leukemia the body's defenses can be overcome by these bacteria and people get serious infections.

Diagnosis

Chronic lymphocytic leukemia is diagnosed in a variety of ways. Very often it is discovered incidentally during a routine examination. The white count is increased by an excessive number of lymphocytes. Chronic lymphocytic leukemia is also often discovered when a person goes to the doctor because of fatigue, sweating, weight loss, or swollen lymph glands. The diagnosis of chronic lymphocytic leukemia is quite simple since all patients have an increased number of lymphocytes in the peripheral blood. There are no other causes of a persistently increased lymphocyte count in older people. Usually a bone marrow examination is done to see whether the lymphocytes are crowding out normal marrow cells. However, the diagnosis of CLL is made by the blood counts and the blood smear.

Prognosis

If you are unfortunate enough to develop a leukemia, CLL is the best one to have. It occurs in middle-aged and older people, and most survive seven to eight years. Many live ten to twenty years with this disease and die of other causes. Good medical care is needed, since bacterial infections are an ever-present threat to life with this disease. A bacterial infection can kill someone with CLL who might otherwise live for many years. Therefore, if you have chronic lymphocytic leukemia and develop fever or chills, you should call your doctor immediately. He should examine you, give you antibiotics, and possibly hospitalize you.

Treatment

Chronic lymphocytic leukemia is treated with chemotherapy, total body irradiation, and occasionally local radiation therapy. Sometimes surgery is needed to remove the spleen. When the diagnosis of chronic lymphocytic leukemia is made, treatment is often not started. People can live for years after diagnosis without specific treatment. Treatment.is reserved for problems. If a person with CLL has bothersome enlargements of lymph nodes or spleen, or is tired, losing weight, and has sweats, he or she is treated. If lymphocytes accumulate in the bone marrow and interfere with the production of red cells, platelets or granulocytes, the patient is treated. A person with chronic lymphocytic leukemia should be followed closely by a hematologist or oncologist, who can decide when treatment should be started.

Large lymph nodes in one area can be treated with local radiation. This has very few side effects. If the disease involves many areas, especially if the bone marrow is "crowded," low-dose, nontoxic chemotherapy or total body irradiation is used. Both can control the disease for a long time.

Who Should Treat You for Chronic Lymphocytic Leukemia? A person with chronic lymphocytic leukemia should be under the care of a board-certified medical oncologist or hematologist. The care of a person with chronic lymphocytic leukemia is quite complex. When the diagnosis is made your doctor must decide whether you need no treatment, local radiation, total body irradiation, or chemotherapy. Only experienced specialists can make these decisions wisely. A trained hematologist or oncologist knows how to treat the infections that are an ever-present threat to life. There is no advantage in going to a large medical center or cancer center, as there are no promising experimental approaches.

C.H., a sixty-five-year-old retired banker, went to his doctor for a yearly physical examination. He felt well and the doctor found nothing abnormal on examination. However, a routine blood count showed an increased number of lymphocytes. His doctor told him that he probably had early chronic lymphocytic leukemia and sent him to a hematologist.

The hematologist reviewed the blood smear and blood counts and did not order any further tests. He explained to C.H. that he probably had an early stage of chronic lymphocytic leukemia. He did not need treatment and could live for years with his disease. However, he had an increased chance of getting serious bacterial infections. Although most people with fever do not have to call a doctor immediately, he warned C.H. to call him if he had any fever or chills. Although C.H. felt well, if he developed an infection, he could die in a matter of hours if he were not treated with antibiotics.

Over the next seven years, C.H. felt well and did not need treatment for his chronic lymphocytic leukemia. However, he had three episodes of pneumonia that were quickly treated with antibiotics. Each of these infections could have killed him if he had not called his doctor and been treated immediately. Over these years his blood count rose to 100,000 but his marrow continued to produce adequate numbers of normal cells. His lymph nodes and spleen started to enlarge but he felt well. At age seventy-two, seven years after the diagnosis of CLL, he died of a stroke. No treatment for his CLL had been needed.

This case illustrates several important points about this disease. (a) It is a chronic disease of middle-aged and elderly people. (b) It is not unusual to die of other causes. C.H. lived seven years with this disease and did not require any treatment for it. (c) C.H. would not have lived for seven years if he had not had his three pneumonia attacks treated immediately. His doctor warned him about infection and he listened. He called his doctor promptly when he developed fever and chills.

W.L. was a seventy-seven-year-old retired painter who went to see his doctor because of a large swelling in the right side of his neck. The doctor found very large lymph nodes in his neck and an enlarged spleen. A blood count showed that he had a white blood cell count of 80,000. (Normal is 4,000–10,000.) Most of the cells were mature lymphocytes. His doctor told him he had chronic lymphocytic leukemia and that he should be cared for by a hematologist.

The hematologist examined W.L. and decided to treat him with local radiation to the right side of his neck because the lymph nodes were so uncomfortable. The lymph nodes completely disappeared with two weeks of radiation. W.L. had no side effects.

He felt well for three more years. Then his red cell, platelet, and granulocyte counts began to fall. The hematologist told him that he needed treatment to control his disease. The CLL lymphocytes were interfering with the production of marrow cells he needed. He was placed on a pill, which he took daily. His blood counts improved and he felt stronger.

Five years after the diagnosis of chronic lymphocytic leukemia, W.L. developed rectal bleeding and constipation. On rectal examination, the hematologist felt a hard mass. W.L. had a second cancer—rectal cancer. He had surgery but died of widespread rectal cancer one year later.

This case illustrates how effective local radiation and systemic chemotherapy can be against chronic lymphocytic leukemia. The local radiation shrank the nodes in W.L.'s neck and the chemotherapy improved his blood counts. Both treatments were given without any side effects. W.L., like many patients with chronic lymphocytic leukemia, died of another problem. Elderly people get cancer frequently, and people with chronic lymphocytic leukemia have an even higher incidence of second cancers than the general population. It is not unusual for a second tumor to claim the life of the person with chronic lymphocytic leukemia.

MULTIPLE MYELOMA

Multiple myeloma most commonly occurs between the ages of fifty and sixty. Approximately 8,000 Americans develop and 5,000 die from this cancer yearly. It is a cancer of plasma cells of the marrow and bone. Plasma cells develop from lymphocytes and produce antibodies to help fight infection. People with multiple myeloma, like those with CLL, are very prone to infection because they do not make antibodies normally.

Diagnosis

Multiple myeloma is usually discovered when people get pain in their bones; the disease affects the bones as well as the bone marrow. Some people are found to have multiple myeloma after they get repeated bacterial infections. Other patients are diagnosed during their routine yearly examinations because of abnormal amounts of protein in their urine or blood that are detected by routine tests.

Prognosis

If not treated effectively, multiple myeloma is a rapidly progressive disease. Without treatment, most people would survive less than one year after they develop bone pain. The disease involves the bone marrow and bones. Without treatment bone pain increases, fractures develop, and people soon become bedridden. In addition, the bone marrow becomes overcrowded with plasma cells and does not produce enough platelets, granulocytes, or red cells. Therefore, infection and bleeding occur.

Fortunately, chemotherapy enables many people with myeloma to live with their disease for years free of pain. About half the people with this disease feel better and live longer with fairly simple nontoxic chemotherapy. Nontoxic chemotherapy in the form of pills can control myeloma for years. Most people respond for approximately two to three years. Treatment helps many people with myeloma to feel better and live longer.

Treatment

Radiation   Radiation is effective treatment for localized bone pain. If there is severe pain initially or if the pain does not respond quickly to drugs, radiation is used. Low doses of radiation to the painful area usually produce dramatic responses with almost no side effects.

Chemotherapy   Chemotherapy is the standard treatment for multiple myeloma. Two or more nontoxic drugs are given by mouth, either on a daily basis or in higher doses for several days each month. About half the patients benefit from treatment. The drugs kill the cancerous plasma cells. Bone pain disappears and the person feels stronger. The person feels well until the myeloma recurs. The average response lasts about two years but can be longer. We have seen people live and feel well with myeloma for five years with nontoxic chemotherapy.

Who Should Treat You for Multiple Myeloma?   Multiple myeloma, like chronic lymphocytic leukemia and chronic myelocytic leukemia, should be treated by a board-certified hematologist or oncologist. There is no need to go to a cancer center, as there are no promising experimental approaches, but you need to be under the care of an experienced and well-trained specialist.

A.N., a previously healthy fifty-eight-year-old dentist, went to his doctor with low back pain. The doctor found no abnormalities on examination except for some tenderness in the lower part of his back. A.N. was given a muscle relaxant and told to rest for several days. Despite resting and taking his muscle relaxant, A.N. returned two weeks later in even more pain. The doctor ordered an x-ray of his back. It showed widespread destruction of bone and was suspicious for cancer. He sent A.N. to a medical oncologist.

The medical oncologist reviewed A.N.'s case and did several tests. He suspected multiple myeloma and therefore did a bone marrow. This showed an increased number of plasma cells. He also found a large amount of abnormal protein in the urine and blood. He diagnosed multiple myeloma.

The oncologist told A.N. about his disease and its treatment. A.N. was started on pills that were given for four days every month. Over three months his back pain slowly disappeared. He continued to take chemotherapy and felt completely well for four and a half years. He was able to work, took several long vacations, and felt well.

Five years after the diagnosis of multiple myeloma, A.N. developed pain again in his back and ribs. He was still taking anticancer drugs. X-rays had previously shown bone healing; now they showed increased destruction of bone. The medical oncologist started other drugs but the disease progressed. A.N. rapidly became bedridden, and he died four months later of pneumonia.

A.N.'s case is fairly representative of people with this disease who respond to chemotherapy. Chemotherapy controls the disease for variable periods of time, but eventually the myeloma recurs. A.N. had five good years with treatment. Without treatment he would have died within a year and would probably never have had a pain-free day.

SUMMARY

Malignant Lymphomas

1. Optimal treatment for Hodgkin's disease and non-Hodgkin's lymphoma requires, at the very least, that the evaluation and the planning and administration of treatment be done by a board-certified radiation oncologist and a medical oncologist.

2. It pays to travel to a large medical center or cancer clinic to receive the best treatment.

Hodgkin's Disease   1. Early Hodgkin's disease is curable with high-dose radiation therapy.

2. Advanced Hodgkin's disease is treated with high-dose combination chemotherapy. This can control and often cure it.

Non-Hodgkin's Lymphoma   1. Early non-Hodgkin's lymphoma is highly curable with high-dose radiation.

2. Unfortunately, over 80 percent of people with non-Hodgkin's lymphoma have advanced or widespread disease.

3. The treatment of nonaggressive advanced non-Hodgkin's lymphomas is low-dose chemotherapy or total body irradiation. People can live for years with nonaggressive lymphomas.

4. The treatment of aggressive widespread advanced non-Hodgkin's lymphoma is high-dose combination chemotherapy. Many patients feel better and live longer with chemotherapy. However, only a small number are cured.

Acute Nonlymphocytic Leukemia

1. Optimal treatment for acute leukemia requires an experienced, board-certified hematologist or oncologist, experienced nurses, and a blood bank that can provide blood products as needed. It is often necessary to travel to a large hospital or cancer center for the best treatment.

2. Young adults with acute leukemia have an 80 percent chance of a complete remission.

3. People over the age of fifty are usually treated with less chemotherapy because they can't tolerate as much toxic therapy as younger people.

4. Chemotherapy for acute leukemia has improved dramatically in the past decade. Still, most remissions only last one to two years.

Chronic Myelocytic Leukemia

1. If you have chronic myelocytic leukemia, you should be under the care of a board-certified hematologist or oncologist. You do not have to travel to a large center for treatment.

2. Chronic myelocytic leukemia is treated with nontoxic therapy taken by mouth.

3. People feel well and can live for years with chronic myelocytic leukemia. Almost inevitably it transforms into an acute phase, called a "blast crisis." This is resistant to treatment and is usually rapidly fatal.

Chronic Lymphocytic Leukemia

1. The person with chronic lymphocytic leukemia should be under the care of a board-certified hematologist or oncologist.

2. People can live for years with this disease. Some live more than twenty years.

3. Treatment may not prolong life but does make people feel better. It is reserved for problems that arise, and therefore you may not need to be treated when the diagnosis is first made.

4. With this disease, severe bacterial infections are a threat to life. Anyone who develops fever or chills that might indicate a serious infection should call the doctor immediately.

Multiple Myeloma

1. Multiple myeloma should be cared for by a board-certified hematologist or oncologist.

2. Multiple myeloma is treated with nontoxic chemotherapy and local radiation.

3. More than half of the patients with this disease will feel better and live longer with chemotherapy.

4. There is no advantage in traveling to a cancer center for treatment, because experimental approaches have not been promising.

19

Head and Neck Cancers

Five percent of all cancer in the United States arises in the mouth (including the tongue and gums), inside the nose and sinuses, and in the larynx, or voice box. Each year, 30,000 Americans develop and approximately 12,000 die from these cancers. They are called head and neck cancers, although they are not really cancers of the head or the neck. These cancers arise in these head areas, invade surrounding normal tissues, and spread mainly to the lymph glands in the neck. Therefore, treatment is directed to the primary site and also to the lymph glands in the neck. It is not surprising that people are more afraid of these cancers than their frequency warrants; indeed, the disfigurement of treatment for advanced head and neck cancers is frightening.

Causes of Head and Neck Cancers

Tobacco and Alcohol Most cancers of the head and neck are preventable. They rarely occur in people who don't use tobacco and/or alcohol heavily. All tobacco products, including cigarettes, pipe tobacco, cigars, and chewing tobacco, contain potent carcinogens. Wherever these carcinogens contact tissue—be it the inside of the mouth, nose, larynx, or lungs—tissue is damaged and cancer may result. For example, in India many people chew a mixture of betel nuts and tobacco. Cancer of the mouth often develops exactly where the betel nut–tobacco mixture was in contact with the tissues—the cheek. Similarly, pipe and cigar smokers are very prone to develop cancer of the lip. Cigarette smokers can develop cancer anyplace within the mouth, nose, and throat.

Tobacco is a more potent carcinogen than alcohol. People who use either in excess are at increased risk for developing cancers of the mouth. The use of both together increases the risk even more.

Early Diagnosis

As with other cancers, cancers of the mouth are easier to treat if they are caught early. Many cancers of the mouth and throat can be detected early. For example, cancers of the lip are readily visible. Any painless ulcer on the lip that doesn't heal in two weeks may be cancer. Likewise, cancers of the larynx cause hoarseness. By warning you of early cancer, hoarseness can save your life. Other cancers, such as those in the back of the tongue or the throat, do not cause early symptoms. By the time pain, bleeding, or an obvious lump develops, the cancer is usually advanced. However, many of these more silent or hidden cancers can also be detected early.

Many Americans see a dentist at least once a year. Dentists can detect early cancers in the mouth and throat. If you are over forty, and especially if you smoke and drink, you should see a dentist each year to check for cancer in the mouth. Programs in dental schools now stress the importance of early cancer diagnosis. Unfortunately, many dentists were not trained to examine the mouth for early cancer and don't routinely do so. When you see your dentist as part of a routine checkup, he should examine the inside of your mouth for cancer. If he doesn't, ask him to. If he will not, we suggest seeing another dentist. The examination for cancer takes no more than one or two minutes. The dentist will look at your gums and the mucous membranes of your mouth, tongue, and throat. He may find cancer early, before it causes symptoms. Early diagnosis can save many lives and can also save many people from disfiguring surgery, the treatment needed for advanced cancers of the head and neck.

LEUKOPLAKIA: A PRECANCEROUS LESION

Cancers of the tongue, lip, and floor of the mouth often develop in areas of leukoplakia. Leukoplakia is not cancer but it can develop into cancer. It appears as white patches or red, inflamed areas in the membranes of the mouth. Your dentist can recognize leukoplakia and refer you to an otolaryngologist (ear, nose, and throat surgeon) for a thorough evaluation. The area must be biopsied and checked regularly for the possible development of cancer. Finally, if you have leukoplakia, you should stop smoking, or the chances of developing cancer in the mouth will be even higher.

Diagnosis

If you have a sore that doesn't heal or a lump that persists in your mouth, it should be biopsied. You should see your doctor, who will send you to an otolaryngologist for evaluation and biopsy. In most areas of the mouth this can be done easily with local anesthesia. If the suspicious area is at the very back of the mouth or in the area of the larynx, the biopsy must be done through an instrument called a laryngoscope. This instrument allows the doctor to look at and biopsy suspicious areas that otherwise could not be reached. These biopsies can be done in a physician's office; no hospitalization is required. If a biopsy of a suspicious area is benign, it should be repeated. It is possible to miss a cancer with one biopsy. If the biopsy shows cancer of the mouth or throat, the otolaryngologist is the doctor best trained to evaluate you further.

The Otolaryngologist: Ear, Nose, and Throat Surgeon   An otolaryngologist is a physician with four years of training in diagnosing and operating for diseases of the ears, nose, and throat. He or she becomes board certified after this training and after passing an oral and written examination. Many otolaryngologists subspecialize their practice; some perform only ear operations, for instance, whereas others specialize in the treatment of cancer. You should be referred to an otolaryngologist who specializes in surgery for head and neck cancer.

Board-certified general surgeons and plastic surgeons also do head and neck cancer surgery. Some surgeons have had specialized training in head and neck cancer at large cancer centers such as Rosewell-Park, Memorial Hospital, or M.D. Anderson Hospital. If you are referred to an otolaryngologist, a general surgeon, or a plastic surgeon, you should ask what kind of training and experience he or she has had in head and neck cancer surgery. If this physician has had training at a cancer center in head and neck surgery, you can be assured that he, or she, is qualified to treat you.

There are two medical societies whose membership is restricted to board-certified surgeons (otolaryngologists, general surgeons, or plastic surgeons) who are experienced and who have a major interest in head and neck surgery: the American Society for Head and Neck Surgery and the Society of Head and Neck Surgeons. A surgeon must have done at least thirty-five head and neck operations during the previous year to qualify for membership in the former society. Ask your surgeon if he or she is a member. If not, ask if any other surgeon in your community is, and consider being referred to that surgeon. Membership in either of these societies means that the surgeon is interested and experienced in surgery for head and neck cancers.

How Large Is the Cancer? Has It Spread?

After the diagnosis is established with a biopsy, it is important to determine how extensive the cancer is. Unless they are extremely far advanced, head and neck cancers rarely spread beyond the lymph glands of the neck. Thus, only a chest x-ray is usually done to look for spread beyond the neck glands. The crucial questions that must be answered are: How extensive is the cancer in the mouth? Has the cancer invaded bone or cartilage? Has the cancer spread to local lymph glands?

The otolaryngologist usually is the physician who determines the extent of the cancer. He will evaluate the extent of the cancer by a careful examination. He must judge its size and whether it moves or is fixed to the surrounding tissue. He will also obtain x-rays of the bones and normal surrounding tissue to determine how extensive the cancer is. He will carefully examine the entire oral cavity to be sure there isn't another cancer present, because people who develop one cancer of the mouth are very likely to develop others. He will also carefully examine the lymph glands in the neck. With head and neck cancer this careful evaluation of the tumor and of the glands in the neck is crucial in making decisions about treatment.

Treatment

Treatment options include surgery, radiation, a combination of both, and occasionally chemotherapy. The aim is to eradicate the cancer with the best cosmetic results.

The Team Approach   People with head and neck cancer should be evaluated by a multidisciplinary team including a surgeon experienced with head and neck cancer and a radiation oncologist. Depending on the size and location of the cancer, a plastic surgeon, an oral surgeon, and/or a speech therapist should also be involved in planning therapy. Decisions are complex, and no one physician, no matter how well trained, can offer the person with head and neck cancer optimal treatment. A team of specialists is needed.

We recommend that a person with head and neck cancer be evaluated for treatment by a team composed of a head and neck cancer surgeon (who may be an otolaryngologist or a general surgeon), a radiation therapist, a plastic surgeon, a dental surgeon who specializes in restorative reconstruction following cancer surgery, and, if needed, a speech therapist. At the very least, you should not have any treatment performed until you have discussed your cancer with both a surgeon and a radiation therapist. A team approach offers the best chance for cure with the best cosmetic result. Many cancer hospitals have clinics for people with head and neck cancers where a team of specialists works together to provide optimal care.

There is still much controversy about whether radiation or surgery should be used to treat some of these cancers. Many early cancers of the head and neck can be cured by either approach. There are advantages and disadvantages with each. It is beyond the scope of this book to discuss the advantages and disadvantages of radiation and surgery for each head and neck cancer. However, you should realize that most surgeons favor surgery and most radiation therapists favor radiation. You should hear both sides of the story and then decide.

The Choice of Treatment   The aim of treatment is to cure the patient with the best functional and cosmetic result possible. Either surgery or radiation or both together is needed. The choice of therapy is determined by the size and location of the cancer and whether it has spread to the lymph glands in the neck.

Smaller cancers can be treated effectively with either surgery or radiation; the choice usually depends upon the location of the cancer. For example, early cancer of the larynx is usually treated with radiation. Either surgery or radiation can cure the cancer but with radiation, the voice is preserved. Likewise, either surgery or radiation can cure early cancer of the lip, but the cosmetic result with surgery is better, so surgery is usually chosen.

The treatment for large cancers is more frightening. In cancer surgery, some surrounding normal tissue must be removed in addition to the cancer to be sure small nests of cancer cells haven't been left behind. Depending upon the location of the cancer, the patient must face removal of half his lower jawbone, his voice box, or some of the muscles and lymph glands on one side of the neck. With advanced head and neck cancer, the person must face and adjust to the threat of death and mutilation of his face.

Surgery   Extensive surgery of the face and mouth is very complicated and interferes with important functions. The primary functions of these organs are chewing, swallowing, talking, and breathing. The operations may have to be done in stages. These functions need to be preserved as much as possible while the operations are being done. A tube may be placed in the stomach to allow the person to eat. A tracheostomy, or tube placed into the neck to allow the person to breathe and to prevent inhalation of food and saliva into the lungs, may also be needed.

Surgery for extensive cancers of the mouth is difficult and takes careful planning. After the surgery to remove the cancer has been done, reconstructive surgery is often needed. Bone grafts, skin grafts, and artificial implants may be needed to re-create normal structures. Months of healing and up to four operations are sometimes necessary. Speech training may also be needed if there has been alteration in the structure of the mouth, tongue, or voice box. The aim is to remove the cancer and have the person look, talk, and eat as normally as possible. We cannot stress too strongly the need for a team of experts for this difficult task.

Maintaining Adequate Nutrition during Treatment Extensive surgery for head and neck cancer, and occasionally radiation, may interfere with eating: the surgery may interfere with chewing or swallowing, and radiation can make the mouth too sore to eat or it can decrease the patient's appetite. People who do not eat do poorly. They heal poorly and are prone to infection.

Doctors often do not realize that their patients are literally starving while undergoing complicated treatment. Regular intravenous solutions do not contain enough calories and provide none of the essential building blocks of body protein, the amino acids. Without adequate nutrition, the body uses its own muscle and fat, and the person feels poorly and heals slowly. Recently, doctors have recognized the value of maintaining adequate nutrition so that the patient can feel better and tolerate treatment better. Therefore, you may receive artificial feedings if you have advanced cancer of the mouth or throat.

Two types of artificial feedings may be needed: intravenous hyperalimentation and intestinal hyperalimentation. If the physician thinks the person will need feedings only for a few weeks, intravenous hyperalimentation—feeding by veins—is a good method. Adequate nutrition can be given in the form of liquid diet supplements. However, intravenous hyperalimentation outside the hospital is complicated, expensive, and dangerous. Infection is a common complication. Thus, intravenous feedings aren't often used if the patient needs months of artificial feedings.

Intestinal hyperalimentation—feeding through the person's own gastrointestinal tract—is done by surgically placing a tube through the abdominal wall under general anesthesia. The patient can feed himself or herself safely at home.

Radiation Radiation is used to treat small cancers of the mouth and throat, and it is used either before or after surgery to treat more advanced cancers. It is also used to control symptoms in people with incurable cancers.

The radiation oncologist and the surgeon must work closely together. They must decide with the patient whether to use surgery, radiation, or both. If they use both, the extent of surgery and radiation must be carefully planned. We cannot advocate either radiation or surgery for any given cancer. Treatment depends upon the size and location of the cancer and to some extent upon the patient's preference. We do strongly suggest that you have a board-certified radiation therapist and a surgeon specializing in head and neck cancer evaluate you. You may also be evaluated by a plastic surgeon and/or an oral surgeon. You can have the advice of these specialists and then decide.

Chemotherapy   Chemotherapy is not very effective treatment for metastatic cancer of the head and neck. Approximately one patient in three will improve temporarily; usually only for a few months. Therefore, we recommend low-dose nontoxic chemotherapy. High-dose, more toxic experimental drug programs are being evaluated, but thus far the results have not been promising.

The role of chemotherapy in treating very advanced head and neck cancers is also currently being evaluated. Chemotherapy is given before or after surgery or radiation. Its value is still unproven, but the results with surgery and/or radiation for very advanced head and neck cancers are so poor that a visit to a major medical or cancer center may be worthwhile.

Prognosis

Doctors use the term *cure* in head and neck cancer if someone lives more than five years after diagnosis with no recurrence. Cancers of the mouth, throat, tongue, and lip usually are cured if they are caught early. The chances for cure decrease as the size of the cancer increases, and they drop sharply if lymph glands in the neck are involved. The cure rate for cancer of the lip is high because it is usually detected early. Cancers of the floor of the mouth and the back of the tongue are much more hidden, are usually diagnosed later, and are less often cured.

Follow-up after Treatment

After you have been treated for any head and neck cancer, no matter how small, you need to be closely followed. The cancer can recur at the original site or show up later in a lymph gland in the neck. Rapid reinstitution of treatment with either radiation or surgery offers the best chance for cure and/or prevention or control of symptoms such as pain. Also, anyone who develops one cancer in the mouth or throat is likely to develop more. Most have used tobacco and alcohol, and all the tissues of the mouth and throat have been exposed. Therefore, even if you have been cured, you should have a thorough examination once a year.

R.B., a sixty-year-old bartender, smoked one and a half packs of cigarettes a day and drank heavily. He had felt but ignored a firm lump under his tongue for over six months. He finally went to his doctor when he felt a hard lump under the right side of his jaw.

His doctor felt both lumps and then told R.B. that he thought he probably had cancer. He referred R.B. to an otolaryngologist at a nearby university hospital who was experienced in head and neck cancer surgery. The otolaryngologist examined him carefully and found a large tumor in R.B.'s mouth and an enlarged lymph gland under his jaw. He told R.B. it probably was cancer. He biopsied the tumor in his office and it showed cancer of the mouth.

The otolaryngologist told R.B. he had cancer and that it was far advanced. The cancer inside the mouth was large, and it had spread to at least one lymph node in the neck. He explained that a few tests were needed to find out whether it had spread to the jawbone or the lungs. Several consultations with other specialists were also needed. Treatment would be decided upon after these tests and consultations.

X-rays of the jaw and chest were normal. R.B. was also evaluated by a radiation oncologist, a plastic surgeon, and an oral surgeon. His case was then discussed by all the specialists, and they agreed on a treatment plan. R.B. had a large cancer and it had spread to the lymph nodes, but cure was still possible. However, he needed extensive and mutilating treatment. A major operation, which involved removing the cancer in the mouth, part of the lower jaw, and the lymph nodes on the right side of the neck, should be done. Then he should receive radiation to the neck after the surgical wound healed. The surgery would be planned by the otolaryngologist, the plastic surgeon, and the oral surgeon together so R.B. would look as normal as possible. The otolaryngologist would do the surgery and the plastic surgeon would operate later to make him look more normal. Nevertheless, his face would be disfigured. The otolaryngologist showed R.B. several pictures of patients who had had this operation.

R.B. went home to think about his situation. He was very upset and depressed. He and his wife talked about the mutilating surgery but both realized that his only other choice was to die from his cancer. After a week, R.B. decided to go ahead with the treatment.

R.B. underwent the radical operation and several weeks later received high-dose radiation therapy to his neck. He then underwent an operation to make his face look more normal. Four years have passed. R.B. is back at work and the cancer hasn't recurred. He is still sensitive about his altered appearance. He visits the otolaryngologist every six months to check for recurrence of the original cancer and for the development of other cancers. He is probably cured. R.B. realizes that he was lucky. Not many people with cancer of the mouth that has spread to the lymph glands in the neck are cured.

R.B. is typical of the person who develops head and neck cancer. He used tobacco and alcohol to excess. But despite ignoring his cancer, he was cured. These cancers tend to grow slowly and spread late. Therefore, the cancer hadn't spread beyond the neck. Still, he had to pay heavily for not going for treatment right away. He needed very extensive and mutilating surgery and radiation. He could easily have died.

This case also illustrates excellent care. R.B. was evaluated by a team of experts. They each saw him and then together planned treatment. If you have a cancer of the head and neck, be sure you are evaluated and treated by such a team.

CANCER OF THE LIP

About 15 percent of head and neck cancers occur on the lip. They usually affect men over the age of forty, and are almost always located on the lower lip. Exposure to sunlight and the use of tobacco both increase the risk for developing cancer of the lip. Pipe and cigar smokers are particularly prone to develop this cancer.

Cancer of the lip starts as a painless ulcer. It can look like a cold sore except it does not heal. All persistent painless sores on the lip should be biopsied. It is very difficult not to notice sores on your lips, so cancer of the lip is usually diagnosed and treated earlier than other cancers of the head and neck. Unless you totally ignore a sore and don't go to a doctor, you will probably be cured.

Treatment

Surgery   Small lip cancers that have not spread to the draining lymph nodes in the neck can be treated simply by surgery. The smaller the cancer, the less normal lip tissue needs to be removed and the better the cosmetic result. Larger cancers of the lip are treated by either surgery or radiation. With large cancers, much of the normal lip must be removed and a plastic surgeon then has to make a new lip. This involves extensive surgery, and the lip will never look completely normal.

When lip cancer has spread to the lymph nodes in the neck, these must be removed by an operation called a radical neck dissection. Part of the jaw must be removed, along with all the lymph nodes on that side of the neck. The jaw must be reconstructed later by a plastic surgeon. Not only is the cosmetic result inferior, but the cure rate, which is 90 percent for small cancers, falls to 50 percent or less.

Radiation   Radiation can be used instead of surgery to cure small lip cancers. Approximately 90 percent are cured. However, surgery is most often used to treat small lip cancers, as the cosmetic result is better. Larger cancers are treated with radiation or surgery. With very large cancers, radiation gives a better cosmetic result and therefore is the preferred treatment.

Radiation for lip cancer, like radiation for other cancers of the head and neck, is given in high doses to a relatively localized area. Side effects include a sore mouth, a loss of sense of taste, dryness of the mouth that may persist for some time, and a general hardening of the irradiated area that is usually permanent.

Six years ago, P.H., a sixty-six-year-old carpenter who worked for years in the hot sun of Arizona, noticed a sore on his lower lip that had failed to heal over several weeks. He went to his family doctor, who examined him and told P.H. the sore should be biopsied. He sent P.H. to an otolaryngologist, who looked at and felt the ulcer and then biopsied it in his office.

P.H. returned three days later and was told that the biopsy showed cancer. Luckily the cancer was very small (one-quarter inch in diameter). He sent P.H. to a radiation oncologist. Then he and the radiation oncologist discussed whether radiation or surgery should be done. Both had a good chance of curing him, but the doctors felt surgery was preferable.

P.H. went back to see the otolaryngologist, who explained the advantages and disadvantages of both approaches and said that both doctors felt surgery was the best treatment. P.H. agreed to have surgery. The surgery was simple; it would mean a few days in the hospital instead of four or more weeks of daily radiation. P.H. spent two days in the hospital and had his cancer cut out and his lip repaired. It is now six years later and the cancer hasn't returned. He is almost certainly cured.

This case is very representative of the usual patient with cancer of the lip. Cancer of the lip is obvious and is usually diagnosed when it is small. P.H. went to his doctor when he noticed a sore that didn't heal. His cancer was small, so he had an excellent chance for cure with either radiation or surgery. He saw both specialists and thought about both treatments. He chose surgery and was cured with a relatively minor operation. He has continued to see his otolaryngologist every six months. P.H. knows that because he smoked a pipe for many years and was exposed to intense sunlight while working as a carpenter, he might develop a second or even a third cancer of the lip.

CANCER OF THE TONGUE

Approximately 15 percent of head and neck cancers arise in the tongue. Cancer of the tongue occurs most often in men over forty who smoke and drink and can arise anyplace in the tongue. The prognosis and the treatment depend upon the location. The further back on the tongue a cancer is located, the smaller the chance for cure, probably because it is more hidden there and so is diagnosed later.

Diagnosis

Cancers of the tongue begin as painless ulcers. They gradually enlarge, and by the time they cause pain or noticeable swelling inside the mouth, they are no longer early, easily curable cancers. In contrast to cancer of the lip, cancer of the tongue frequently has metastasized to the lymph nodes of the neck by the time it is diagnosed.

Cancer of the tongue can be diagnosed early. If your dentist carefully examines the inside of your mouth for cancer, he or she can detect early tongue cancer and save your life. Any suspicious lesion should be biopsied, usually by an otolaryngologist.

Evaluating the Extent of the Disease

Once cancer has been diagnosed, the local extent of the disease is determined. A careful examination of the cancer by feeling the tongue and nearby areas, feeling the lymph glands in the neck, and obtaining x-rays of the nearby bones will show the extent of the cancer. A chest x-ray is the only test needed for spread of the cancer.

Treatment

Surgery and Radiation   Surgery and radiation are both used to treat this cancer. The tongue is a very important organ. We need it for two vital functions, to speak and to swallow. Therefore, in planning treatment every attempt is made to preserve as much tongue function as possible. However, unless the cancer is diagnosed when it is small, curative treatment involves fairly radical surgery and/or high-dose radiation. The chances for cure depend upon the location and size of the cancer and whether it has spread to the lymph nodes in the neck. Cancers toward the front of the tongue are more often cured than those toward the back. About half are cured if the lymph nodes in the neck are not involved, but only 15 percent with spread to these glands.

Small cancers of the front part of the tongue can be treated by surgery or radiation. The functional result is quite good with either treatment. Larger cancers require extensive surgery, with or without radiation. If the cancer is in the middle or back of the tongue, radiation is the standard treatment. Surgery, a radical operation removing a large part of the tongue along with part of the jawbone and the neck nodes, leaves major problems with speech, swallowing, and facial deformity. Months of rehabilitation are needed to train the person to speak and swallow.

R.W., a sixty-four-year-old man who smoked and drank heavily, developed pain inside his mouth and felt a lump on his tongue. He went to see his doctor, who found a large, ulcerated, firm tumor in the front of his tongue. The doctor sent R.W. to an otolaryngologist, who examined him carefully and then biopsied the tumor. The biopsy showed cancer. X-rays of the mouth and jawbone did not show spread to the bones. R.W. was also examined by a radiation oncologist and a plastic surgeon.

The otolaryngologist told R.W. that he had advanced tongue cancer. Although the lymph glands in the neck were not enlarged, there was a good chance that they were involved with cancer. The three specialists agreed that a radical operation with removal of much of his tongue, part of his lower jaw, and the glands in his neck was necessary to offer him the best chance for cure. Even so, the chances were no better than fifty-fifty. R.W. decided to accept the operation.

Three months after the operation with the help of a rehabilitation and speech therapist, R.W. was again able to eat and to talk understandably. His face was reconstructed by a plastic surgeon and, unless you looked closely, he appeared normal. He was lucky to have a close family and many friends who helped him get through the difficulties he faced.

Two years later, the cancer recurred in his mouth. He was treated with radiation therapy, which controlled the cancer for an additional year and a half. It recurred again. This time, low-dose chemotherapy was given by a medical oncologist. He did not respond. He died four and a half years after diagnosis from progressive malnutrition and pneumonia.

P.W., a seventy-year-old heavy smoker and drinker, saw his dentist every year. The dentist noticed a small ulcer in the middle of his tongue that seemed firm and was approximately one-half inch in diameter. He immediately sent P.W. to an otolaryngologist, who did a biopsy, which showed cancer.

P.W. was seen by a radiation oncologist and a plastic surgeon. When he saw the otolaryngologist again, he was told that he had an early cancer of the tongue. It could be treated with either radiation or surgery and could be cured. Radiation was preferable. Over a period of five weeks, R.W. received radiation to the tongue, surrounding areas, and the right side of his neck. He developed a sore mouth and throat but continued to eat while he was treated. Six years after radiation, he is well and cured of his cancer. His only long-term side effect is some dryness of his mouth.

Unfortunately, cancer of the tongue is already advanced if you wait for it to cause pain or problems in swallowing or speaking. The chances for cure are only 15–20 percent. Despite very aggressive treatment, R.W. died. He had a preventable cancer (since the cancer was probably related to his smoking and drinking), and it could have been diagnosed early by a dentist. If his cancer had been diagnosed early before it caused symptoms, he probably would have been cured like P.W.

CANCER OF THE FLOOR OF THE MOUTH

Fifteen percent of head and neck cancers occur in the floor of the mouth. As with other mouth cancers, cancer of the floor of the mouth develops in people who smoke and drink heavily. Because it is one of the more hidden areas of the mouth, cancer here is often found only when it has spread to the lymph glands in the neck. However, it can be diagnosed early.

Early Diagnosis

Early diagnosis is possible if your dentist or physician examines your mouth carefully. He or she can find this cancer when it is still small. Otherwise no symptoms occur until the cancer is fairly large and has often spread to lymph nodes in the neck. Any suspicious lesion should be biopsied. Staging, or evaluating the extent, of cancer of the floor of the mouth is the same as that discussed for cancer of the tongue.

Treatment

The treatment for this cancer is similar to that for cancer of the tongue. The overall cure rate is about 35 percent. Small cancers that do not involve the jawbone can be controlled with radiation therapy. The cure rate with early cancer is about 60 percent. However, the majority of victims have large cancers that have spread to the jawbone and the lymph nodes in the neck. Therefore, a radical operation involving removal of part of the lower jaw and the lymph glands in the neck, similar to that for cancer of the tongue, is usually needed. If you smoke or drink heavily, be sure you are examined yearly by your doctor or dentist.

CANCER OF THE BUCCAL MUCOSA (INSIDE OF THE CHEEK)

Ten percent of cancers of the mouth start in the cheeks. A lump in the cheek is usually the first sign of this cancer. Sometimes it may bleed. This cancer grows slowly and spreads relatively late. The staging evaluation and standard treatment are essentially identical to the procedures outlined for cancer of the tongue. Radiation therapy is used for very small lesions that have not spread to the lymph nodes in the neck, although surgery is an accepted alternative. For larger cancers that have spread to the nodes in the neck, radical surgery is the standard treatment. Approximately 45 percent of patients are cured.

CANCER OF THE GINGIVA (GUMS)

Cancer of the gums is relatively rare, and usually occurs in the lower gums. It shows up as a painful ulcer and may cause difficulty if dentures are worn. After a biopsy has confirmed the diagnosis, x-rays of the jaw are done to see if the bone is involved. If so, the chances for cure are slim.

The treatment for this cancer consists of radiation followed by surgical removal of part of the lower jaw. If the cancer is on the upper gums, radiation or surgery alone is more often used. About 35 percent of patients are cured. Early diagnosis improves the chance for cure: 70 percent of early gum cancer is cured.

CANCER OF THE OROPHARYNX (THROAT)

The oropharynx includes the areas of the tonsils and back walls of the mouth. Unfortunately, cancers arising here do not produce early symptoms. When pain on swallowing or pain sensed in the ear occurs, the cancer is advanced. Enlarged lymph nodes in the neck may be the first sign of these cancers.

Diagnosis

The evaluation for this cancer involves a laryngoscope, an instrument that allows the physician to look at and biopsy lesions at the back of the throat. A laryngoscope is also used to visualize the larynx and vocal cords located deep in the throat.

After a biopsy has been performed to confirm the diagnosis, x-rays to evaluate the extent of the tumor are taken. Cancers arising in the oropharynx tend to be more malignant and to metastasize earlier than other cancers of the mouth. They are diagnosed late, and their cure rate of 20 percent reflects this.

Treatment

Radiation is used more often than surgery to treat cancer of the oropharynx. Sometimes radiation is used to treat the primary cancer and surgery to treat the lymph nodes in the neck.

CANCER OF THE HYPOPHARYNX

The hypopharynx is the area behind and below the back of the tongue. Symptoms of cancer here are pain or difficulty in swallowing, due to obstruction of the food passage, and shortness of breath, due to obstruction of the upper airway. The hypopharynx cannot be seen without either a laryngoscope or the use of indirect laryngoscopy. The latter technique uses a mirror to look down the back of the throat. Cancer of the hypopharynx spreads early to lymph nodes in the neck. A laryngoscopic biopsy is needed to make the diagnosis.

Treatment

Treatment most often involves a combination of radiation and surgery. For people with advanced cancers, radiation alone may be used, not for cure but to control pain and to relieve obstruction of the airway or the esophagus. Because this cancer is not noticeable until quite late and because it can spread early, the overall cure rate is less than 15 percent. Early diagnosis is not feasible because your dentist cannot see these cancers.

CANCER OF THE LARYNX (VOICE BOX)

Cancer of the larynx occurs predominantly in men who smoke and drink. Fortunately, it is often diagnosed early because hoarseness is an early symptom. Hoarseness that persists for more than one or two weeks should prompt an examination for early laryngeal cancer.

Diagnosis

Since the vocal cord area cannot be seen or felt directly, indirect laryngoscopy is used to look at this area. If anything suspicious is seen, a biopsy needs to be done with a laryngoscope. A qualified otolaryngologist should perform this examination. He or she will biopsy the suspicious area and assess the size or extent of the cancer. If the biopsy shows cancer, x-rays of the area are needed. However, the laryngoscopic examination is the most important test for staging this cancer. Treatment depends upon where the cancer develops and its extent.

Treatment

Small cancers are usually treated with radiation alone. It offers a high cure rate, and speech is preserved. However, with larger cancers, surgery is necessary. This usually means removal of the larynx. If your larynx is removed, you lose your ability to talk. Speech rehabilitation is of obvious importance so you can learn to speak again by esophageal speech or by using a mechanical or electric voice box. If lymph node metastases are present in the neck, they are usually treated by surgery—a so-called radical neck dissection.

Prognosis

The cure rate with laryngeal cancer is 80 percent with small cancers. Even with more advanced cancers, 60 percent of patients are cured.

Rehabilitation

Radiation usually leaves the voice intact, a partial removal of the larynx causes some hoarseness, and a total laryngectomy results in complete loss of speech. Obviously, any treatment that affects a person's ability to speak is devastating. The person must adjust to a major change in his self-image and ability to communicate. He must be taught how to speak using his esophagus or a mechanical larynx. A mechanical larynx is a device that converts air motion into sound. It is held up to the hole in the neck left when the larynx was removed. Speech with this is easy to understand but has no normal inflections. It is extremely important to have a speech therapist see the patient before the operation and discuss rehabilitation. This will help the person who will awaken from anesthesia and have to learn to speak again.

The person who has a laryngectomy needs all the help he can get to adjust. Following this operation, he will have a permanent opening or stoma in his neck and will not be able to speak naturally. Fortunately, with determination and help he can learn to speak again. There is a nationwide network of volunteers to help a patient adjust to life after losing his voice box. These groups help the new laryngectomy patient learn to talk, shower, and face life again. The volunteers have all had laryngectomies. They can answer the many questions the patient has and are living proof that one can live and talk after this operation. If your doctor requests a volunteer, he or she will visit you, bring a kit and brochures, and ask you to join the club.

These volunteer organizations go under the names of the Lost Chord Club, New Voice Club, or the Anamilo Club. They are usually affiliated with the International Association of Laryngectomies, an agency separate from but supported by the American Cancer Society. Finally, the American Cancer Society will provide free instruction in esophageal speech.

CANCER OF THE NASOPHARYNX

Cancer of the nasopharynx is extremely rare in the United States; it occurs most often in the Chinese population. It is usually discovered when it causes obstruction of the nasal passages or damages nerves that pass nearby. This cancer is very malignant and spreads quite early. In fact, 75 percent of people at diagnosis have involvement of the lymph nodes in the neck. Staging work-up includes x-rays of the bones of the sinuses and skull, a chest x-ray, and often a liver scan.

This cancer is treated with high-dose radiation to the primary cancer and the lymph nodes in both sides of the neck. Few patients are cured because this disease is so malignant: one patient out of ten lives five years. Most die from cancer that spreads into the brain and skull.

SUMMARY

1. Many cancers of the head and neck can be diagnosed early if the mouth is carefully examined during yearly dental examinations. Most can be prevented. These cancers are related to the immoderate use of tobacco and alcohol. Cancer of the lip is also related to intense exposure to sunlight.

2. Head and neck cancers grow slowly and first spread to the lymph glands in the neck. The chance for cure is higher if the cancer is small and has not spread; the cosmetic and functional results are also better.

3. Surgery, radiation, or a combination of both is used to treat head and neck cancers. The aim of treatment is to eradicate both the cancer at the primary site and any metastases to lymph nodes in the neck. It is important not only to cure the cancer but also to obtain as good a cosmetic and functional result as possible.

4. The role of chemotherapy in the initial treatment of head and neck cancers has yet to be defined. Experimental results using chemotherapy before radiation and/or surgery for advanced but still localized cancers are encouraging.

5. For optimal results, a person with head and neck cancer should be

evaluated by a team of physicians with training and experience in treating these cancers. The team should include a surgeon (an otolaryngologist or a general surgeon), a radiation oncologist, a plastic surgeon, and a dental surgeon. A chemotherapist should also be consulted if the cancer is very advanced.

6. It is important that your surgeon be experienced in surgery for head and neck cancers. Otolaryngologists, general surgeons, and even plastic surgeons are trained to do this type of surgery. You must ask questions to make sure that your surgeon is qualified to treat you. If you live in a small community, it may pay you to visit a major cancer center for initial treatment.

7. Chemotherapy is of limited value for metastatic disease, but it offers temporary improvement to some. Therefore, we suggest either low-dose, nontoxic therapy or no therapy at all.

8. All people with one head and neck cancer should be followed closely for signs of cancer recurrence. They also need regular examinations to detect new cancers.

20

Thyroid Cancer

The thyroid gland is located in the neck below the larynx and "Adam's apple." It produces thyroid hormone, which helps regulate many body functions including the rate of metabolism. There are many common nonmalignant thyroid gland diseases that result in enlargement of this gland. Thyroid cancer is quite rare. Therefore, if you are told your thyroid is enlarged, you need not immediately fear that you have thyroid cancer. Most likely you have one of the noncancerous thyroid diseases briefly discussed in this chapter.

Thyroid cancer occurs in all age groups but is most common between the ages of thirty and sixty. As with other thyroid diseases, cancer occurs more often in women than in men. It is rare and accounts for less than 1 percent of cancer deaths in the United States. Most thyroid cancer is fairly slow growing and spreads, or metastasizes, late in its course. Often these cancers are still localized to the thyroid itself when diagnosed and are curable with surgery.

Even the person with metastatic or incurable thyroid cancer should not give up hope. One can often live for many years with metastatic thyroid cancer. It usually grows slowly and it can often be controlled for many years with treatment by radioactive iodine and thyroid hormone.

Thyroid cancer may become more common in the near future, because of the widespread, inappropriate use of radiation to the neck during the 1940s and 1950s. Radiation to the thyroid increases the risk for cancer as well as for other types of thyroid disease.

Causes: Radiation

The United States set up a study center in Hiroshima and Nagasaki to examine the effects of atomic bomb radiation upon the people who survived the bombing. By determining how far from the center of the blast the survivors were, it was possible to calculate the approximate dose of radiation they received. Within ten years after the bomb blast, survivors showed a radiation dose–dependent increase in thyroid cancer. Unfortunately, the data on the atomic bomb survivors began appearing only after approximately 2 million American children had already been exposed to neck radiation for everything from enlarged tonsils and adenoids to acne, and to treat a supposedly enlarged but actually normal gland called the thymus. The thymus gland is a lymph gland in the upper chest that has important regulatory functions for the body's immune system. It is normally large in childhood and becomes smaller as one gets older. Years ago doctors thought the thymus caused a variety of childhood illnesses. If it was large, they prescribed radiation.

Radiation, like other carcinogens, increases the risk for cancer only after a long latent period. The risk remains elevated for years. Radiation to the thyroid increases the frequency of thyroid cancer from five to more than forty years after the radiation.

What Should You Do If You Have Been Exposed to Radiation?

In 1977, the United States Department of Health, Education and Welfare issued a bulletin asking all physicians to examine carefully the thyroid glands of all people who had received radiation to the neck during childhood. HEW recommended that this be performed yearly. Some experts think that technetium thyroid scans on a regular basis are also indicated in this high-risk group of people. Radiation exposure causes other thyroid diseases that are benign and must be distinguished from cancer.

If you are one of the many who received neck radiation as a child, you should tell your physician. He or she should check you regularly for the development of thyroid enlargement. This may signal the development of an early, curable thyroid cancer.

NONCANCEROUS THYROID CONDITIONS OR ABNORMALITIES

Your physician may use several medical terms to describe thyroid conditions. We will define a few of the more common conditions. A goiter is any enlargement of the thyroid gland. If the gland is evenly enlarged, one need not fear cancer.

A thyroid nodule is a growth in the thyroid gland that may be benign or malignant. The nodule may or may not function as normal thyroid tissue. If it does function and produces thyroid hormone, the nodule may lead to hyperthyroidism, or overfunctioning of the thyroid gland. This condition causes nervousness, inability to tolerate warm weather, weight loss, a rapid pulse, and generalized weakness. Thyroid nodules that function as thyroid tissue are almost always benign.

A nonfunctioning (cold) thyroid nodule may be either cystic (fluid filled) and benign or solid and possibly malignant. Almost half of nonfunctioning single thyroid nodules are cancerous. Cancer is even more likely if you received radiation.

It is obvious that an enlarged thyroid must be evaluated by an experienced physician to determine if cancer is present. If an abnormality is suspicious for cancer, a surgical biopsy must be obtained.

Diagnosis

Any doctor can examine your thyroid and detect enlargement. However, if your thyroid is abnormal you should be referred to one of several types of physicians who have special training and experience with thyroid diseases. This physician may be: an internist called an endocrinologist, who specializes in treating hormonal disorders; a general surgeon or a head and neck surgeon, who has a special interest in thyroid disease; or a specialist in nuclear medicine. In some communities the nuclear medicine doctor is the most expert. In others, it may be the endocrinologist or the surgeon.

The Evaluation for Possible Thyroid Cancer

If your family doctor or one of these specialists examines your thyroid and finds it abnormal, further thyroid tests are needed to make sure cancer is not present. This is especially important for people who received radiation to the neck in childhood.

Thyroid Scans

The most useful single test to evaluate thyroid disease is a thyroid scan. A small amount of radioactive technetium is injected into a vein. The thyroid gland picks up and concentrates this material. Then a camera sensitive to small amounts of radioactivity is placed over the thyroid and a picture of the pattern of radioactivity over the thyroid gland is obtained. With a normal thyroid gland, there is a fairly uniform pattern of radioactivity over the whole gland, as all the tissue is normally functioning thyroid tissue.

If a technetium scan is abnormal, a radioactive iodine scan may need to be done. The thyroid gland picks up and concentrates iodine. Radioactive iodine thus gives a very accurate picture of the thyroid. However, unlike technetium scans, iodine scans themselves expose the thyroid to a significant dose of radiation. They should not be done repeatedly without a good indication.

Radioactive iodine scans will show whether nodules on the thyroid gland are functional (hot) and noncancerous or nonfunctional (cold) and possibly cancerous. A nodule that is functional concentrates the radioactive iodine and shows radioactivity with the scanning camera. In contrast, a cold nodule or cyst shows up as an area without radioactivity.

Ultrasound Examinations: How to Tell If a Cold Nodule Is Cystic

Ultrasound examination of the thyroid, like ultrasound examination of the abdomen, does not require injections or other painful procedures. An ultrasound probe is placed over the surface of the thyroid and transmits and receives sound waves. A picture of the sound waves appears on a television screen and is photographed. The physician is able to interpret these pictures and decide whether or not an area is fluid filled (cystic) or solid.

The ultrasound examination is an important test in evaluating a person with a cold thyroid nodule. It tells whether or not the nodule is cystic or solid. If a cold nodule is cystic, it is unlikely to be cancerous. If, however, a cold nodule is solid, cancer is present about 50 percent of the time.

Management of the Nonfunctional (Cold) Solid Thyroid Nodule

Cold solid nodules occurring in a large diseased thyroid gland (multinodular goiter) are less likely to be cancer than if the nodules occurred in an otherwise normal gland. Individuals with these should be given thyroid hormone, and the thyroid gland will usually shrink. If it does not, surgery is necessary to be sure cancer is not present.

If a person has a single solid cold nodule, thyroid hormone is also often given. If the nodule decreases in size or disappears, the patient can be observed at increasingly infrequent intervals and should continue to receive thyroid hormone indefinitely. If the nodule persists or enlarges, it must be biopsied to make sure it is not cancer.

If someone who has had neck radiation develops a cold solid nodule, he or she should have surgery and not receive a trial of thyroid hormone. The chance that the nodule is due to thyroid cancer is too great.

Diagnosis

Thyroid cancer is found in an unsuspecting person during a routine neck examination about 30 percent of the time. Most often it is found after someone notices an increase in the size of his or her neck. The shirt collar size may increase. A person may notice that his or her neck bulges. More rarely, hoarseness, difficulty swallowing, pain, or shortness of breath due to pressure on the trachea (windpipe) are the first symptoms. These are all serious warning signs for thyroid cancer as well as for other cancers in the neck area. Therefore, if you have any of these signs, you should see a doctor immediately.

Most thyroid cancers are slow-growing tumors. They remain localized to the thyroid for up to several years before they metastasize. Thyroid cancer first spreads to the nearby lymph glands in the neck. However, it also spreads to the bones and the lungs. It is important to diagnose this cancer before it has spread. Thyroid cancer localized to the thyroid can be cured with surgery. Thyroid cancer that has spread to the lymph glands of the neck is less often cured. Once the disease spreads beyond the lymph glands to other parts of the body, it cannot be cured with surgery. Despite its slow progression, thyroid cancer can kill you.

THYROID CANCER

There are several types of thyroid cancer. From the most benign to the most malignant, they are: papillary or papillary-follicular, follicular, and anaplastic. Papillary thyroid cancer is the most common type. Fortunately, about 80 percent of people with papillary or mixed papillary-follicular cancer are cured. In fact, if the cancer is localized to the thyroid, almost 100 percent will be cured. Follicular thyroid cancer is somewhat more malignant. It spreads to other organs earlier, and therefore the cure rate is lower. Anaplastic thyroid cancer is both rare and highly malignant. Few people with anaplastic carcinoma are cured. Most die within a year.

Treatment

Surgery   Surgery is the standard initial treatment for thyroid cancer. An operation called a total thyroidectomy, which involves the removal of the thyroid gland, is usually done. The lymph nodes of the neck on the side of the cancer are also removed. There is some controversy about whether surgery need be this extensive. Some surgeons do a subtotal thyroidectomy, that is, they only remove part of the thyroid. This leaves some normal thyroid tissue in the neck. Some surgeons also question the necessity of removing the lymph nodes if they are not enlarged.

Complications. There are some serious problems associated with thyroid surgery. An operation may result in a decrease or lack of function of the thyroid gland, which leads to hypothyroidism. Lifetime thyroid hormone treatment is necessary if your thyroid is removed. All people who have had a total thyroidectomy need thyroid hormone for the rest of their lives.

There are four small glands called parathyroid glands located within the thyroid tissue that may be inadvertently removed or damaged during the operation. These glands control the body's calcium balance. If they are removed, hypoparathyroidism results. The calcium in the blood falls and causes disturbing and serious symptoms such as muscle twitching and seizures. Hypoparathyroid individuals need to take supplements of vitamin D and calcium.

Surgery can also damage and cause paralysis of a nerve called the recurrent laryngeal. This nerve goes to the voice box, and damage to it leads to permanent hoarseness.

Who should do your thyroid surgery?   It is important that the surgeon who performs your thyroid surgery be experienced and do these operations frequently. Surgeons performing only one or two thyroidectomies a year incur more complications than do surgeons who perform many. In most communities, one or two surgeons do most of the thyroid surgery; you should ask for a referral to one for your surgery. It is quite reasonable for you to ask your doctor who is the best thyroid surgeon in your community. Finally, when you see the surgeon, ask if he or she does many thyroid operations. Ask how many thyroidectomies he or she has done in the past year. You will be better off if your operation is done by a board-certified general surgeon who does thyroidectomies frequently.

Radiation   Radiation therapy has almost no role in the primary treatment of papillary or follicular thyroid cancer. However, it may help control anaplastic thyroid cancer.

Treatment of Metastatic Thyroid Cancer

Radioactive Iodine   One of the advances in the treatment of widespread thyroid cancer is the use of radioactive iodine. Papillary or follicular cancers may act like normal thyroid tissue. They pick up and concentrate iodine. This can be tested with a total body radioactive iodine scan. If the cancer concentrates radioactive iodine, it will show up with this test. These cancers can be treated with high-dose radioactive iodine.

First, to treat metastatic thyroid cancer, normal thyroid tissue is destroyed with a low dose of radioactive iodine. No thyroid hormone is given. Without thyroid hormone replacement and without a functioning thyroid, the body will produce increased amounts of another hormone that regulates the thyroid called thyroid-stimulating hormone. The high level of thyroid-stimulating hormone stimulates the tumor tissue to take up and concentrate iodine.

Then a large dose of radioactive iodine is given every three to four weeks until the tumor no longer takes it up. This can be checked with a scanning camera. The radioactive iodine gives a localized but very high dose of radiation to the tumor. Almost no radiation to normal tissue occurs. This treatment can control thyroid cancer metastases for years. Sometimes it is curative.

After the treatment with radioactive iodine is finished, the person is placed on replacement doses of thyroid, since there is no functioning thyroid gland left. The side effects with this treatment are minimal; unlike regular radiation therapy, the tumor tissue receives almost all the radiation. The side effects from radioactive iodine treatment include mild radiation sickness (loss of appetite, some nausea, and vomiting), and rarely mild bone marrow depression. The one possibly serious long-term effect of any radiation including radioactive iodine is the increased risk of a second cancer.

The physician who uses radioactive iodine to treat metastatic thyroid cancer is usually an endocrinologist. This is a doctor who has received specialized training in the management of thyroid disease. Some medical oncologists also may use radioactive iodine. Many physicians in the new specialty of nuclear medicine are also qualified to treat thyroid cancer. This type of treatment can be administered in any good community hospital where there is a well-trained specialist available.

Thyroid Hormone Treatment   Thyroid cancer that functions like normal thyroid tissue can sometimes be controlled with oral thyroid hormone. This occurs most often with papillary or follicular cancers. Thyroid hormone replacement suppresses the levels of thyroid-stimulating hormone in the body. Just as normal thyroid tissue is stimulated by thyroid-stimulating hormone, so are many papillary and follicular thyroid cancers. Therefore, when thyroid hormone is given, the tumor shrinks. This is simple and often effective treatment for some thyroid cancers. It can control metastatic thyroid cancer for many years in some people.

Chemotherapy   Chemotherapy with anticancer drugs offers only temporary improvement to about 20 percent of people with advanced or metastatic thyroid cancer. We recommend that people with metastatic thyroid cancer that is not controlled by radioactive iodine or thyroid hormone take fairly nontoxic chemotherapy. The standard drug is Adriamycin. This drug will help about one in five who take it. But usually it only works for a short period of time. We do not recommend taking experimental, high-dose chemotherapy, as there are no promising experimental drugs for thyroid cancer at present.

Most thyroid cancers are slow growing, and therefore the chance for cure is quite good with surgery. People with widespread papillary or follicular thyroid cancer should not give up. It is possible to live many years with metastatic cancer. The disease itself may grow very slowly, and it can often be controlled with radioactive iodine and thyroid hormone. It is not too unusual for patients to live ten to twenty years with metastatic disease. Unfortunately, the picture for anaplastic cancer is quite different. Almost all people die within a year of diagnosis of this very aggressive tumor. Luckily it is much less common than the others.

A.L., a forty-five-year-old housewife, had received multiple radiation treatments for acne as a teenager. At age forty, she noticed her thyroid gland enlarging. She went to her family doctor, who examined her and sent her to an endocrinologist. He examined her and obtained a thyroid scan. Afterward he told her she probably had a benign condition called a multinodular goiter. Her thyroid gland was enlarged and had multiple nodules. He said that the gland would probably shrink with thyroid hormone treatment. She was started on two tablets of thyroid hormone per day and saw the endocrinologist every two months.

Atfer two months there was some decrease in the size of her thyroid gland, but the endocrinologist felt one firm nodule on the left side of the gland that had not decreased in size. Therefore, he obtained another thyroid scan. This scan showed that the nodule he felt was "cold," that is, it did not concentrate radioactive iodine. He next obtained an ultrasound, which showed that the nodule was solid and not fluid filled.

The endocrinologist told her that she might have cancer, especially with her history of radiation exposure in the past. A.L. was very frightened. Several pepole in her family had died from cancer. She had often fantasized her own death from it. Her doctor reassured her that early thyroid cancer was almost always cured by an operation.

The endocrinologist sent A.L. to the general surgeon who did most of the thyroid surgery in this community. He explained the need for surgery, and she and her husband agreed. She was admitted to the hospital and surgery was done. A large thyroid gland was partially removed along with the "cold" nodule. Fortunately, A.L. did not have cancer; the nodule was benign. She was very relieved. She has done quite well since then and continues to take thyroid hormone.

A.L.'s case was managed well. She had a multinodular goiter, a common benign condition, and therefore was treated with thyroid hormone. However, one nodule did not shrink. In fact, it appeared to grow despite the thyroid hormone. Tests showed that the nodule was nonfunctional, and therefore could be a cancer. A.L.'s history of radiation increased the chance that she had cancer. Although she did not develop thyroid cancer, the radiation for acne probably contributed to the development of her multinodular goiter. Radiation causes not only thyroid cancer but also a variety of other benign but often troublesome thyroid diseases.

In summary, A.L. had excellent care. She had her thyroid abnormality promptly diagnosed and correctly treated with thyroid hormone. She underwent prompt surgery when a "cold" nodule was discovered. Her surgery was done by the surgeon in the community most experienced in thyroidectomies. In the hands of an experienced surgeon, the operation is safe and complications are rare.

R.S., a sixty-three-year-old accountant, had not received neck radiation as a child. He noticed a rapidly growing lump in his neck and saw his doctor when he developed hoarseness and trouble breathing. His family physician found a large lump in the area of his thyroid that pushed his trachea to the right. R.S. was given an immediate appointment with a head and neck surgeon, who examined him and then admitted him to the hospital.

Examination of his vocal cords with a mirror (indirect laryngoscopy) showed that one of them was paralyzed, causing the hoarseness. To R.S.'s doctor this meant that a growth, usually cancerous, had invaded the recurrent laryngeal nerve and caused paralysis of the vocal cord. This is almost always a sign of incurability both for lung cancer and for cancers in the neck.

On the following day, an exploratory operation of the neck was performed. The surgeon did a biopsy for a frozen section so that a preliminary diagnosis could be made while R.S. was still under anesthesia. The pathologist found an anaplastic thyroid cancer. This is the most malignant type of thyroid cancer. The surgeon quite correctly determined that cure was impossible. Even extensive surgery was futile for symptom control. He therefore stopped, closed the incision, and sent R.S. to the recovery room.

The following day, R.S. was told he had thyroid cancer, that it was incurable, and that he needed radiation or chemotherapy for relief of symptoms caused by the tumor. He saw a radiation therapist, who told him that radiation might help him but could not cure him. R.S. also saw a medical oncologist, who agreed with the radiation oncologist. He told R.S. that chemotherapy should be tried only if radiation failed to control the tumor.

R.S. and his wife were both in a state of shock. He had been well, or thought he was well, only a few weeks ago. Now he faced death in a matter of weeks.

R.S. started radiation therapy, and within two weeks the tumor became smaller and he was breathing more comfortably. The only side effect from the radiation was a sore throat. During the four weeks that R.S. received radiation to the thyroid and surrounding neck region, the tumor shrank. He felt better for about three months. Then, the tumor started to grow and he noticed increasing difficulty breathing again.

He was sent to see the medical oncologist, who told him that chemotherapy might give him temporary relief. A recently introduced drug, Adriamycin, could temporarily shrink some thyroid cancers but could not cure them. He agreed to take chemotherapy and was given Adriamycin by intravenous injection on two occasions three weeks apart. The cancer continued to grow.

R.S. knew the end was near. He wrote a will and settled his financial affairs as best he could. He wrote out detailed instructions for his funeral and had long discussions with his wife about their life together and his impending death. One day he did not wake up. He had died peacefully in his sleep when the cancer eroded into his carotid artery, which then bled into his neck. It probably happened over a period of several minutes and he died with minimal suffering.

Luckily, anaplastic cancer of the thyroid is rare. It is rapidly progressive and rarely responds to treatment. Most people are dead from this disease in a year or two. Many, in fact, die within several months. Unlike the other thyroid cancers, anaplastic thyroid cancer usually causes symptoms because it invades nearby normal structures. Therefore, like R.S., people have symptoms such as hoarseness or trouble swallowing or breathing. R.S.'s symptoms, lack of response to treatment, and short survival are typical of this cancer.

SUMMARY

1. Radiation to the neck used to be commonly given to children for a number of trivial problems. It increases the risk for the development of thyroid cancer between five and forty years later.

2. If you have been exposed to radiation as a child, you should have your thyroid gland examined yearly. Some experts think that you should also have regular technetium thyroid scans.

3. Thyroid cancer presents with enlargement of the thyroid gland. Symptoms are rare.

4. Lumps or nodules that are not functional, that is, they do not concentrate iodine, are called "cold" nodules. A thyroid scan determines if a lump or nodule is cold.

5. A cold nodule cannot be ignored; it may be cancer. If you have not had radiation exposure, thyroid hormone can be used. If the nodule either shrinks or disappears, surgery is not indicated. If the nodule persists or enlarges, it must be biopsied to make sure it is not cancer.

6. If a cold nodule develops in someone with a history of radiation exposure, immediate surgery is necessary to determine if it is cancer.

7. Surgery is the standard treatment for thyroid cancer. Most thyroid cancers are slow growing and late spreading. Therefore, they are often cured by surgery.

8. The treatment of metastatic papillary or follicular thyroid cancer is often very effective. The metastatic cancer can function like normal thyroid tissue by picking up and concentrating iodine.

9. Functional metastatic thyroid cancer can be controlled for long periods of time with radioactive iodine. Simple thyroid hormone replacement in high doses can also control functional metastases.

10. Chemotherapy is relatively ineffective for thyroid cancer. Approximately 20 percent of patients will respond temporarily to Adriamycin. It should only be used after radioactive iodine and thyroid hormone have been tried without effect.

21

Soft Tissue and Bone Sarcomas

Sarcomas are uncommon cancers that arise from bones and from the mass of soft tissue (supportive structures) located between the organs and the skin. Fat, fibrous tissue, nerves, muscles, bones, and several other structures can give rise to these cancers. Although these tissues comprise 60 percent of our body weight, only 1.3 percent of all cancers arise from these tissues. Many nonmalignant tumors arise from these tissues, but any tumor called a sarcoma is malignant. The word *sarcoma* is derived from the Greek words *sarc* and *omo*, which together mean fleshy tumor. Indeed, these tumors fit the description well.

Soft Tissue Sarcomas

Soft tissue sarcomas arise from fat, muscle, fibruous tissues, and even blood vessels. There are over fifty types of soft tissue sarcoma, and their names correspond to the tissues from which they arise. Accordingly, sarcomas from fibrous tissue are called fibrosarcomas, those arising from fat are named liposarcomas, those arising from muscle are either rhabdomyosarcomas or leiomyosarcomas—the list is endless. They share many characteristics and are treated quite similarly. Benign tumors from these tissues are named fibromas, lipomas, leiomyomas, etc. If you have a fleshy tumor with one of these names without the word sarcoma, you do not have cancer.

Causes

There is no known cause for most soft tissue sarcomas, but some occur in scars and in areas that have been irradiated. For example, women may develop sarcomas many years after a mastectomy and irradiation for breast cancer.

Diagnosis

Most of these tumors are noticed because a mass or lump develops. Occasionally sarcomas become large enough to impinge upon nearby structures such as nerves and cause pain. Sarcomas are firm to hard lumps that are usually not tender. Any mass under the skin or in a muscle that persists and does not go away in a few weeks should be evaluated by a physician and should be biopsied to determine if it is benign or malignant.

Biopsy of the Suspicious Lump   People should be referred to general surgeons for biopsies of suspicious lumps under the skin or in muscles. It is important for the surgeon to obtain enough of the tissue for the pathologist to determine two important things: (1) is the mass benign or malignant? and (2) if it is malignant, how malignant? Therefore, a biopsy obtained by inserting a needle into the mass, a so-called needle biopsy, is inadequate. A small mass should be excised completely and a large mass should have a large biopsy taken for pathologic examination.

Soft tissue sarcomas are graded from 1 to 5 by the pathologist. Grade 1 is a sarcoma that does not look very malignant under the microscope, and grade 5 is a highly malignant sarcoma. Usually there is a good correlation between the grade of the sarcoma and how it behaves clinically. Low-grade sarcomas usually grow slowly and don't metastasize, while high-grade ones tend to grow more quickly and spread to other organs. Therefore, the pathologist helps guide the physicians who perform the actual treatment by telling them how the cancer is likely to behave, how much treatment is necessary, and what the chances are for cure.

Has the Tumor Spread?

After a tumor biopsy shows a sarcoma, your physician will determine the extent of the cancer. X-rays of the area are obtained and arteriography if possible. For an arteriogram, a needle is inserted under local anesthesia into the artery feeding the tumor. A radio-opaque dye is rapidly injected and a series of x-rays is taken. This test helps the surgeon by outlining the blood supply and often the local extent of the cancer. A bone scan also will often help determine the extent of the tumor by indicating whether it has invaded nearby bone. A chest x-ray will show whether the cancer has metastasized to the lungs, a common site for sarcomas to spread. If the sarcoma is large or if it looks very malignant (high grade), a liver scan is usually also obtained. If the cancer has spread to the lungs or liver, then extensive surgery is fruitless.

Treatment

The standard treatment of soft tissue sarcomas is surgery. Recently the combination of less extensive surgery and radiation has been evaluated and shows promise. Chemotherapy to treat suspected metastases (adjuvant chemotherapy) is still an experimental and unproven approach. Many oncologists will use adjuvant chemotherapy for highly malignant sarcomas because the likelihood of microscopic metastases to other organs is high.

Many soft tissue sarcomas grow slowly and appear to be not very malignant (low grade) under the microscope. These are sometimes inadequately removed by the surgeon, because he or the patient wishes to minimize the amount of normal tissue damaged or removed, with an unfortunate result. The sarcoma recurs, and with each recurrence the chance for cure decreases. When a sarcoma recurs, it is often more malignant than it was at the onset. Metastases are more common and, if present, the chances for cure are lost. Surgery for all soft tissue sarcomas, even those that are small and low grade, involves removal of the tumor and much of the surrounding normal tissues, as they often contain microscopic deposits of tumor cells.

C.W., a forty-nine-year-old waitress, noticed a lump in her right thigh that persisted for several months. She eventually went to her doctor, who felt a firm lump in the right thigh muscle. He sent her to a general surgeon, who examined her, obtained x-rays, and then told her that she would need a biopsy. He told her it could be a benign or malignant tumor. A biopsy was done in the outpatient clinic under local anesthesia, and it revealed a grade 1 fibrosarcoma.

The surgeon told C.W. that she had a malignant tumor called a fibrosarcoma, but that the chances for cure were very good. The cancer was not very large and did not look very malignant under the microscope. He recommended that she have extensive surgery to her right thigh, which would be deforming and might leave her with a limp. She would receive rehabilitation therapy after surgery but her leg probably wouldn't ever be normal again. However, this radical surgical approach offered her a very good chance for cure.

C.W. thought about the treatment her doctor advised but then went to another, less experienced surgeon, who advised a more limited operation. She decided upon the lesser operation. He removed the whole tumor but very little surrounding normal tissue. Three years after this inadequate surgery, the cancer recurred in the same area. Biopsy showed a grade 4 fibrosarcoma, a far more malignant tumor. A chest x-ray, liver scan, and abdominal ultrasound did not show any metastases.

This time C.W. was more frightened. She returned to her first surgeon and underwent a radical operation followed by radiation therapy. She was undergoing rehabilitation and was improving when, six months later, a chest x-ray showed that the sarcoma had spread to her lungs and a bone scan showed that it had also spread to bones. She was given combination chemotherapy with severe side effects; however, the lung metastases decreased in size for six months. Then the tumors started to grow again and she died three months later of progressive fibrosarcoma in the lungs and bone.

C.W.'s history is all too common. Low-grade, small sarcomas are frequently not adequately treated when they can be cured. The sarcoma is not entirely removed because this would involve removing many normal structures. Many surgeons are not trained in cancer surgery and only rarely see people with these uncommon tumors. They do not realize that soft tissue sarcomas spread far beyond the obvious tumor into muscles and other surrounding structures. C.W. almost certainly could have been cured initially. For obvious and understandable reasons, she did not accept radical surgery early enough. She had radical treatment only when it was too late to cure her.

Surgery   Radical surgery is the established treatment for soft tissue sarcomas. This involves removing the obvious sarcoma and a good deal of the normal surrounding tissue such as fat, muscle, nerves, and even bone. It is necessary because the tumor tends to spread microscopically into these surrounding tissues, and all the tumor cells must be removed if the person is to be cured.

Surgery with Radiation   Recent studies have evaluated the combination of less radical surgery to remove the bulk of the cancer with high-dose radiation therapy to treat the area around the cancer. The early results are promising. If these results do show that this approach is as good as surgery, we will be able to treat people with fewer side effects. Perhaps if C.W. had been offered combined treatment—less extensive surgery and high-dose radiation—she would have accepted it and been cured. Many surgeons, however, do not know of or accept the results with surgery and radiation, and so do not offer the combination to their patients with sarcomas.

In summary, either radical surgery alone or less radical surgery with high-dose radiation therapy given to the tumor and draining lymph nodes should be the treatment for soft tissue sarcomas, no matter how small or low grade the tumor is.

Adjuvant Chemotherapy   The use of adjuvant chemotherapy after treatment of the local cancer is still experimental and unproven for soft tissue sarcomas. These are fairly rare cancers and have an uneven natural history depending on the grade and site of origin. Therefore, it has been difficult to show whether chemotherapy in conjunction with local eradication of the sarcoma is of benefit. Many oncologists recommend chemotherapy for high-grade and large sarcomas, where the chances for cure with local treatment are low.

Chemotherapy for Metastatic Sarcoma   If the sarcoma is already widespread, surgery rarely helps. Chemotherapy is used to treat widespread metastases and radiation to treat local problems such as bone pain. Chemotherapy is moderately effective against soft tissue sarcomas. Combinations of drugs will cause at least 50 percent of soft tissue sarcomas to decrease in size. People who respond feel better and may live longer. However, the chemotherapy does not cure people with metastases.

Who Should Treat You?   If you have a soft tissue sarcoma, you should initially be evaluated for treatment by a team of physicians that includes a board-certified surgeon who specializes in cancer surgery, a radiation therapist, and a medical oncologist. This team approach may require you to travel to a major medical center.

FIBROSARCOMA

Fibrosarcomas are among the most common soft tissue sarcomas. They occur most often between the ages of twenty and fifty, and they arise almost anywhere. Common places for these cancers to start are the leg, the arm, the head, and the trunk of the body. Fibrosarcomas start from normal fibrous connective tissue. They spread locally and through the blood stream to other sites. The lungs are a favorite site of metastases.

Has the Cancer Spread?

Evaluation for spread of fibrosarcoma should include the tests mentioned earlier to determine the extent of the primary cancer (bone scan, arteriogram) and a chest x-ray and liver scan to look for metastases.

Treatment

The treatment is radical surgery or surgery and radiation. Chemotherapy may be given after surgery and/or radiation for people with very malignant fibrosarcomas to destroy presumed microscopic nests of cancer cells in the lungs and other organs. We suggest that a medical oncologist be consulted for an opinion as to whether chemotherapy should be tried. We recommend chemotherapy if there is better than a 50 percent chance of recurrence, although adjuvant chemotherapy for these tumors isn't of proven benefit.

Prognosis

The odds for cure depend upon the size and pathologic grade of the tumor, as these two factors correlate with the chance of spread to other organs. Small tumors of low grade have a 60–70 percent chance for cure, but larger tumors, especially if high grade, have a much lower cure rate.

LIPOSARCOMA

Liposarcomas arise from fat, are almost as common as fibrosarcomas, and occur commonly in middle-aged people. They can attain tremendous size, especially if they occur in the abdomen. The staging and treatment are the same as described for fibrosarcomas. The prognosis, or chance for cure, is also like that of fibrosarcoma. Tumors of low grade have a high cure rate and tumors of high grade a low cure rate. Overall, about 30 percent are cured. Many people also have nonmalignant fatty tumors called lipomas. These require no treatment.

RHABDOMYOSARCOMA

Rhabdomyosarcomas are tumors that arise from muscles and occur most often in middle-aged adults. These sarcomas are staged and treated much like the other two—with extensive surgery or surgery and radiation. As with other soft tissue sarcomas, the grade and the size of the tumor play a big role in determining the prognosis.

EMBRYONAL RHABDOMYOSARCOMA

Embryonal rhabdomyosarcoma is extremely rare in adults. This tumor occurs primarily in children and is discussed in chapter 23, "Cancer in Children." The treatment for it involves surgically removing as much of the cancer as possible and then giving high-dose radiation and chemotherapy. The cure rate for this cancer has been increased significantly with this approach.

UNDIFFERENTIATED SARCOMAS

Approximately 20 percent of sarcomas are unclassified, that is, the pathologist cannot tell from which tissue the cancer arose. The sarcoma looks so abnormal under the microscope that it does not resemble the tissue from which it arose. These sarcomas are highly malignant. The principles of staging and treatment are the same as those discussed for other sarcomas.

Sarcomas from Bone and Cartilage

Bone cancers are also sarcomas. These cancers are growths arising from normal bone that destroy the surrounding bone tissue and frequently spread to other parts of the body. Bone cancer is relatively rare and accounts for less than 1 percent of all cancers in the United States. Unfortunately, it is more common in children between the ages of five and fifteen. Factors contributing to the development of bone cancer include a variety of abnormalities that cause irritation or stimulation to bones. These include chronic bone infection (osteomyelitis), fractures, Paget's disease of bone, and exposure to radiation.

The most common bone cancer is osteogenic sarcoma, a cancer arising from bone-forming cells. Chondrosarcoma, another common sarcoma, develops from cartilage. Ewing's sarcoma arises from the bone marrow. However, the most common cancer affecting bone is not primary bone cancer but cancer that metastasizes, or spreads, to bone. Cancer of the prostate, breast, and lung, malignant melanoma, and other cancers often spread to bone. In this chapter we will discuss only cancers that arise from bones themselves and not cancers that arise in other organs and spread to bone.

Diagnosis

Primary bone cancers most often arise in an arm or leg. As one might expect, cancers in bone are noticed because they cause pain and swelling. The disease may weaken the bone and thus cause a fracture. Cancerous bone can break with only trivial injuries. Often the person relates the pain or swelling to a minor injury. However, instead of getting better, it gets worse.

The first step in evaluating any bone abnormality is to obtain x-rays. X-rays are indicated if a bone is persistently painful or swollen. While the x-ray cannot definitely tell what is wrong, it will often strongly indicate whether the problem is due to a malignant or benign tumor or merely to an injury. Aside from the x-ray, the age of the person, the location of the bone, and the symptoms can suggest not only whether the symptoms are from cancer but also whether the cancer is primary or metastatic. Bone sarcomas arise in younger people, tend to be larger, cause more fractures, and damage surrounding bone much more than do benign bone tumors.

The Orthopedic Surgeon

No matter how classic the symptoms and x-rays are for a benign or malignant tumor, a biopsy is always necessary. The biopsy should be done by an orthopedic surgeon. This is a doctor who has had four years of training in diseases of the bones and joints. The board-certified orthopedic surgeon has completed four years of training in this specialty and has successfully completed an examination. He or she is the surgeon best trained to evaluate and treat bone cancer.

The Biopsy

It is extremely important that the orthopedic surgeon confer with the radiologist and decide which area of the tumor to biopsy. A biopsy should never be obtained prior to adequate x-ray studies. Also, if the biopsy is not diagnostic or shows only benign changes but the x-rays are suggestive of cancer, the biopsy must be repeated. Pathologic interpretation of bone tumor biopsies can be difficult. Therefore, the biopsy and the operation, if needed, are usually done at different times. Surgery is done after the biopsy has been adequately examined by the pathologist. This is a different procedure from that used in other cancers—for example, in breast cancer, where the biopsy can be interpreted in a matter of minutes (by frozen sections) and definitive surgery can be done at the time of the biopsy.

Treatment

The Team Approach   Optimal management of both benign and malignant bone tumors should involve a multidisciplinary approach from the outset. A board-certified radiologist, a specialist in diagnostic x-rays, a board-certified orthopedic surgeon, and a board-certified pathologist must all work together. The radiologist must take enough x-rays of the bone to guide the orthopedic surgeon, who will biopsy an area of the tumor that has the highest chance of enabling the pathologist to decide whether the tumor is malignant or benign.

If the biopsy is benign, the orthopedic surgeon can adequately treat the tumor. If the biopsy shows bone cancer, a multidisciplinary approach is necessary to plan and deliver the best treatment. This team should include an orthopedic surgeon, a radiation oncologist, a medical oncologist, and a pathologist. If an extremity must be amputated, an expert in rehabilitation is also necessary. Bone cancers often require surgery, radiation, and chemotherapy. Therefore, bone sarcomas are best treated in major medical centers. Radical surgery, high-dose radiation, or a combination of both are necessary. More often than not chemotherapy is also used. The exact therapy will depend upon the location and type of the cancer. The larger and more malignant the cancer, the more aggressive the treatment.

The Need for Adjuvant Chemotherapy   Many bone cancers have spread microscopically to other parts of the body by the time they are diagnosed. Therefore, chemotherapy is often given in addition to surgery and/or radiation to treat these suspected microscopic metastases. A medical or pediatric oncologist should be involved when treatment is planned.

If all three types of treatment are to be used, they must be planned very carefully. Radiation and chemotherapy can each interfere with the healing of surgical wounds; when chemotherapy is added, more side effects occur in tissues receiving radiation. In summary, the best treatment requires specialists in all three areas of treatment. Furthermore, they must be involved from the beginning so that each of the treatments can be used for optimal antitumor effect with the fewest side effects and the least mutual interference.

BENIGN BONE TUMORS

The most common benign bone tumors are osteochondromas, osteomas, enchondromas or chondromas, chondroblastomas, osteoid osteomas, benign osteoblastomas, and giant cell tumors. Benign bone tumors need treatment because they cause pain and can destroy enough bone tissue to cause the bone to break.

MALIGNANT CHANGE IN BENIGN BONE TUMORS

Aside from causing symptoms, these benign bone tumors can change into malignant tumors if not treated. For example, osteochondromas and enchondromas or chondromas may transform into chondrosarcoma, and giant cell tumors may become malignant giant cell tumors. Therefore, benign tumors should be removed and/or followed very closely by an orthopedic surgeon so that they can be treated early if they transform and become malignant. The development of pain or an increase in tumor size are signs of possible malignancy. If you have either of these symptoms, you should see your orthopedic surgeon immediately.

Treatment

Benign bone tumors are treated by surgically scooping out the tumor. If the tumor is large, a bone graft may be needed. Radiation and chemotherapy have no place in the treatment of these tumors.

Has the Malignant Bone Tumor Spread?

If the bone tumor is malignant, further evaluation or staging depends upon the type of bone cancer. Bone cancers are well supplied by blood vessels and spread early through the blood stream. They metastasize to distant organs such as the lungs, liver, and other bones more often than to the local lymph nodes. Details of tests that are indicated for the different bone cancers are outlined later in this chapter, but a few examples will be given to explain why certain tests are done. When bone cancer starts in an arm or leg, arteriography is useful to determine the extent of the cancer and its blood supply. Bone cancers have a very rich blood supply, and this test helps the surgeon to identify the real extent of the tumor. Osteogenic sarcoma (a bone-forming cancer) often spreads to the lungs. Therefore, a chest x-ray and a more sensitive x-ray of the lungs called a tomogram should always be obtained before surgery. Lung x-rays are the key staging test for this cancer. Ewing's sarcoma also spreads often to the lungs, and to other bones as well, so in addition to chest x-rays and tomograms of the lungs, a bone scan should always be done. The behavior and location of the cancer determines which tests should be obtained.

OSTEOGENIC SARCOMA

Diagnosis and Staging

This cancer starts most commonly in the legs or arms. It comes from the cells that actually make bone, and areas of the cancer contain bone. Therefore, bone shows up on x-ray, and a simple x-ray of the lump can suggest the diagnosis. It is highly malignant and spreads very early through the blood stream to other areas, especially to the lungs. Prior to treatment, the physician must find out how far the cancer extends. X-rays of the involved area, and an arteriogram of the arm or leg, will help evaluate the local extent of the tumor, and x-rays of the chest, including lung tomograms and a bone scan, are done to look for metastases. Osteogenic sarcoma is also discussed in chapter 23, "Cancer in Children," since it usually afflicts children and adolescents.

Treatment

Surgery   Until recently, the only treatment for osteogenic sarcoma was radical surgery, usually an amputation of the affected limb. Although amputation ensured removal of the primary area of the sarcoma, the cure rate was very low. Only 10–15 percent of people were cured because the cancer had usually already spread to the lungs. Even if the chest x-rays were normal at the time of surgery, within one year most people had died of lung metastases. Therefore, the treatment was changed.

Adjuvant Chemotherapy   Surgery, followed by one to two years of adjuvant chemotherapy, is now used to treat the small nests of cancer cells that have escaped through the blood stream to the lungs and other sites. This combined approach thus far has proven very successful; people treated with adjuvant chemotherapy right after surgery have had a much lower recurrence rate than people treated only with surgery. The use of adjuvant chemotherapy has increased the cure rate from 15 to 40–50 percent.

Saving the Limb

Some centers recently have attempted to obtain the same improved results without amputation. Their approach has been to use first chemotherapy and/or radiation to shrink the tumor and then less extensive surgery. This approach is still experimental and unproven; more experience and time are needed to see if it is as effective as amputation.

Rehabilitation

Surgery for osteosarcoma almost always requires an amputation. Most osteosarcoma victims are young, and may have more difficulty than an older person adjusting to the loss of an arm or leg. Psychological support and active rehabilitation are needed if the person is to adjust to his cancer and to the loss of a limb. Large medical centers or cancer centers often offer the best support for these patients.

Cancer centers have pioneered new approaches to rehabilitation. In the past, amputations were performed but artificial legs were not used for several months. Recently, a temporary artificial limb has been installed at the time of surgery, so the patient awakens with the artificial leg in place. He or she can walk soon after surgery, which is a great psychological boost. In addition, the wound heals faster with the artificial leg in place. About two months after surgery the temporary limb is removed and the patient is fitted with a permanent one. Most people cannot tell that a person has an artificial leg unless they are told. Walking can be almost normal.

METASTATIC OSTEOSARCOMA

People with osteogenic sarcoma who are not cured and who develop spread to their lungs can be treated by chemotherapy, radiation, or surgical removal of small numbers of metastases. Chemotherapy is moderately effective against this cancer: about 50 percent of people with osteosarcoma respond temporarily. Recently, the combination of surgical removal of the metastases and chemotherapy has been tried. Fortunately, most of the metastases to the lungs are located just beneath the surface of the lungs and, therefore, can be removed quite easily with surgery. This approach is promising but more time is needed to evaluate how effective it really is.

In summary, the treatment for osteosarcoma is complex and demands a team of experts. Treatment should be done in a cancer center or at least a major medical center. The cure rate has been doubled by the use of adjuvant chemotherapy. More information on this cancer is included in chapter 23, "Cancer in Children."

EWING'S SARCOMA

Ewing's sarcoma is the second most common tumor of bone and, like osteogenic sarcoma, almost always occurs in younger people. Therefore, it is discussed in detail in the chapter on childhood cancer. Like osteogenic sarcoma, it is a very malignant cancer that usually has spread to distant sites by the time of diagnosis. The staging workup includes the tests mentioned for osteogenic sarcoma. In addition, a liver scan and a brain scan are often obtained.

Treatment

The treatment for Ewing's sarcoma differs somewhat from that for osteosarcoma because this tumor is fairly radiosensitive. Instead of surgery, radiation in very high doses (5000 to 7000R) is used to treat the primary site of cancer and chemotherapy is given to treat the microscopic nests of cancer cells that have already spread to other parts of the body. When radiation alone was used, only 10–15 percent of people were cured. The rest developed metastases in other organs and died. New treatment programs using radiation and one to two years of adjuvant chemotherapy are yielding promising results. As with osteogenic sarcoma, adjuvant chemotherapy has increased the cure rate significantly. At present 40–50 percent are cured.

In summary, all people with Ewing's sarcoma should be treated with a combination of high-dose radiation and chemotherapy for a long period of time. The treatment should at least be started in a cancer center where expert radiation and medical oncologists who specialize in the treatment of this rare cancer are available.

CHONDROSARCOMA

Chondrosarcoma, unlike osteosarcoma and Ewing's sarcoma, occurs most often in middle-aged adults. It is much less malignant than the other bone tumors. It grows more slowly and rarely spreads to distant sites. Therefore, treatment is simpler and more often successful. Two benign bone tumors, osteochondromas and enchondroma or chondroma, both may develop into chondrosarcoma. Approximately 1 percent of solitary osteochondromas and 20 percent of multiple osteochondromas, an inherited condition, will eventually turn into chondrosarcoma. Therefore, these two benign tumors should always be removed surgically to prevent development of chondrosarcoma.

Diagnosis and Treatment

Chondrosarcomas can develop within any bone. They usually occur in the arms, the legs, and the bones of the trunk. Staging for this cancer involves tests to find out the extent of the primary tumor. These include x-rays and sometimes arteriography. The treatment for this cancer is surgery. Occasionally, if the cancer is large, an amputation is necessary. Most often removal of the chondrosarcoma and some surrounding normal bone is sufficient. Depending upon the location, a bone graft may be needed. In some cases an artificial replacement for a joint is required. A common error in treatment of the cancer has been to do inadequate surgery. H.B.'s case illustrates the difference between curative and non-curative surgery.

H.B., a fifty-seven-year-old farmer, noticed swelling of his right knee. He waited for it to get better for one year. Instead, it got larger and more painful. He finally saw his family doctor. The doctor felt a hard lump and took an x-ray, which showed a tumor. He sent H.B. to see an orthopedic surgeon at a nearby large hospital. Many more x-rays were taken, and H.B. was examined carefully. The orthopedist told H.B. that he most probably had a malignant bone tumor and that a biopsy needed to be done. The orthopedic surgeon and the radiologist discussed which area to biopsy. Under spinal anesthesia, a biopsy was obtained in the operating room, and it showed a chondrosarcoma.

H.B. was told that an extensive operation including replacement of his knee joint was necessary. This would probably leave him with a useful knee but the orthopedic surgeon couldn't guarantee it. Less surgery would not ensure removal of all the cancer. H.B. thought about this for several weeks and finally decided to have the surgery. The orthopedic surgeon did an adequate operation to cure the cancer. The replacement of the knee joint was also done. Four years have passed and H.B. is alive and well, still working as a farmer. Although this is the way chondrosarcomas should be treated, too often the patient and his physician compromise, with disastrous results.

If H.B. had decided against radical surgery, he might not have been cured. Perhaps after thinking about the radical surgery that was recommended and the possibility of not ever being able to work as a farmer again, he decided to take a chance. Even though the surgeon told him that he might die with a lesser operation, H.B. was adamant. Therefore, a limited operation followed by low-dose radiation was used to preserve his knee.

H.B. was happy and remained well for two years. During the two years he saw his orthopedist four times a year. He had x-rays done each time, and they were normal. Then he started to develop pain around his knee. X-rays showed recurrent chondrosarcoma. This time H.B. was frightened and agreed to have extensive surgery with a knee replacement. He found he could function fairly well with the artificial knee. However, one year after the second operation, metastases appeared in his lung and, despite chemotherapy, he died several months later.

Only you can decide whether to follow your doctor's advice. He can present the facts about your disease and try to advise you accordingly. H.B.'s story is retold often with chondrosarcomas and even more often with soft tissue sarcomas. Any time a cancer is not completely removed and regrows, the chance for cure falls dramatically. In the first case, H.B.'s doctor was adamant and strongly recommended the correct treatment. Sometimes the doctors themselves compromise, and their patients lose the chance for cure.

SUMMARY

Soft Tissue Sarcomas

1. Soft tissue sarcomas are uncommon cancers; they represent less than 0.5 percent of all cancers in the United States.

2. Any suspicious lump under the skin or in a muscle should be biopsied as soon as possible to determine if it is benign or malignant.

3. The evaluation of soft tissue sarcoma involves determining the extent of the cancer. X-rays of the area and a chest x-ray are needed. Arteriography may be required. Depending upon the type, size, and grade of the tumor, additional tests may be necessary, such as a bone scan and/or liver scan.

4. Optimal treatment requires a multidisciplinary team consisting of a board-certified general surgeon experienced in cancer surgery, a radiation oncologist, and a medical oncologist. Since you may only have one chance for cure, the initial treatment should be planned by experts. Travel to a larger hospital or cancer center if this expert care is not available in your community.

5. Extensive surgery or less extensive surgery and high-dose radiation therapy is needed to eradicate the tumor reliably. A common and unfortunate error is not to treat an early sarcoma aggressively enough. The sarcoma can then recur and the chance for cure may be lost. Though not of proven benefit, adjuvant chemotherapy may be used if the tumor is large and looks very malignant under the microscope.

6. The main treatment of metastatic soft tissue sarcoma is chemotherapy. This should be planned by a medical oncologist. Radiation therapy is used to treat local problems such as painful bone metastases. Occasionally, surgical removal of a single lung metastases is helpful.

Sarcomas from Bone

1. Bone cancers are relatively rare; they occur more often in children and teenagers than adults.

2. A benign bone tumor can be treated by an orthopedic surgeon alone. For optimal management of a suspected bone cancer, a team consisting of an orthopedic surgeon, a radiologist, and a pathologist is needed. Bone cancers should be evaluated in major medical centers.

3. Treatment of malignant bone cancer calls for a multidisciplinary team approach: an orthopedic surgeon, a radiation oncologist, a medical oncologist, a pathologist, and often a specialist in rehabilitation all should be involved from the start.

4. Osteogenic sarcoma is treated by surgery and adjuvant chemotherapy. The treatment of Ewing's sarcoma is nonsurgical: high-dose radiation is given to the primary tumor along with adjuvant chemotherapy. The treatment of chondrosarcoma is extensive surgery alone.

5. When an amputation is required, a rehabilitation medicine specialist should be consulted early. Psychological support should also be readily available to help the amputee adjust. The rehabilitation team should also include trained professional psychologists or social workers.

22

Lung Cancer

Lung cancer was uncommon in the United States prior to 1930. It became a common cancer in men in the 1930s, twenty years after the First World War, when Americans first started to smoke cigarettes heavily. In the past two decades an increasing number of women have smoked cigarettes and, as expected, the incidence of lung cancer in American women has climbed alarmingly and is rapidly approaching the incidence in American men. Lung cancer is very rare in nonsmoking, nonindustrialized societies. Nonsmokers who live in unpolluted areas only rarely get lung cancer.

Other environmental carcinogens in addition to cigarette smoke probably contribute to the high incidence of lung cancer in this country. The carcinogens that have been associated with lung cancer include asbestos, arsenic, nickel, chromium, and radioactive elements such as radon and plutonium. These are most commonly encountered in factories and mines, but the air in the vicinity of these factories and mines is also contaminated. Not only the workers, but also their families and the people who live near these factories are more likely to get lung cancer. For example, the air in the vicinity of copper smelting plants has a high concentration of arsenic, and the incidence of lung cancer is increased in nonworkers who live downwind of the plant.

Exposure to a second carcinogen makes smoking cigarettes more likely to lead to lung cancer. This is because when two or more carcinogens such as asbestos or arsenic and tobacco are combined, the effect is more than just additive. The incidence of lung cancer skyrockets with such combined exposure. Therefore, if you are exposed as a worker to any of the above substances, it is especially important that you do not smoke. If you do, your chances of developing lung cancer will be much greater than those of other smokers. You are not always able to control all the carcinogens that contribute to the development of lung cancer, but you can avoid the most important, cigarette smoke.

Lung cancer at present is the most common cancer and the leading cause of cancer deaths among American men, and it is rapidly becoming almost as common among women. Each year, approximately 90,000 Americans develop and 80,000 die from lung cancer. It accounts for one-fourth of all cancer deaths in American men. Although the incidence at present is four times higher in men than women, there is no reason to think that the incidence in women will not approach and equal that of men in the next several decades because of the increasing number of women who smoke cigarettes.

The Facts about Smoking and Lung Cancer Are Incontrovertible

—Smoking definitely causes lung cancer. Data on male smokers indicate that they have a twenty-five-fold increase in the most common type of lung cancer (squamous cell cancer of the lung) and a twentyfold increase in the most malignant type of lung cancer (oat cell or small cell carcinoma) when compared to nonsmokers.

—The effect of smoking is dose related; thus, low tar and nicotine cigarettes are probably beneficial if you must smoke.

—Approximately ten years after a person has stopped smoking, his or her chances of developing lung cancer decrease to close to that of a nonsmoker. Therefore, even if you have smoked heavily, it pays to stop. The lung can repair damage caused by the carcinogens in tobacco smoke.

—Certain people may have a genetic tendency to develop lung cancer when exposed to carcinogens. They have a greater quantity of an enzyme called aryl-hydrocarbon decarboxylase, which metabolizes tobacco smoke to the active carcinogen and puts those people with high levels of the enzyme at greater risk for the development of lung cancer. Therefore, if your father, mother, or sibling smoked cigarettes and developed lung cancer, you may have a greater tendency to develop lung cancer if you also smoke.

—If you are exposed to coal dust or other cancer-causing substances such as asbestos, arsenic, nickel, or uranium, you are very likely to get lung cancer if you also smoke.

—Cigarette smoking not only increases your chances of getting lung cancer, but it also increases the risk of several other cancers, including cancers of the mouth, throat, bladder, and possibly pancreas and breast.

It is obvious how we feel about cigarette smoking. If you are a smoker and do not feel you can stop, at least try to cut down on the number of cigarettes you smoke each day and switch to a low tar–low nicotine cigarette. It is only fair to tell you that if you develop lung cancer, your chances for surviving are abysmal.

Lung Cancer Cannot Usually Be Diagnosed Early

Many studies have shown that there is no currently available method capable of detecting lung cancer early enough to improve survival. Regular chest x-rays and physical examinations do not usually detect lung cancer early and therefore do not increase the cure rate for this cancer. Chest x-rays are too insensitive. It is usually not possible for the radiologist to see small, curable cancers on chest x-rays.

One of the reasons why lung cancer cannot be diagnosed early is that the lungs and bronchi are inaccessible. Therefore, no equivalent to a Pap smear for cervical cancer is available. When sputum is available for cytologic examination under the microscope, it may be helpful; however, people do not usually cough up sputum with very early lung cancers, so often it is not possible to obtain adequate screening specimens. Moreover, even if an early lung cancer is found by sputum cytology, it is sometimes not possible to find with either chest x-rays or bronchoscopy. A lung cancer must be more than one-half inch in diameter to be seen on x-ray. So even if a very small lung cancer is found by examining your sputum for cancer cells it may not be possible to find that cancer and remove it surgically. You must wait until it grows large enough to be seen on your chest x-ray. In short, early diagnosis of lung cancer is not usually possible with current techniques.

Cancers of the lung are usually quite advanced by the time they are diagnosed. Usually they have already metastasized, or spread, cannot be completely removed by surgery, and are thus incurable. Over the past several decades there has been no improvement in the cure rate. Only 5–10 percent of people live more than five years after they develop lung cancer; most people are dead within one to two years.

Diagnosis

Most lung cancer develops in people who smoke heavily. The usual first symptoms are a worsening of existing chest symptoms. Many heavy smokers already have such symptoms as chronic cough, sputum production, and chest pains. These may be due to the chronic lung disease and bronchial infections related to cigarette smoking. However, if any of the above symptoms develop or worsen, you should see your doctor, who will try to find out if you have lung cancer.

This can usually be done without an operation. First, a chest-x-ray is taken, which can show a shadow or mass in the lung. If the x-ray is normal, no further tests for lung cancer are useful. If a shadow is seen, the next step is to find out whether the shadow is due to lung cancer.

Most of the time this can be done by collecting several samples of sputum and examining them for malignant cells. In 75 percent of cases the pathologist can find the cancer cells in the sputum if lung cancer is present. However, if the sputum cytologies are negative, the next diagnostic test is a bronchoscopy. A major improvement has been the recent development of the flexible fiberoptic bronchoscope, which is smaller, more flexible, and therefore much easier to tolerate than the older rigid metal bronchoscopes. Bronchoscopic examination is performed under light sedation with the throat sprayed with a local anesthetic to prevent gagging. The bronchoscope is placed through the mouth and down through the bronchial tree to the suspicious area in the lung. The physician can look directly through the bronchoscope to see if cancer is present in the bronchus and obtain tiny biopsies of any suspicious areas. Almost all people with lung cancer can be diagnosed by either sputum cytology or bronchoscopy.

There are two important subtypes of lung cancer. Seventy percent of people develop squamous cell carcinoma, adenocarcinoma, or large cell carcinoma of the lung, and 30 percent have small carcinoma, also called oat cell cancer, of the lung. Squamous cell carcinoma, adenocarcinoma, and large cell carcinoma are evaluated and treated the same way, and therefore will be discussed together. They are often referred to as non–small (oat) cell lung cancers. Small cell lung cancer is evaluated and treated differently from the other types and is discussed separately.

NON–OAT CELL LUNG CANCER (SQUAMOUS CELL, ADENO, AND LARGE CELL CANCERS OF THE LUNG): CAN THE CANCER BE SURGICALLY REMOVED?

Once lung cancer has been diagnosed, the next important step is to evaluate the extent of the cancer. The questions are: is it localized? can it be surgically removed? It is important to do a careful and complete evaluation because surgery for lung cancer is major surgery with an appreciable risk and only a few people can be cured. Therefore, if a test can be done that is safe and tells the surgeon that a patient will not be cured by surgery because the cancer is too advanced, the patient can be saved from unnecessary major surgery.

Here are some figures that explain why so many tests should be obtained before surgery is undertaken. Out of every 100 people who have non–oat cell lung cancer, only 50 will be found suitable for operation. For the other 50, tests show that cancer has spread beyond the lung and therefore cannot be entirely removed by surgery. Operable patients are those whose disease is still possibly curable after tests have been performed looking for spread and who are in good enough condition to undergo major surgery. However, out of these 50, or half of the original 100 who undergo surgery, only half have their cancer completely removed. Therefore, only 25 percent of patients who have non–oat cell lung cancer can even have a chance for cure. Of these, only approximately one-third are cured. Thus, only 5–10 percent of all patients with non–oat cell cancer are cured by surgery. Obviously, it pays to find out before surgery that cure is impossible and therefore to avoid the risks, the costs, and the time spent in the hospital.

The tests usually obtained before surgery include a liver scan and a bone scan to detect metastases to these organs. If these are normal, many surgeons will perform a scalene node biopsy. The scalene lymph nodes are located in the left lower part of the neck, and in about 20 percent of persons with lung cancer, cancer is found in these nodes even if they are not enlarged.

If the scalene node biopsy is normal, the next and very important test is mediastinoscopy. This test is usually done under general anesthesia. A small incision is made below the neck and a tube inserted so that the physician may directly examine and biopsy lymph nodes surrounding the roots of the lungs. If cancer is found in these lymph glands, the disease is incurable. Mediastinoscopy is a very important test because approximately 25 percent of patients who undergo this procedure are found to have metastases to the lymph nodes, and therefore are not curable by surgery. To put it another way, 25 out of every 100 patients who undergo mediastinoscopy are spared major surgery that cannot help them. When these tests are finished, there is enough information to decide whether or not to operate.

Treatment

Surgery Surgery is the only curative method of therapy for lung cancer at present. However, only 50 percent of people with non–oat cell lung cancer are candidates for surgery. The other 50 percent have disease that is so extensive that it cannot be removed by surgery. Also, before surgery can be performed with potentially curable cancer, it is important to assess the state of the lungs by pulmonary function tests. The question now is: can the patient tolerate removal of a lung or part of a lung? For these tests you are asked to breathe into a cylinder that measures your lung function and tells your physician whether or not you can survive cancer surgery. Most people who develop lung cancer are not young and have smoked for years. They usually have chronic lung disease. Therefore, it is not too uncommon for someone not to be able to undergo surgery even if the cancer is potentially curable. Surgery should only be done if there is no evidence of spread of the cancer beyond the lung and if lung function is good enough to survive surgery.

The board-certified thoracic surgeon.   Surgery for lung cancer involves removing part of a lung (lobectomy) or the whole lung (pneumonectomy) and should be performed by an experienced, board-certified thoracic surgeon. A thoracic surgeon has had training in general surgery and in addition two years of specialized training in chest surgery. Most middle-sized and larger communities have a board-certified thoracic surgeon. Your family physician or internist will probably refer you to one.

Five to ten percent of people who undergo surgery for lung cancer will die from direct complications of the surgery. Therefore, you should not only try to get the best surgeon available, but you should not undergo surgery without the previously described tests. If surgery cannot cure you, it will not prolong your life.

Radiation For the majority of people whose cancer cannot be surgically removed, cure is impossible and the aim of treatment should be to relieve or prevent symptoms such as pain, pneumonia, or coughing up blood from the lung. Although radiation plays the key role in preventing and treating these problems, it only rarely prolongs life. The use of radiation in non–oat cell lung cancer must be tailored to fit each person's situation. In some cases radiation is not indicated, but most will require some radiation sooner or later. Radiation is used to shrink the cancer in the lung if it is pressing on and obstructing the bronchial tubes. An obstructed bronchial tube can lead to pneumonia. Radiation is also used to shrink the cancer in the lung if it is causing pain or bloody sputum. Radiation can usually control these problems and make the patient much more comfortable.

Radiation to the lungs is usually given over a three- to four-week period and is relatively nontoxic. One side effect is temporary irritation of the esophagus, or swallowing tube, which may make it difficult or painful to eat. People may also lose their sense of taste, and their appetite may decrease temporarily.

Radiation is extremely useful in controlling pain due to metastases to bone, a common problem in lung cancer. It also relieves symptoms from metastases to the brain such as severe headaches. (See chapter 17, "Brain Tumors.") Radiation is used to control problems or symptoms, but does not usually prolong life. Therefore, whenever possible, low doses of radiation are given over a short period of time. The object is to control problems with as little cost in time, money, and side effects as possible. For example, radiation for painful bone metastases is given over a two-week period and almost always successfully relieves pain with no side effects. Radiation for brain metastases is also given over two to three weeks. Temporary hair loss is the only usual side effect.

In summary, the judicious use of radiation plays a key role in controlling problems of lung cancer but usually does not prolong life.

Chemotherapy Chemotherapy for squamous cell, adeno, and non–oat cell types of lung cancer is relatively ineffective. It does not offer a chance for cure. About 20 percent of people will improve, usually for short periods of time (months), with moderate doses of chemotherapy. Your chances of responding to chemotherapy do increase somewhat if you take higher doses of combination chemotherapy, but so do the side effects, and the responses to more aggressive chemotherapy are usually short. Since the aim of therapy is to make you feel better or to control problems, the advantages and disadvantages of treatment must be carefully balanced. For example, if your cancer shrinks or gets smaller for three months but you are sick much of the time from the chemotherapy, and in fact lose weight and feel weaker because of the chemotherapy, you have not benefited from the treatment even though it controlled the growth of your cancer. We know that what we advise is difficult to accept. We suggest that, if you have non–oat cell lung cancer, you take either low-dose, nontoxic chemotherapy or no chemotherapy.

If you feel the need to try something that might give you more hope, there are experimental treatment programs available throughout the country. Thus far, these experimental regimens have not prolonged life and are very toxic. However, some people may be helped. Above all, we feel you should have the facts and make your own well-informed choice.

F.R., a forty-six-year-old schoolteacher, had smoked one to two packs of cigarettes each day since he had entered the army during the Korean War at age eighteen. He had always been in good health, was married, and had two children, ages fourteen and sixteen. As part of his employment health examination, he had yearly chest x-rays. An abnormality was noted on one of these chest x-rays, and he was referred to a community hospital. He felt entirely well and had a normal physical examination. However his chest x-ray did show a 1½-by-2½ inch shadow in his right lung that was very suspicious for lung cancer. F.R. was asked to expectorate his sputum into a cup so that it could be sent for microscopic examination. Six specimens were collected and examined, but they were all normal. Therefore, he underwent bronchoscopy. His doctors were able to examine the bronchial tree and with a tiny forceps biopsy the area of the lung shadow. The biopsy showed squamous cell carcinoma of the lung. Next, F.R. had a liver and spleen scans, which were normal, and a scalene node biopsy and mediastinoscopy, which did not show cancer. Because the cancer appeared localized, he underwent surgery (lobectomy), and a small lung cancer was removed, along with some surrounding lung tissue. Pathologic examination of the specimen showed no evidence of cancer cells at the edges of the resected tissue. The lymph nodes were also normal. Therefore, the entire cancer was removed. F.R. was told he had a reasonable chance of having been cured, and he recuperated promptly and was back at work in two weeks.

F.R. felt well for the next four months but then began to notice right-sided headaches that were worst in the morning. He thought little of this for about one week, but as the headaches became increasingly severe, he went back to see his doctor. After examining him, his doctor ordered a brain scan, which is capable of detecting the presence of cancer that has spread to the brain. Indeed, his scan showed three separate abnormalities, all highly suspicious for cancer. He was immediately placed on a drug (Decadron) that reduced the brain swelling, and he was referred to a radiation oncologist, who administered radiation for a two-week period. His headaches disappeared completely, and the only side effects from the radiation were minimal mouth soreness and the loss of his hair (which grew back normally over the next few months).

He felt well again, returned to work, and resumed most of his other usual activities for the next eight months. Then he developed pain in his right hip, and a bone scan showed spread to this area. Again, a two-week course of radiation to the right hip completely controlled the bone pain without any side effects.

F.R. again felt well, but this time only for two and a half months. He began to lose his appetite, felt tired, and had fullness in his abdomen. His doctor found spread to his liver. F.R. was sent to a medical oncologist, who had to tell him that chemotherapy was not very effective for lung cancer. F.R. thought about his options and he decided to take low-dose, nontoxic chemotherapy. He was given a single drug for several weeks but the cancer progressed, and he died eight weeks later from pneumonia due to his weakened state.

What happened to F.R. happens all too commonly with lung cancer. His tests showed no spread and his cancer was completely removed. But F.R. was not cured because the cancer had indeed spread. Although better and better tests have been developed to look for metastases, they still have limits. F.R. had a bone scan and liver scan that were normal, and yet metastases must have been present at the time of surgery. They were too small to be detected. Unfortunately, even if your cancer can be resected, your chances for cure are still not good. F.R.'s case does highlight how effective radiation can be in controlling symptoms. His bone pain and his headaches were totally controlled with very low doses of radiation, allowing him to live almost a year feeling well most of the time.

SMALL CELL (OAT CELL) CARCINOMA OF THE LUNG

Small cell carcinoma of the lung is different from the other subtypes of lung cancer. The important differences are:

—Oat cell carcinoma of the lung is a very rapidly growing and early metastasizing cancer. By the time it is diagnosed, metastases to other parts of the body have occurred in moɩe than 95 percent of patients. Therefore, oat cell carcinoma is almost never cured, even if the cancer in the lung is completely eradicated. In almost all cases it has already spread beyond the lung.

—Oat cell carcinoma is very responsive or sensitive to radiation therapy. Radiation can completely eradicate local deposits of this cancer. Therefore, there is no place for surgery in the treatment of oat cell carcinoma.

—Chemotherapy is effective in the treatment of oat cell carcinoma, though not for other types of lung cancer. Several drugs are effective against this cancer, and they work even better if used together. Combination chemotherapy (the use of two or more anticancer drugs together) for oat cell carcinoma helps more than two-thirds of people. They will feel better and also live longer. Thus, chemotherapy is a key treatment for oat cell carcinoma. Radiation is often being used as a supplement, but surgery has no place in the treatment of this type of lung cancer.

Diagnosis and Testing for Metastases

The diagnosis of oat cell carcinoma is made exactly as with the other types of lung cancer—by sputum cytologies or bronchoscopy. However, the process of testing for metastases is different from that for non–oat cell cancers. The object of these tests is to decide how best to use chemotherapy and radiation and not to decide if surgery should be done. Therefore, mediastinoscopy and scalene node biopsy need not be done. We repeat, surgery has no place in the treatment of this disease. After the diagnosis of oat cell cancer, the next step is a thorough search for metastases. A liver scan, bone scan, brain scan, and bone marrow biopsy are usually obtained. Because oat cell carcinoma spreads more rapidly than other types of lung cancer, more tests are needed to look for these metastases.

In summary, then, the tests done to evaluate the extent of this type of cancer concentrate on the search for metastases to other organs rather than looking for local spread to the lymph nodes in the area of the lung.

Treatment

Chemotherapy and supplemental radiotherapy are the mainstays of treatment for oat cell cancer. If no metastases are found, radiation is given to control the cancer in the lung and nearby lymph nodes, and chemotherapy is used to treat the presumed metastases. More than 95 percent of patients harbor microscopic deposits of tumor in other organs and need systemic treatment with chemotherapy. The combination of high-dose chemotherapy and radiation can cure some of these people. If the tests show spread to the liver, bones, brain, or other organs, chemotherapy is used as the main treatment and radiation is only used as a supplement to control the cancer when chemotherapy is not effective.

The treatment for oat cell carcinoma of the lung is more complicated than that for other subtypes, since chemotherapy and radiation are often used together. In order to do this, the treatments must be coordinated. Therefore, it is important that you be evaluated by both a radiation oncologist and a medical oncologist, who together should plan your treatment. Because many of the side effects from radiation and chemotherapy are similar, the treatments must be coordinated so that side effects or toxicity are minimized. For instance, both radiation and chemotherapy damage the bone marrow, resulting in low blood counts; one cannot use full doses of radiation and chemotherapy if one wants to use both together.

Many new drugs and combinations are under evaluation. In general, we use high doses of combination chemotherapy because this benefits most patients: they will feel better and live longer because of treatment. However, because we are using high doses of drugs, there are many side effects, including fatigue, nausea, vomiting, temporary hair loss, and depression of bone marrow function. The last causes lowered blood counts, which can lead to bleeding and the danger of serious infections. Although you can expect to have side effects from therapy, most often you will ultimately feel better and live longer because the treatment is so effective.

Modern chemotherapy for oat cell cancer is the only significant advance in the treatment of lung cancer in the past two decades. Prior to modern chemotherapy, most people with this disease died within three months. Now, some people are cured and many live one or more years.

J.S., a forty-two-year-old automobile salesman, had smoked two packs of cigarettes a day for over twenty years. He noticed an increasing cough, fatigue, and a decreased appetite. By the time he went to see his physician, he had lost eighteen pounds and was feeling so badly that he was unable to get through a day of work. His physician found an enlarged liver. His chest x-ray showed a small shadow in the middle of the left lung with enlarged lymph nodes in the area around the heart, called the mediastinum. J.S. was admitted to the hospital for evaluation. Sputum cytology showed oat cell cancer. Because his liver was enlarged, a liver scan was obtained, and it showed several areas that were almost certainly involved with cancer.

J.S. was sent to a medical oncologist for cancer chemotherapy, since the disease had spread to his liver and radiation to his lung would not have helped him. The medical oncologist explained to J.S. that drugs would have a good chance of helping him but that cure was probably impossible. J.S. started treatment with a combination of three drugs. Within two weeks he felt much stronger. He was hungry again and was gaining weight. His liver decreased to normal size, and his chest x-ray showed disappearance of the cancer. Within five weeks he was back to work, feeling much better. He was treated every three weeks with this drug combination and had only mild side effects. He would be tired and lose his appetite during the evening on the day he received the drugs. He lost his hair and started to wear a wig. But the rest of the time he felt well. Nine months later J.S. again began to feel tired and lost his appetite. A chest x-ray showed that his cancer had begun to grow again. Despite the use of other drugs, the disease grew quickly, and he died of pneumonia one year after the diagnosis had been made.

This case illustrates several very typical points about oat cell cancer. Oat cell cancer of the lung grows very quickly and has almost always spread beyond the lungs by the time it is diagnosed. This was the case with J.S., who had liver metastases when first seen. Because the disease is widespread, it cannot be controlled with surgery or radiation alone, and thus chemotherapy is the mainstay of treatment. Most people benefit from chemotherapy. Without drugs, J.S. would have died within a month or two, but with therapy he lived many months longer and felt well. It is also obvious that modern chemotherapy isn't good enough, since most people have their disease controlled for only about one year. The main point about oat cell carcinoma is not that people do better with it than with other types of lung cancer, but that therapy, mainly chemotherapy and radiation, can help most people. This is not true for non–oat cell lung cancer.

This is the only type of lung cancer for which new and more aggressive types of therapy make sense. The more intensive the chemotherapy used, the better your chance of responding and the longer you will probably live. The chemotherapy should be administered by or at least directed by a board-certified medical oncologist. Some people may wish to travel to major medical centers that offer experimental treatment for this disease so that they many benefit from the most recent advances in therapy. It is worth traveling to the nearest medical center that has a board-certified radiation therapist and a medical oncologist. Treatment can be planned that often may be administered by your family physician or an internist in your own community.

What, then, is to be done about this terrible disease? Lung cancer can be prevented. All we have to do is convince people not to expose themselves to carcinogens. The American Cancer Society is currently conducting a major campaign to convince teenagers not to smoke. People should be encouraged to give up smoking, to cut down on smoking, or to switch to low tar and nicotine cigarettes. Research into carinogen-free tobacco should be encouraged. The government could mount massive education campaigns and use punitive taxation to fund research into carcinogenesis and the development of a noncarcinogenic tobacco. It has been estimated that cigarette-induced illness, which includes not only many cancers but heart disease and many vascular diseases, accounts for 20–30 percent of our annual expenditures in this country for health care. This is a greater share than alcohol-induced illness. With our astronomical annual budget for health care, some money could be well spent if it were diverted to research aimed at preventing tobacco-induced diseases.

Lung cancer, then, remains a terrible disease that is for the most part self-inflicted. It often has its origins early in life, when at age twelve to sixteen a young person, in an effort to emulate his or her parents or peers and to appear more mature, lights the first cigarette. We as physicians and you as readers have little control over the individual who chooses to smoke. We must, however, exert control over our environment. We must control involuntary exposure to carcinogens such as asbestos and smoke from other people's cigarettes.

SUMMARY

1. Cigarette smoking is the major cause of lung cancer. The risk increases the more you smoke, the longer you have been smoking, and the higher the tar content of your cigarettes. It pays to stop smoking, because ten years after discontinuation of cigarette smoking, your risk decreases to that of nonsmokers.

2. Other carcinogens associated with an increased risk of lung cancer are asbestos, arsenic, nickel, chromium, and radioactive elements. Exposure to those carcinogens is most common in factories and mines.

3. It is impossible to diagnose most lung cancers early. Nevertheless, if you are a heavy smoker, it pays to have a chest x-ray once or twice a year, because occasionally a small and still curable lung cancer may be found.

4. The usual symptoms of lung cancer occur fairly late in the disease and include chest pain, bloody sputum, a persistent cough, and shortness of breath. If you smoke cigarettes and have any of these symptoms, you should see your doctor.

5. The chances of cure if you have lung cancer are extremely small. Between 5 and 10 percent of patients with non–oat cell lung cancer are cured with surgery, and less than 5 percent with oat cell carcinoma are cured with radiation and chemotherapy.

6. The treatment of non–oat cell lung cancers (in which we include squamous cell carcinoma, adenocarcinoma, and large cell carcinoma of the lung) is surgery, if the tumor is curable. Surgery offers the only chance for cure with these types of lung cancer.

7. Radiation can be useful to control specific problems or symptoms such as pain due to metastases.

8. Chemotherapy for non–oat cell lung cancer is relatively noneffective. Therefore, we recommend either no chemotherapy or low-dose chemotherapy. There is no evidence that high-dose chemotherapy is of any benefit for these subtypes of lung cancer.

9. Treatment for non–oat cell lung cancer is available even in many smaller community hospitals. It is of questionable benefit to travel to major cancer centers for experimental therapy. A board-certified thoracic surgeon should perform the operation if one can be done. Radiotherapy should be given by a board-certified radiation oncologist.

10. The basic treatment for oat cell carcinoma of the lung is combination chemotherapy, which will make most patients feel better and prolong life. Nevertheless, chemotherapy is not usually curative for this disease.

11. Radiation is also very useful for oat cell cancer. It controls local problems such as pain and can relieve symptoms that don't respond to chemotherapy.

12. If you have oat cell cancer you should be treated by, or at least have your care planned by, a board-certified medical oncologist and a board-certified radiation oncologist.

23

Cancer in Children

Although cancer is much less common in children than in adults, it is the second most common cause of death between the ages of one and fifteen. Only accidents claim more lives than cancer in American children. Approximately 6,000 children develop cancer and 3,000 die from it each year. The main message of this chapter is that children with cancer should be treated or have treatment planned at a major medical center, usually a children's hospital in a large city or a cancer center. There are two very important reasons for this.

First, childhood cancers are very malignant and are rapidly fatal unless treated successfully. Fortunately, there have been striking advances in the treatment of most childhood cancers. With modern therapy, prolonged survival and cures are now possible with most types of childhood cancer. But the treatment is complicated and can require a combination of surgery, radiation, and chemotherapy. Thus, a team of specialists experienced and trained in the treatment of childhood cancer is necessary. These specialists are usually found only in cancer centers or large children's hospitals.

Children with cancer need specialists trained and experienced in the evaluation and treatment of childhood cancers. The surgery should be done by a surgeon who has received formal training in children's surgery in addition to training in adult surgery. Such surgeons usually don't restrict their practice only to children except at very large medical centers. Surgeons who have this training and who have also passed a test become board-certified pediatric general surgeons, thoracic surgeons, or urologists. Likewise, a pediatric oncologist is a pediatrician, or children's doctor, who has received several years of additional training in the treatment of childhood cancer with chemotherapy. After this training and passing a test, he or she becomes a board-certified pediatric oncologist. There are no formal training programs in pediatric radiation therapy, so there is no test for board certification. There are, however, radiation oncologists who have experience in treating children with radiation at large children's hospitals or cancer centers. Most childhood cancers need to be treated with surgery, radiation, and chemotherapy to cure them. Treatment is extremely complex, as all three treatments must be carefully integrated for the best results. You want a team of specialists in childhood cancer to evaluate, plan, and at least start treatment if your child has cancer.

The second reason to go to a large medical center is for the psychological help it can offer. The psychological impact upon the family whose child has cancer is extremely difficult to describe. The parents must face the possibility of their child's suffering and dying from cancer. In addition, the whole family structure is altered. The parents must often concentrate on the sick child and ignore other children. In fact, every aspect of family life and normal interactions is altered. Most families need help to get through this severe crisis. The children's hospitals and cancer centers that specialize in the treatment of childhood malignancies offer psychological support to the family and to the child with cancer. This support is not available in most communities.

The nurses and doctors in major children's hospitals are used to dealing with children with cancer and with their families. In addition, there are social workers, psychologists, and psychiatrists available to help. Finally, there are other families whose children have cancer. This offers the opportunity for families to talk together and find that they are not alone with their burden. Even for the children, it helps to see other children with similar problems. They feel less singled out than if they are the only child with cancer in a small community hospital.

Therefore, both for the best medical treatment and for the psychological support, the place for a child with cancer to be is a large center that treats many children with cancer. These centers have the specialists in surgery, radiation, and chemotherapy who can offer your child the best modern medical care and the psychological support that most families need to survive this terrible crisis.

Childhood cancer differs significantly from cancer in adults in a number of ways: Cancer in children arises from a few organs or sites. More than 90 percent of all childhood cancers arise from the blood and lymph, the nervous system, the bones and connective tissues, the kidneys, and the eyes. Cancers from these organs are relatively uncommon in adults and, likewise, the common cancers in adults (such as cancer of the breast, colon and rectum, lung, uterus, cervix, and skin) are extremely rare in children.

Childhood cancers are usually very malignant. They grow fast and spread, or metastasize, widely to other parts of the body quite early. Without effective treatment survival tends to be short.

Fortunately the most striking advances in cancer treatment have occurred in the treatment of childhood cancers. Twenty years ago, almost all children with cancer died, usually within one year. At present, up to half of the children with cancer can now be cured with the best therapy. Similar advances in the treatment of most adult cancers have not occurred. The factors responsible for the remarkable progress in treating childhood cancers are:

—These cancers respond to many different anticancer drugs.

—These cancers also usually respond well to radiation therapy.

—There is a centrally organized, well-run group of medical centers that concentrate on treating children with cancer and have dedicated themselves to offering the best treatment to children with cancer. They test the effectiveness of new treatments with experimental studies. Medical centers such as St. Jude's in Tennessee, Children's Hospital in Philadelphia, Sloan Kettering in New York, and many others have participated in studies that have shown the path to better treatment. Of course, since there is a long way to go before all children can be cured, these studies continue. Although half the children are currently cured, half still die of cancer.

Studies are also in progress to determine whether too much treatment is being used for some cancers. Chemotherapy, radiation, and surgery all have unwanted side effects, especially in children. It is important to find out if less chemotherapy, radiation, or surgery can be used so that the side effects of therapy are decreased without decreasing the number of children who are cured.

Adjuvant chemotherapy, that is, chemotherapy to treat assumed but unproven tiny metastases after surgery, and/or irradiation is of proven value in several childhood cancers, including Ewing's sarcoma, osteogenic sarcoma, Wilms' tumor, and rhabdomyosarcoma. Adjuvant chemotherapy definitely increases the number of children who are cured with these cancers. In contrast, its value in adult tumors is largely unproven. In fact, only in menstruating women with breast cancer that involves lymph nodes has adjuvant chemotherapy been shown to be of probable value.

We, therefore, recommend that children with cancer be evaluated and treated or have treatment planned at a large children's hospital or cancer center. The chances for cure are much greater if the child receives the best treatment. Children are often evaluated and treatment is planned and started at a medical center. It can then be continued in a smaller community. This enables the child to be treated in or near his home. The best treatment can be given with minimal cost and dislocation for the child and the family.

Psychological Aspects of Childhood Cancer

There is probably no situation more difficult for parents to face than the dreadful possibility of their child's suffering and dying from cancer or any other illness. Parents and other children may have more difficulty emotionally handling the child's illness than the child himself.

Divorces may occur among parents of children with cancer. Many studies show that disease, as any other stress, worsens problems that have long existed between the husband and the wife. The child with cancer doesn't cause a close relationship to rupture. Those who were close often become closer; those who were having problems often have more, and this may lead to separation or divorce.

Brothers and sisters often have great difficulty dealing with the attention the parents give to the sick child at their expense. They can become angry and feel guilty about their anger. They may also feel guilty that their brother or sister got cancer. These feelings may take years to deal with and recover from. Counseling is usually necessary for the parents, the healthy children, and the child with cancer.

To compound the problem, the family must also often face economic hardship. Cancer is an expensive illness, and cancer in children can be even more expensive than cancer in adults. Often the family and child must travel to a distant city to a large medical center. Therefore, not only must hospital bills be met, but also motel or hotel rooms, which are not covered by health insurance. In addition, at least one parent may have to give up a job. Since both parents work in almost 50 percent of American families, the loss of the income of one parent and often a decrease in income from the other add to the financial woes. Special schools and/or tutors are necessary to allow the child with cancer to remain at the same grade level as his classmates. These are sometimes supplied by the school system but private schools may become necessary. Thus, in addition to the psychological affront caused by the child with cancer, a financial crisis is precipitated. No family can deal with this situation easily.

The hospital or medical center that routinely treats many children with cancer offers many services to help the family cope with this stressful situation. Usually both individual and group therapy are available for the parents and other children. There is also the opportunity to meet other families in the same situation. This is not merely helpful, it is often necessary for the family to survive. Discussion groups between parents and children with cancer are often formed and the parents and the children are encouraged to talk freely about what is happening with the child and the child's cancer. Parents are encouraged to interact with the parents of other children with cancer and to discuss common problems. Parents can discuss with others how to deal with their feelings about their child who may undergo mutilating surgery, toxic radiation, and chemotherapy. They can also share their fears about the death of their child. The very meaning of death for the family members and the child is frequently discussed. Just being able to talk about these problems and knowing that others are facing them, or have faced them and have survived, is extremely important. A national group, the Candlelighters, has been formed by these parents to help each other.

Children are not very different from adults. When they have a serious illness, they fear death and are usually aware of their impending death. It is almost impossible to hide the gravity of cancer from children. When in the hospital they see other children with cancer dying. Children discuss their illness with other children and with the staff. We think this is healthy. We feel that the children should feel free to talk with their parents, their brothers and sisters, other children, and the hospital staff.

Children with cancer must face their illnesses. In a large childhood cancer center there are doctors, nurses, social workers, and others who are experienced and feel at ease in helping the child face the disease, the treatment, and possible death.

It is important that the child continue to feel part of the family and not hide his fears from his parents to avoid upsetting them. Similarly, parents should not hide their fears. The child with cancer and his family must feel free to communicate during this stressful time. The doctors, nurses, and others on the staff at these large medical centers can often help such communication. Surprisingly, many families become closer and more intimate, and they remember in a positive way this stressful period even if the child dies. It can be a time of solidification of relationships between the husband and wife, between the parents and the other children, as well as between the parents and the ill child.

Six childhood cancers will be discussed in this chapter: Wilms' tumor, neuroblastoma, rhabdomyosarcoma, Ewing's sarcoma, osteogenic sarcoma, and acute lymphocytic leukemia. In the past almost all children with these cancers died. Now, with therapy, the survival of most of these cancers has been significantly prolonged and more children are cured. Brain tumors, which are not uncommon in childhood, are discussed in chapter 17. Malignant lymphomas in children, which include non-Hodgkin's lymphoma and Hodgkin's disease, are discussed in chapter 18.

WILMS' TUMOR

Wilms' tumor is a kidney tumor of children. In the United States, approximately 500 children a year develop this cancer, which represents about 7 percent of cancer in children. This is a cancer of early childhood and has even occurred in utero. More than half the cases occur before age four and 90 percent before age eight. The tumor can arise from any portion of either kidney. It often attains great size by the time it is diagnosed due to rapid growth and bleeding within the tumor. At the time of discovery it may weigh up to ten pounds. Occasionally, the tumor can be so large that it fills half of the abdomen. About 10 percent of the children have both kidneys involved. There is an increased incidence of Wilms' tumor in children with developmental anomalies such as hemihypertrophy, a condition in which one half of the body is larger than the other, and a variety of urinary tract malformations.

Diagnosis

Wilms' tumor is diagnosed when it has grown large enough to be felt by a parent while bathing or dressing a child or by a pediatrician or family doctor doing a routine checkup. As a rule, the child has no symptoms whatsoever, though some have abdominal pain, fevers, high blood pressure, or blood in the urine. Signs of more advanced Wilms' tumor are weight loss, loss of appetite, and tiredness or lack of pep. These symptoms may mean the child has metastatic disease.

If you feel that your child's abdomen is swollen and the swelling persists for more than several days, you should take the child to your pediatrician or family doctor. If, on examining the child, he also feels that a mass or lump is present in the abdomen, he should send the child immediately to a major medical center, to a children's cancer center, or to a large hospital for further evaluation and treatment.

The evaluation should be done quickly. First an intravenous pyelogram, an x-ray of the kidney, is obtained. This will show whether the tumor arises from the kidney. If it does, the tumor is most likely a Wilms' tumor. A chest x-ray, bone scan, and liver scan are also usually obtained to test for spread to other organs.

Treatment

The treatment of Wilms' tumor consists of surgery, radiation, and chemotherapy used together to treat all of the cancer cells. Surgery, often with radiation, is used to treat the cancer in the abdomen. In the past radiation was given to all children after surgery. However, recent studies have shown that radiation isn't needed in all children; for example, children under two who have tumors completely removed by surgery do as well with surgery alone. Chemotherapy is used in all children to kill cancer cells that have spread to other parts of the body.

At surgery the surgeon will remove as much of the tumor as possible. He, or she, also looks at the other kidney, the liver, and the rest of the abdomen for possible metastases. If the tumor is too large to be removed by surgery, either chemotherapy or radiation must be given first to shrink the tumor. In most cases, surgical removal of most or all of the tumor is possible. Radiation, directed to the area of the tumor, is usually given after surgery. Approximately three to four weeks of radiation is administered. Chemotherapy is started at the same time and continued for one to one and a half years. This treats cancer cells that may have spread to other parts of the body.

The cure rate for Wilms' tumor has improved significantly with the combined approach. Approximately 40 percent of children were cured with surgery alone and perhaps 10 percent more when radiation was used with surgery. However, with the addition of chemotherapy to treat cancer cells that have already spread, approximately 80 percent of children are now cured. This was the first cancer in which the use of chemotherapy in conjunction with surgery and/or radiation was tried and found to be of definite benefit. Chemotherapy in Wilms' tumor increased the number of children who were cured by eliminating microscopic deposits of cancer cells in the lungs, liver, and elsewhere.

Mrs. Jones took her two-year-old son, Edward, to the pediatrician when she noticed that his abdomen was enlarged. The pediatrician felt a large, hard mass in Edward's abdomen that he believed was probably cancer, either Wilms' tumor or neuroblastoma. He told Mrs. Jones about his suspicion that Edward might have cancer and advised her to take him to a large children's hospital 300 miles away. Mrs. Jones was in a panic. After talking with her husband, she and her son went that evening to the hospital that the pediatrician had recommended.

Edward was examined by several doctors that evening and the next morning had a series of tests. An intravenous pyelogram showed that the mass arose from the kidney and was almost certainly a Wilms' tumor. Other tests to evaluate whether the cancer had spread to other organs included a chest x-ray, a liver scan, and a bone scan, which were normal.

The pediatric surgeon had a long talk with Mrs. Jones to explain her son's condition. Edward almost certainly had a Wilms' tumor. It was a very large tumor but probably was still localized to the abdomen. She was told that this was a malignant tumor but that with modern treatment (which included removing as much of the tumor as possible with surgery, radiating the area of tumor, and giving chemotherapy for two years) there was a good chance of a cure.

Mrs. Jones talked with her husband, and they agreed to the operation. The next day Edward was taken to surgery and a two-pound tumor arising from the right kidney was removed. The surgeons found no spread of the tumor in the abdomen but pathologic examination of the kidney tumor and surrounding tissues showed that the tumor had not been completely cut out.

Edward recovered quickly from surgery, as most children do. Over the next several days, Mrs. Jones found out more about Wilms' tumor. She gradually came to understand that radiation and chemotherapy, although time consuming, costly, and unpleasant, offered him the best chance for cure. She had several talks with Edward's physicians and was given some pamphlets to read about Wilms' tumor that had been prepared specifically for parents of children who have this cancer. She talked on the phone several times to her husband, and both agreed that Edward should get the treatment the doctors recommended—radiation and chemotherapy.

Edward received radiation over a three-week period of time with almost no side effects. In fact, he recovered from his operation, left the hospital, and lived with his mother in a motel while the radiation was completed. He was also started on chemotherapy while still receiving radiation. The chemotherapy did make him ill. He had trouble eating and vomited several times. The nausea and vomiting disappeared several days after the chemotherapy was completed. Five weeks after arriving at the children's hospital, he was ready to go home again. He had had surgery, recovered, and received radiation. He had begun a long course of chemotherapy and all was going well. Tests showed no evidence of metastases and Edward was getting stronger by the day.

Edward went back to his hometown and received chemotherapy for five days every three months over a year and a half. The drugs were given by his pediatrician with guidance from the pediatric oncologist at the cancer hospital where Edward was first treated. Edward lived an almost normal life. During the days he got chemotherapy—five days every three months—he felt tired and occasionally vomited. Between these times, he felt well and was a very active child.

He returned to the large children's hospital every six months for a checkup. Finally, after a year and a half of chemotherapy, he had his last checkup. Extensive tests for Wilms' tumor where negative. His parents were told he had a good chance for cure but it was too early to tell.

Over the next two years all went well. Edward felt well and the tumor did not recur. The doctors told Mr. and Mrs. Jones that Edward was almost certainly cured. Wilms' cancer, like most other cancers in children, recurs quickly after treatment is stopped if the cancer is not cured. At long last the parents relaxed. They no longer looked at Edward and wondered if he would be with them for long.

This case illustrates some very important points about Wilms' tumor and the treatment of childhood tumors. The pediatrician wisely sent the family and child to a large center where a pediatric surgeon, a radiation oncologist, and a pediatric oncologist were available to evaluate Edward and plan his treatment. Although the treatment was aggressive and had many side effects, children are strong. Most children can take a lot of therapy and still function quite well. During most of the eighteen months Edward was treated, he felt normal. Edward, like 80 percent of children with Wilms' tumor, was cured. He will probably have a normal life span.

The treatment of Wilms' tumor has improved dramatically over the past decade. Surgery, radiation, and chemotherapy used together cure approximately 80 percent of the children. However, questions still remain that can only be answered by therapeutic trials. For instance, does every child with Wilms' tumor need so much therapy? Some children don't need radiation because surgery and chemotherapy are sufficient treatment. This is an important issue because all of the treatments have side effects. Radiation and chemotherapy are both carcinogenic, that is, they may cause second cancers. If possible, it is better to use one and not both in the same patient. On the other hand, perhaps children with more extensive Wilms' tumor need more chemotherapy than the usual vincristine and actinomycin D. Perhaps children with very extensive or a particular histologic type of Wilms' tumor should receive three or four drugs rather than just two. Trials are still in progress in attempt to improve treatment. If your child has Wilms' tumor, you may well be asked if you would allow your child to enter a clinical trial to evaluate one of these questions. These trials are usually well thought out and will offer your child good medical care, regardless of which treatment is chosen.

NEUROBLASTOMA

Neuroblastoma is another highly malignant tumor of children. It accounts for about 9 percent of childhood cancer. It most commonly occurs in infants and very young children and is rare over the age of thirteen. In fact, 50 percent of afflicted children are under two and 85 percent are under five. Neuroblastomas arise from remnants of embryonic or developmental nervous tissue and can occur anywhere in the body between the neck and the lower back. Most commonly, it arises in the abdomen. This is a highly malignant cancer that invades the local surrounding normal tissue and also spreads widely to other areas such as the bones, liver, skin, bone marrow, and lungs. In addition, it often secretes hormones called catecholamines that are normally produced by the adrenal gland. This may produce such symptoms as sweating, flushing, fast heart rate, anxiety or nervousness, and high blood pressure.

The first symptoms of neuroblastoma are due to the growth of the original tumor, to metastases, or to excessive secretion of catecholamines. Neuroblastomas are often discovered because of an abdominal mass, much like Wilms' tumor, or a neck mass. Many children are brought to the pediatrician because of fever, weakness, weight loss, excessive sweating, and other symptoms due either to metastases or to the secretion of catecholamines. Metastases can also cause bone pain or noticeable lumps in the skin.

Diagnosis

The evaluation for neuroblastoma depends on its presentation. In children who have an abdominal or neck mass as the first sign, an x-ray of the mass is done. More than half have calcifications in the tumor that can be seen on x-ray and that are almost diagnostic for this cancer. If neuroblastoma is suspected, one can also test the urine for breakdown products of catecholamines. The combination of a cancer in a young child and a positive urine test for catecholamines is diagnostic for neuroblastoma.

If the mass is abdominal, several tests are indicated. An intravenous pyelogram will demonstrate that the mass does not arise from the kidney and therefore is not a Wilms' tumor. Likewise, if the child's first symptom is bone pain, x-rays and bone scans are done, followed by a biopsy of the involved area. Neuroblastoma, unlike many other tumors, presents in many different ways, and the diagnostic workup and evaluation of the extent of the disease depend upon how it shows itself.

Evaluating the Extent of the Disease

For children who do not have obvious widespread metastases, it is very important to find out how much the tumor has spread before embarking on treatment. If the child presents with an abdominal or neck mass, a few tests, including a bone scan, a liver scan, a chest x-ray, and a bone marrow biopsy, are done to evaluate spread to other organs. With neuroblastoma, spread to other organs has already occurred in 50–70 percent of children when it is first discovered.

Prognosis

Age is an important prognostic factor. Young children do much better than older children. For example, a child born with neuroblastoma has almost a 100 percent chance of being cured, a child under the age of one has a 50 percent chance of cure, and a child older than two has only a 20 percent chance of cure. There are two reasons why younger children do better. Often they have localized tumors that can be removed by surgery. Young children are also cured because the tumor is less malignant. For example, children under the age of one can have widespread metastases to the bone marrow, liver, or skin (called stage 4-S disease). They don't usually die. Often the doctors merely observe the children and the tumor goes away without treatment. Other children need chemotherapy. In summary, neuroblastoma acts quite differently in young children from the way it acts in older children.

Treatment

The treatment of neuroblastoma depends upon the extent of the disease and the age of the child. Surgery, radiation, and chemotherapy are utilized depending on the extent of the cancer and also the age of the patient. Neuroblastoma is much harder to cure than Wilms' tumor. The disease is often widespread when it is discovered, and chemotherapy is not as effective for this cancer.

Surgical removal of neuroblastomas that are still localized is the treatment of choice. Radiation is usually administered to the bed of the cancer if all the tumor could not be removed. However, neuroblastomas are only moderately radiosensitive, that is, radiation will not reliably eradicate neuroblastomas, and often only temporarily controls the tumor. The use of chemotherapy to treat and eradicate microscopic metastases in children who initially have localized cancers is currently being tested. Thus, children with localized tumors are routinely treated with surgery and often also with radiation.

For the large majority of children with neuroblastoma who have metastases to other organs such as the bones or liver, chemotherapy is used. Chemotherapy is not very effective against this tumor. It only offers temporary improvement in children with metastases. Most children with extensive neuroblastomas, if they are over the age of two, eventually die of the disease. We must await the development of more effective anticancer drugs before we can cure more of these children.

Overall, only 30 percent of children with neuroblastoma are cured. The cure rate depends on the age of the child when the tumor is first discovered and on the extent of the disease. Young children tend to have localized neuroblastoma and older children more widespread disease. Therefore, these two prognostic factors often go hand in hand.

There are some intriguing features about this tumor that may lead to better treatment in the future. Infants and very young children who develop neuroblastoma sometimes do not die of their disease because the cancer matures into a benign tumor called a ganglioneuroma. This almost never occurs in older children. In addition, neuroblastomas can undergo spontaneous regression, which is the shrinkage and even disappearance of the tumor without treatment. In one book that documents 176 spontaneous regressions of cancer, 29, or 17 percent, occurred in young children with neuroblastoma. If your child is under two and has a neuroblastoma, there is hope even if the tumor is widespread. Unfortunately, if your child is older and the neuroblastoma is widespread, it is unlikely that it can be cured even with the most advanced treatment.

A six-month-old infant was taken to the pediatrician because she had become very irritable and had lost four pounds. The pediatrician felt a hard lump in the child's abdomen. He got an x-ray, which showed calcification in the mass. He suspected the child had a neuroblastoma and told the parents the bad news.

The family and child were referred to a nearby city that had a large children's hospital. There, a urine test showed increased amounts of catecholamine breakdown products, proving that the tumor was neuroblastoma. A series of tests were done that showed that the tumor had not spread. The parents were told the chance of cure was good. Neuroblastoma in an infant, especially if the tumor is localized, has a high chance for cure.

Two days after arriving at the children's hospital, a laparotomy was performed and the mass was entirely removed. Pathologic examination of the specimen showed that the entire tumor had been removed. There was normal tissue at the edge of the resected specimen. The doctor told the parents no further treatment was needed.

The parents took their child home and, over two years, periodic checks showed no recurrence of tumor. The doctor then told the parents that their child was almost certainly cured because neuroblastoma is a fast-growing tumor and usually recurs quickly.

Neuroblastoma is often cured when it occurs in an infant or young child. This case illustrates the effective treatment of a localized neuroblastoma with surgery. The pediatrician wisely referred the family and child to a large center. Diagnostic tests were performed and appropriate specialists were available to treat the tumor properly.

Fred was a seven-year-old boy who complained of pain in his lower back that persisted for several weeks. At first his mother thought it was a bruise, but she became more concerned when the pain did not go away, and she took him to see his pediatrician. The pediatrician found that Fred was indeed tender in one area of his back and also felt a mass in his abdomen. An x-ray of the back showed destruction of bone that suggested cancer. An x-ray of the abdomen showed the mass was calcified. The pediatrician suspected neuroblastoma.

She sent Fred to the nearby children's hospital, where further tests were done. An intravenous pyelogram showed that the abdominal mass was separate from the kidney, and a urine test showed increased amounts of catecholamine breakdown products. Fred had neuroblastoma. Additional tests included a bone marrow biopsy (which showed spread to the bone marrow), a liver scan (which was normal), and a bone scan (which showed several areas of bone involvement in addition to the back). Fred had stage 4, or widespread, neuroblastoma. The prognosis is grim with metastases in children older than two. The pediatrician told Fred's parents that their child would probably die from his cancer.

Fred had a widespread malignant tumor. Chances for cure were very, very small no matter what was done. His parents couldn't believe it. Their previously healthy son was in pain and would probably die soon. The doctors advised trying chemotherapy to control the widespread disease. They had to tell Fred's parents that chemotherapy was likely to be toxic and was unlikely to control the disease very long. Nevertheless, it might prolong his life. His parents agonized over the situation. Should they allow their son to undergo chemotherapy just to live a little longer? They decided at least to try and see what would happen.

Fred received several drugs in combination, and this worked. The bone pain disappeared, the mass in the abdomen became smaller, and he felt better. He received chemotherapy on an intermittent basis for several months. He was able to return to school but he was weaker than normal. Then the bone pain returned and the mass grew larger in his abdomen. He died six months after diagnosis of widespread neuroblastoma.

Neuroblastoma in children over the age of two is very malignant. Only 15–20 percent of children older than two survive. It is difficult to advise parents of children who have cancer and can't be cured. The chemotherapy could not cure their child, it could only give him some time and, of importance, make him more comfortable for awhile. Nevertheless, it is difficult to say how useful several months or even a year is for the child or the parent.

In summary, neuroblastoma shows itself in a variety of ways, but more than half the children have an abdominal mass. After the disease is diagnosed by a biopsy, further tests depend partially on the presentation. Treatment can effectively control or cure many neuroblastomas in children under the age of two but few in children over two. Better treatment awaits the development of more effective anticancer drugs.

RHABDOMYOSARCOMA

Rhabdomyosarcoma is a highly malignant cancer that arises from primitive muscle cells and is the fifth most common cancer in children. There is no known cause, no association with other diseases, and no known familial tendency. There has been remarkable progress in the treatment of this very malignant tumor in the past decade. The number of children cured with this cancer has increased from a dismal 15 percent to 50 percent.

In the past, children were treated with surgery and radiation. Few were cured because the tumor recurred in other organs such as the liver or lungs. Over the last ten years, chemotherapy has been added to surgery and radiation. Surgery and radiation are used to treat the original site of tumor and chemotherapy to treat cancer cells that spread to other parts of the body. With rhabdomyosarcoma, as with Wilms' tumor, adjuvant chemotherapy has been successful. More children are saved.

Diagnosis

This cancer can arise anyplace, but it generally occurs in areas of the head and neck, in the genitourinary tract, or in the arms or legs. The symptoms from this cancer, of course, depend upon where it arises. Because of the unusual symptoms as well as the rarity of this tumor, it is often misdiagnosed. For example, it can occur as a swelling around the eye like a simple eyelid infection, inside the nose causing a bloody nasal discharge like nasal polyps, in the middle ear like a chronic ear infection, or in a muscle as a lump like a muscle bruise. Rhabdomyosarcoma is rare, while infections and muscle bruises are common in children. Nevertheless, if a lump or mass persists, it deserves attention. You, as parents, should take your child to a pediatrician and he or she should have a biopsy of any persistent lump to make sure it is not cancer.

When rhabdomyosarcoma is diagnosed, the child should immediately be referred to a major cancer center. At that center a team of experts including pediatric surgeons, radiation oncologists, and pediatric oncologists will first evaluate the extent of the child's disease and then determine the right treatment.

Determining the Extent of the Disease

Tests are needed to find out how far the tumor has spread in the local area. For example, an intravenous pyelogram, a barium enema, and cystoscopy are done if the rhabdomyosarcoma starts in the genitourinary tract. Likewise, x-ray of the bone, a brain scan, and a spinal tap to examine the spinal fluid are useful for a rhabdomyosarcoma that begins in the head or neck. Because rhabdomyosarcoma metastasizes widely, before treatment is begun an extensive search for metastases is also needed. The tests needed are a bone scan, a liver scan, a bone marrow biopsy, and a chest x-ray.

Treatment

Surgery and Radiation   Treatment for rhabdomyosarcoma consists of surgery, radiation, and chemotherapy. Surgery and radiation are used to treat the main body of tumor. Surgery is used to remove as much of the tumor as possible. Every effort is made to save as much normal tissue as possible and to give a good cosmetic result. The object is to cure the child and allow him or her to live as normally as possible. Radiation is then given to the bed of the tumor to kill any tumor cells not removed at surgery.

Chemotherapy   Chemotherapy is usually given for one and a half to two years. It is used to treat the microscopic metastases in other organs that doctors assume are present. Without chemotherapy, 85 percent of children will develop recurrences of the cancer in sites far from the original area of tumor. Anticancer drugs used for rhabdomyosarcoma are vincristine, cyclophosphamide, and actinomycin D. When surgery and radiation were used, at best 15 percent of children were cured. By contrast, when chemotherapy was added almost one-half of the children were cured.

The chance for cure depends greatly on how much the cancer has spread. Approximately 80 percent of children are cured with localized cancer that can be completely removed surgically; 50 percent are cured with localized tumors that can't be completely removed; but only 10–20 percent of children who have widespread disease live more than two years. The number of children who are cured has increased dramatically with the use of chemotherapy but there is obviously still much room for progress.

Timmy, a healthy twelve-year-old seventh grader, was playing football with some friends when he fell on his left arm. He ignored it at first but showed it to his mother when it was still painful and swollen two weeks later. His mother felt the swelling and told him it was a bruise. The swelling continued over the next two weeks, and his mother became alarmed and took him to see his pediatrician. He examined Timmy's arm and suspected a tumor. An x-ray of the arm was taken, and Timmy was admitted to the nearby community hospital for a biopsy.

The pediatrician told Timmy's parents that he thought Timmy had a tumor but that only a biopsy could tell. Timmy's parents were shocked. It was beyond their wildest fears that one of their children might have a potentially fatal disease.

A small biopsy was performed by an orthopedic surgeon the next day under local anesthesia, and the pathologist informed the pediatrician that Timmy had a malignant tumor. It was almost certainly a sarcoma, but he was unsure of the exact type and wanted the slides to be seen by other pathologists who were experts in childhood tumors. The pediatrician met with Timmy's mother and father and told them that their child had a highly malignant tumor and strongly recommended that they take the child to a children's cancer center 200 miles from their hometown. After initial shock and disbelief, they decided to take Timmy to the cancer center.

What should they tell Timmy? The pediatrician, although not an expert on childhood cancers, told the parents that they should tell him at least that he had a cancerous condition that was going to need long-term treatment. He thought the parents should not bring up the possibility of death but should attempt to deal honestly with the questions that Timmy asked.

That evening Timmy's parents told him what was in store. His first and only question was, "Am I going to die?" His mother began to cry and his father, barely in control, said, "We have faith in God. You will receive the best treatment from your doctor, but we are not sure." The father arranged for a leave of absence from his job and the whole family drove to the medical center.

Timmy was admitted, examined by the intern, a resident, and a fellow (all physicians in training), and by an older physician who was the attending doctor and in charge of children on Timmy's ward in the hospital.

Timmy went through a bewildering series of tests that included a bone scan, a liver scan, a bone marrow biopsy, and a chest x-ray. The nurses were extremely friendly and helpful. Before each test was performed, they explained what could be expected from the test, how it was done, and what Timmy would feel. He was allowed and encouraged to ask questions. The results of the tests showed no evidence of cancer aside from the lump on his upper arm.

A pediatric general surgeon, a radiation oncologist, and a pediatric oncologist all were consulted and examined him. They planned his treatment at a weekly meeting where the treatments for all new children with cancer in the hospital were discussed. Timmy had the benefit of many doctors' experience and training in cancer treatment.

They decided that Timmy should undergo an operation on his arm to remove as much of the tumor as possible without actually amputating his arm. After surgery, radiation would be given to the arm to kill cancer cells left behind. Then he would start one and a half years of chemotherapy to kill cancer cells that had probably spread to other parts of his body. Five years earlier Timmy would have needed his whole arm and shoulder amputated. Modern treatment is directed not only to improving the number of children cured but also to doing so with as little harm to the child as possible.

Timmy was scared. Would he ever be able to play football again? Would he be able to continue school? He was now afraid of what might happen to him because of treatment. The tests had come out well and his doctors were able to assure Timmy and his parents that he had a very good chance for cure. While in the hospital his parents met with other parents of children in similar situations. They began to realize how much of their lives in the next two years would be devoted to caring for their child. Talking with other people in the same situation, however, made the prospects much less frightening. They met parents whose children had been treated and were doing well and some whose children were probably cured.

Timmy's operation took four hours. The surgeon came out to talk to the parents after he was finished. He said he had only been able to remove part of the tumor because it was deeply invading the muscles of the upper arm and shoulder. The pathologist found the tumor to be an embryonal rhabdomyosarcoma. Radiation therapy was started two days after surgery and chemotherapy was started soon thereafter. Timmy received radiation to his arm and to the armpit where the lymph nodes nearest the tumor were located. The radiation did not make him sick since it was directed to a small area of his body. The only short-term side effect was a slight burn to the skin. Later, the tissue of his arm became harder than normal. He also received a combination of three anticancer drugs every four weeks for two years. These drugs did make him very nauseated, but he was only sick for two or three days each month. He also lost all his hair and was very embarrassed. His parents bought him a wig to wear in public. His hair grew back six months after he started treatment. It is strange and not well understood why hair regrows while someone continues taking treatment.

During Timmy's six-week stay in the hospital, tutors set up a program for him so that he would not fall behind his classmates in school. When the radiation was finished, arrangements were made to continue chemotherapy in his hometown. Often, once a treatment plan is formulated and begun, it can be continued by doctors in smaller communities.

Timmy continued to receive chemotherapy over the next year and a half and, except for the few days of nausea and vomiting from the chemotherapy each month, he was able to live a fairly normal life. He missed very few days of school and joined in most of the activities he had enjoyed before he developed cancer.

The radiation and surgery left his arm very weak. He could barely pick up a pen and could not do more than simple motions when he first returned to his hometown. He had muscle wasting and was unable to lift his arm above his head. He worked hard with a physical therapist at his community hospital and slowly but surely his arm became stronger.

As time went on and there was no evidence of tumor recurrence, both he and his parents became more and more optimistic that the tumor was cured. The depression that had hung like a cloud above the whole family slowly began to lift. Every four months Timmy returned to the cancer center for a checkup, and each time he got a clean bill of health; no tumor recurrence was found. Finally the day arrived for his two-year checkup. The family went back to the cancer center and again Timmy was put through a battery of tests like those he had when he was first diagnosed. No evidence of recurrence was found. His doctor, with a smile on his face, told Timmy and his parents that there was a good chance that he was cured. He did tell them they would have to wait several years to be sure, but the odds were in Timmy's favor.

It has now been six years since Timmy had cancer. His disease has not relapsed, and he has just finished high school. The only apparent ill effects of his treatment are that his left arm is weak and smaller than normal. However, he has learned to compensate for this quite well, and was even a track star at his high school.

Increasing numbers of children like Timmy have been cured of previously devastating rhabdomyosarcoma. Timmy benefited greatly from a team of experts who planned treatment to control his cancer. Surgery and radiation were used to control the cancer in his arm without amputation; they were able to leave him with a weakened but still functional arm. Chemotherapy was given for a year and a half to kill the microscopic deposits of tumor. Without chemotherapy, Timmy would most likely have died from recurrent cancer in his liver, lungs, or elsewhere.

The story of rhabdomyosarcoma is a success story. Many more children are being cured now than were ten years ago. However, questions are still being asked, and therefore clinical trials are still in progress. For example, is it possible to obtain the same cure rate in children with localized or early stages of rhabdomyosarcoma with surgery and chemotherapy but omitting radiation? This is an important question, since these treatments are toxic to the child. For example, if Timmy did not need radiation but could have been treated with chemotherapy and surgery, he might have a more functional arm. On the other hand, children with widespread rhabdomyosarcoma have a low cure rate at present. Therefore, newer combinations of drugs are being tested to see whether they are more effective than the standard treatment of vincristine, Cytoxan, and actinomycin. Thus, although treatment has improved dramatically, doctors still have much to learn about tailoring the treatment to the extent of the disease.

EWING'S SARCOMA

Ewing's sarcoma is a highly malignant bone cancer of children. It occurs most often between the ages of five and sixteen and is extremely rare after the age of thirty. This tumor can arise in any bone but most commonly occurs in the femur (the thigh bone), the pelvic bones, and the shoulder. Ewing's sarcoma, much like rhabdomyosarcoma, is a very malignant cancer; more than 90 percent of the time it has already metastasized widely when it is discovered.

As you might expect, this tumor is discovered because children complain of painful swelling in a bone or because swelling is noticed by their parents. When the child is taken to the pediatrician, he or she will obtain x-rays of the painful, swollen bone. These show a destructive process in the bone, which indicates a tumor. The diagnosis is confirmed by a biopsy of the bone. Occasionally the pathologist will be unable to tell whether the tumor is Ewing's sarcoma or some other tumor such as neuroblastoma or a lymphoma. A second biopsy may be needed, or the slides may have to be sent to another pathologist who is an expert in this area to determine what cancer is present. This is very important, since different cancers are treated somewhat differently and have different prognoses.

Once the diagnosis is made, a series of tests are performed to determine whether the tumor has spread. A bone scan, a liver scan, a chest x-ray, lung tomograms, and a bone marrow biopsy all should be obtained. Once the tests have been done, it is time to initiate treatment.

Treatment

Treatment consists of a combination of radiation and occasionally surgery to treat the local cancer and chemotherapy to treat the metastases that are present in most children. We know that most children with this cancer have microscopic metastases, since in the past 80 percent or more developed recurrent cancer in the lungs, bones, or other organs after radiation had eradicated the original site of cancer. Routinely, radiation in very high doses is used to treat the original site of the tumor. The value of surgery in addition to radiation is being studied for Ewing's sarcoma of the pelvis, since it has been difficult to eradicate the disease in this bone with radiation alone. However, most often radiation alone is utilized to eradicate or control the original area of tumor.

Chemotherapy   All children with Ewing's sarcoma should also receive a prolonged course of chemotherapy much like that for Wilms' tumor and rhabdomyosarcoma. Chemotherapy is used even if tests show no obvious spread because when radiation is used alone, more than 85 percent of children have recurrence of the disease in other areas of the body, mainly in the lungs, liver, and other bones. The use of radiation and chemotherapy together has improved survival and increased the cure rate for Ewing's sarcoma, much as it has for rhabdomyosarcoma and Wilms' tumor.

The prognosis in Ewing's sarcoma is still not good, but it has improved in the last ten years. In the past only 10–15 percent of children with this disease were alive and well five years after diagnosis. With the addition of aggressive chemotherapy, the cure rate has increased from a dismal 10–15 percent to 40–50 percent. As more effective drugs are developed to treat this cancer, we can expect the cure rate to improve further. Because Ewing's sarcoma is so malignant and because the use of chemotherapy and high-dose radiation together improves the survival and the cure rate, children with this disease should be treated in childhood cancer centers. These centers specialize in the treatment of these rare tumors and offer each child with Ewing's sarcoma the best chance for cure.

OSTEOGENIC SARCOMA

Osteosarcoma is a malignant tumor characterized by the formation of bone, and it is the most common malignant bone cancer in children and adolescents. It occurs most commonly during childhood growth spurts and is slightly more common in boys than girls. Children affected are usually between the ages of ten and twenty-five. Osteosarcoma most commonly arises in the bones of the legs—the femur (thigh bone) or the tibia (shin bone)—and in the humerus, the base of the upper arm.

Osteosarcoma is normally brought to the attention of the physician because a child has persistent pain and swelling in a bone. Pain or swelling lasting more than one to two weeks in a child should not be attributed to an injury. Rather, it should be evaluated by a doctor. Until recently, 85 percent of children with this disease treated with just amputation of the extremity affected by the cancer died within two years. Fortunately, more are now cured with the use of chemotherapy in combination with surgery.

Diagnosis

When bone cancer is suspected in a child because of persistent bone pain or swelling, the pediatrician should obtain an x-ray of the suspicious area. If the x-ray shows abnormalities suspicious of bone cancer, the child should be referred to an orthopedic surgeon, who specializes in the diseases of bones and who is experienced in obtaining bone biopsies. The x-rays tell the orthopedic surgeon where to biopsy. Often he or she will order additional x-rays of the area before obtaining a biopsy. The x-ray of the bone will not only show an abnormality but also can show changes that are very suspicious of osteogenic sarcoma. If the biopsy shows osteogenic sarcoma, referral to a large children's hospital or major cancer center is important even if it means traveling several hundred miles from the child's hometown.

Evaluating the Extent of the Disease

The first step at the cancer center or children's hospital will be to evaluate the extent of the disease. A chest x-ray and tomograms of the lungs, a bone scan, and a liver scan will be obtained. After these tests, a treatment plan will be devised.

Treatment

Surgery   Treatment for osteogenic sarcoma has changed dramatically in the past decade. Up until the 1970s, surgery was the mainstay of treatment. An amputation of the affected limb was usually performed. Unfortunately, usually within several months, lung metastases appeared and, despite the use of chemotherapy, the child died within a matter of months or years. Osteogenic sarcoma, like most childhood cancers, is extremely malignant and has often metastasized widely by the time it is diagnosed. Even if all tests are normal and show no metastases, microscopic deposits of tumor are usually present in other parts of the body. Therefore, even if the entire cancer is removed by amputation, microscopic deposits elsewhere grow and kill the child.

Chemotherapy   A major advance in the treatment of this disease has occurred with the availability and use of modern chemotherapy. Clinical trials begun early in the 1970s have shown that children treated with intensive long-term chemotherapy live longer and have a better chance for cure than children who had amputation as their only treatment. With amputation alone, the cure rate is approximately 15 percent, while with amputation and chemotherapy approximately 40–50 percent of children are being cured. The results with adjuvant chemotherapy are much like those obtained for childhood rhabdomyosarcoma, Wilms' tumor, and Ewing's sarcoma.

Treatment programs for osteogenic sarcoma should be carried out at large children's hospitals or cancer centers where specialists are available that include orthopedic surgeons experienced in operating on children, pediatric oncologists, and a rehabilitation team that can motivate and train the child to be active and live with the amputation of an arm or leg.

The treatment of osteogenic sarcoma currently involves surgery and chemotherapy. The possibility of obtaining the same cure rate and avoiding amputation of a leg or arm is being evaluated. High-dose radiation and/or chemotherapy are being used to shrink the cancer and then surgery is used to remove the tumor, and the bone is then repaired with a bone graft. This approach is still experimental but is promising. As with other childhood cancers, the best treatment is available at large children's hospitals or cancer centers where there are experienced specialists dedicated to the treatment of childhood tumors. The child with osteogenic sarcoma must face, in addition to long-term chemotherapy, amputation of one of his extremities. Therefore, the child needs intensive rehabilitation, which is rarely available at most community hospitals. Osteogenic sarcoma is also discussed in chapter 21, "Soft Tissue and Bone Sarcomas."

ACUTE LYMPHOCYTIC LEUKEMIA (ALL)

Acute lymphocytic leukemia, or ALL, as it is called by physicians, is the most common cancer of children: one of three children with cancer has ALL. Its peak incidence is between the ages of two and seven, and it is relatively uncommon after the age of fifteen. The prognosis and treatment of acute lymphocytic leukemia in children differ significantly from those of acute nonlymphocytic leukemia in the adult and are, therefore, described in this chapter. Children with acute lymphocytic leukemia can be cured with far less toxic therapy than that needed to treat adults with acute nonlymphocytic leukemia.

Leukemia is a cancer that arises from the blood-forming tissues called the bone marrow, which is located inside bones. The leukemic cells accumulate in the bone marrow and in the blood. The bone marrow normally produces red blood cells, which deliver oxygen to body tissues, white blood cells called granulocytes or polys, which fight infections, and platelets, which are important in controlling and preventing bleeding. The symptoms of leukemia usually result from a lack of these normal cells.

Diagnosis

Children may tire easily or just not feel well due to a lack of red blood cells. They may have fever or infections due to a lack of normal white cells, or they may bruise easily or have nosebleeds due to a lack of platelets. Occasionally leukemia is diagnosed because parents notice abdominal swelling due to enlargement of the liver or spleen. Sometimes persistently swollen lymph nodes worry the parents, who then bring the child to the pediatrician. Some children have bone pain from leukemia. The diagnosis is easy if the pediatrician suspects that something is wrong. A routine blood count will almost always suggest or establish the diagnosis. The blood count will usually reveal anemia (a lack of red cells), thrombocytopenia (a lack of platelets), and either a low white blood cell count due to lack of normal white blood cells or a high white cell count with a large number of leukemic cells present in the blood. The pediatrician usually suspects leukemia with these blood abnormalities even if leukemic cells are not present and should refer the child to a pediatric oncologist or hematologist for a bone marrow examination.

A bone marrow examination is obtained by inserting a small needle into a bone, usually the hip, after anesthetizing the area with the same type of local anesthesia that a dentist uses. The procedure is somewhat painful but takes only about two minutes. If leukemia is present, a bone marrow examination will almost always show it. Leukemia is not difficult to diagnose.

Treatment

Once the diagnosis of acute lymphocytic leukemia is made, the child should immediately be referred to a cancer center or children's hospital. Modern treatment has improved the survival dramatically and cures many children. Twenty years ago almost all children died within weeks or months of the diagnosis. At present, with chemotherapy, approximately 50–70 percent of children will live five years and close to 50 percent of children are cured. At the children's hopsital or cancer center, the diagnosis will first be confirmed by experts who will review the bone marrow specimen and blood smears.

Treatment will usually be started within a day or two. The child will have to face two to four years of treatment directed by the doctors at the cancer center. Both the parents and children will be educated about this disease, its treatment, and how other children and parents have fared. Once treatment is under way, the specialists at the cancer center or children's hospital can often send the child back to his or her own community for completion of treatment.

Many communities now have a pediatric oncologist, a hematologist, or at least a pediatrician who is interested and has had some training in the treatment of childhood tumors. Usually the specialist at these large centers knows of other physicians who can treat your child adequately. If at all possible, most of the treatment will be completed by a physician in your area. However, your child's life depends on receiving the best treatment available. Therefore, you should not accept treatment in your community without at least a consultation at a cancer center or large children's hospital. Community-based treatment should be done only if the specialist at the large center feels that there is a pediatrician available with sufficient knowledge and interest in this disease to treat it adequately in conjunction with him.

The treatment for ALL is aimed at curing the child. There are basically three phases of treatment. First, induction therapy rids the bone marrow, the blood, and the rest of the child's body of identifiable leukemia cells. When and if this is accomplished, the child again appears normal and is said to be in complete remission. The bone marrow and blood look entirely normal. However, this does not mean that the child is cured.

There are still microscopic deposits of leukemia present but these are too small to be seen even under a microscope.

The next phase of treatment involves therapy aimed at killing any leukemia cells that are residing in the brain and spinal cord—a common site of recurrence. Many of the drugs used to treat acute leukemia do not enter the brain tissue and cerebrospinal fluid in good concentrations. Therefore, drugs must be placed directly into the spinal fluid. The brain is usually also treated with radiation to kill any leukemia cells that are present in these areas. This phase is called central nervous system (or CNS) prophylaxis. It is normally started soon after the child enters complete remission with chemotherapy.

Finally, children receive maintenance therapy, which consists of two to four years of chemotherapy to treat the microscopic deposits of leukemia that remain after the child enters complete remission. After maintenance therapy is stopped, the child is closely observed for signs of recurrence, with blood counts and bone marrow examinations.

Thus, children with acute leukemia must undergo long-term treatments that are extremely trying to the child and the parents. However, 40–50 percent of children are now being cured of what was thought only a decade ago to be a rapidly fatal disease.

Induction Induction therapy is the descriptive term for the initial treatment of acute lymphocytic leukemia. Two drugs, vincristine and prednisone, are most often used. Over a matter of weeks, these two drugs will put more than 90 percent of children into complete remission. Prednisone is given as a pill several times a day and vincristine is given once a week as an injection. The toxicity from this treatment is much less than with most other types of chemotherapy. There is usually minimal or no nausea. A disturbing side effect of vincristine is nerve damage, though this gets better after the drug is stopped. The child will often feel tingling in his arms and legs and the doctors will have to watch closely for any muscle weakness that signals that this drug should not be used anymore. Prednisone will cause the child's appetite to be increased and his face to become puffy or fat, but this is also only temporary.

If the child feels well enough, treatment is given in the doctor's office or outpatient clinic. Therefore, the child can often leave the hospital and stay at home or in a motel. During this phase, the physicians will very closely watch the child's blood count because he may need blood transfusions for anemia, or platelet transfusions to prevent bleeding because the platelet count becomes dangerously low. The child may have to be hospitalized for fever or for infections resulting from a lack of white blood cells, which normally fight infection.

By the end of one month of treatment, more than 90 percent of children are in complete remission. Their bone marrow contains no recognizable signs of leukemia, their blood counts are normal again, and they feel much better. Induction therapy for acute lymphocytic leukemia is, therefore, not only very effective in inducing complete remissions but also not difficult for the child to take. However, it requires very close observation by a pediatric oncologist to prevent and treat complications.

Central Nervous System Treatment   Once the child is in complete remission, the next phase of treatment is directed at the brain and spinal cord. Without this treatment, more than half the children with acute lymphocytic leukemia will develop recurrence in the brain and spinal cord while still having no leukemia in other parts of the body. Although recurrence in the brain can be controlled with radiation and drugs such as methotrexate given by spinal tap, the leukemia can't be eradicated and so eventually recurs. Therefore, the chance for cure is usually lost. Clinical trials pioneered by St. Jude's Hospital in Tennessee were conducted to see if treating the brain early (prophylactically) before the disease appeared would be effective. These trials showed that treatment of the brain and spinal cord with radiation and methotrexate prevented relapse in the brain most of the time.

Therefore, this stage of treatment—central nervous system prophylaxis, or CNS—is now a standard and essential part of the approach to children with acute lymphocytic leukemia. The standard treatment for the central nervous system consists of radiation to the head and weekly injections of methotrexate given by spinal punctures over a period of one to two months. It is not pleasant for the child, his parents, or the physician to have to administer the methotrexate by spinal taps. However, the anxiety over the procedure is usually worse than the procedure itself. In well-practiced hands, spinal taps are not very painful and can be performed quickly. If the first spinal tap and administration of methotrexate can be done smoothly, the child sees it is not so bad. Radiation to the head, which is administered over several weeks, causes temporary hair loss and also can cause temporary lethargy or sleepiness.

Maintenance Therapy   After CNS prophylaxis, the child is placed on maintenance therapy. The drugs used vary but usually are given in moderate doses, so they rarely cause noticeable side effects and the child is able to function fairly normally during this period of time. He or she can go to school and engage in most activities. During this phase, bone marrow examinations are still needed every month or two to check for relapse. This is often the most upsetting aspect of the treatment program. Many children come to fear bone marrow examinations much more than the treatment itself.

Maintenance treatment can be given by a pediatrician or pediatric oncologist in a smaller community so that the child and family will not be dislocated during this long period of time. Visits back to the cancer center are indicated periodically to check on the progress of treatment. Most treatment programs also call for more intensive treatments periodically, which often are administered at the larger center. These are aimed at eradicating any remaining tumor cells not being killed by the maintenance drugs.

At the end of approximately two to four years of treatment, all chemotherapy is stopped if the leukemia hasn't recurred, and the child is watched carefully. This must seem like a lot of treatment for a small child to take, and it is. However, chances for cure are very good if the child goes through this complete program and is in remission at the end.

One of the major unresolved problems with this disease is infection during remission. The drugs and radiation given to cure the disease lower the body's defenses, and the child becomes susceptible to overwhelming life-threatening infections from viruses, fungi, and some bacteria and to an unusual infection known as pneumocystis, which produces a treatable but sometimes fatal type of pneumonia. Therefore, even the child with acute lymphocytic leukemia in complete remission must be watched closely, and early treatment of infections is necessary. It is important to call or take the child to the doctor for any fever, sore throat, or cough that you could safely treat yourself in a healthy child. The child with acute leukemia being treated does not have the normal defenses against infection and not only develops unusual infections that need special treatment but becomes very sick with everyday bacterial infections that are not serious in a healthy child.

It is most important to protect these children from common childhood viral illnesses such as chickenpox. Chickenpox in a child with acute leukemia can cause fatal pneumonia. Recently some antiviral drugs have been developed that show some progress in the treatment of life-threatening viral disease in these children. However, parents of children with acute leukemia must always live in fear that their child will be exposed to childhood illnesses and die. This causes major complications if there are other children in the house who are exposed to these illnesses at school or from their friends.

A difficult compromise must be reached between treating the leukemic child as normal and protecting him from hazards in the environment. Certainly it is difficult enough for a child and his family to face the treatment needed to cure acute leukemia. We do not, therefore, recommend that the child be isolated from his friends and schoolmates. However, we do think that, as far as possible, he must be protected from diseases such as chickenpox.

If leukemia recurs, second, third, and even fourth complete remissions can be obtained. However, the remissions tend to be progressively shorter, and few children who develop recurrent leukemia live more than two years after the first recurrence. Some children will be considered for a procedure called bone marrow transplantation if they have a brother or sister whose tissue type (HLA type) is identical to theirs. This is a dangerous and difficult procedure, but approximately 10–15 percent of the children whose leukemia has recurred can be cured by it. Bone marrow transplantation will be discussed in more detail in chapter 24, "Experimental Treatment for Cancer."

Even for the child who is eventually cured, this is a devastating disease. The family must live with the knowledge that even though he has been in remission for four or five years, their child may still die of leukemia. In addition, he may develop an infection and die. Great stresses are placed on the marriage. Interactions between the parents and with the other healthy children are changed. A child with a disease like leukemia is singled out; he knows he is different from other children. His parents may become overprotective and overindulge him. Very often this will lead to controlling and unpleasant behavior by the child. The child with leukemia does need special attention but he also needs to be treated in many ways like a healthy child. For example, he needs discipline like any other child. How do you punish your child who may die of leukemia? Very often family counseling can help you cope better with your child in these circumstances.

We believe that it is a myth that families usually become closer with life-threatening illness of a child. That can happen but often it becomes a major source of friction. Parents often blame each other. Occasionally one parent is emotionally totally unable to deal with a sick child, and the full burden of care, nurture, and discipline of the child is left to the other parent. A leukemic child will exacerbate any problems that were present in the marriage before. A close relationship may become even closer but a shaky one is in trouble and divorce is not uncommon. A sensitive physician can recognize emotional problems within a family surrounding the child's illness and assist the family in obtaining supportive help either through associations of families of children with leukemia or through professional counselors.

In summary, treatment of acute lymphocytic leukemia in childhood is very difficult for the child and family. Usually the child is hospitalized only at the onset when the diagnosis is made; the rest of the treatment can be administered outside of the hospital. Still, during the two to four years of treatment, the child will receive many drugs and procedures such as spinal taps, drawing of blood, and bone marrows, all of which are painful. There is also the threat of the leukemia's recurring and therefore the threat of death hanging over the parents and the child. However, the chance for cure has improved dramatically. Fifty percent of the children are now being cured, which was unheard of only a decade ago. There is hope for children with acute lymphocytic leukemia. The following case history illustrates several important aspects of acute lymphocytic leukemia. Although this particular child was not cured, many others are.

C.O. was four years old when his acute leukemia was diagnosed. He had been in good health until that age. His mother first noticed that he seemed tired most of the time and no longer wanted to play with other children. He spent much of the time watching television and falling asleep. She also noticed that he had several swollen glands in his neck and that he appeared pale. His father was a physician but he completely denied that the child could be ill. However, his mother suspected that he was seriously ill and, after three visits to a pediatrician, a blood count was performed and the diagnosis of acute lymphocytic leukemia was obvious.

The child was referred to a medical center 200 miles from where the family was living. The boy had a six-year-old sister, who stayed with her father while C.O. and his mother went to the medical center. This center included an excellent children's hospital with facilities for parents to sleep in the child's room and an understanding staff, who explained everything, both to the child and his mother. His mother's exposure to medicine through her spouse led her to expect the worst. She went to the medical library and read all she could about this disease.

The child was treated with vincristine and prednisone. During the treatment he stayed with his mother in a motel and saw his physicians several times a week. They gave him drugs and checked him for infections and for whether he needed blood transfusions. His blood counts improved over the next four weeks and a bone marrow examination at the end of one month of treatment showed that he was in complete remission.

Despite his feeling better, C.O. became increasingly disturbed by the painful bone marrow examinations. He came to hate procedures such as blood drawing and bone marrow exams much more than the treatment itself. The doctors and nurses were understanding but explained why they had to be performed. C.O.'s reaction was not unusual. These tests are painful to some extent and the child with a serious illness is angry. Why should he be sick and be hurt by doctors when his parents and his friends are okay? Why don't his parents protect him?

Next C.O. was given radiation to his head. This is frightening to a child because he has to be in a room by himself with a big radiation machine. Also, if he is younger, like C.O., he is strapped down to the table. He cried during the entire first treatment but then realized it did not hurt. Over the next two weeks radiation treatment went smoothly. C.O. was taking pills by mouth and an injection once a week. The only unpleasant parts of the treatment were the spinal taps done once a week to give methotrexate into the spinal fluid and the monthly bone marrow examinations.

After six weeks, the mother and the child both returned home to be treated by a pediatrician who lived in their town. This pediatrician treated C.O. with so-called maintenance therapy, which was not very toxic. C.O. and his family felt better. His energy slowly returned and he appeared to be a healthy, normal child except for his bald head. He was told that his hair would regrow in a matter of months.

After the family was reunited, the boy's parents had long conversations, discussing their fears, their hopes, and plans for the future. They discussed how they would handle their daughter and the child with leukemia. Both children were told that C.O. had leukemia and that this was a bad disease that required treatment for several years. The possibility of death was not discussed. They tried to treat him much as they had before he became ill with leukemia. They also tried to give extra attention to their healthy daughter to compensate for the attention they knew they must be giving to the sick child.

C.O. did well for one and a half years. He received maintenance chemotherapy with few side effects. At times he felt tired with treatments, and he still needed blood counts and bone marrow examinations on a periodic basis. Every six months the family made trips to the medical center, where he received more intensive treatment that did make him sick. Two years had passed from the day of diagnosis and C.O. was in the second grade. The family was cautiously optimistic that he was one of the children who are cured.

Then he developed an enlargement of one of his testicles. Both parents knew that this almost had to be recurrence of leukemia. They drove all night and reached the medical center the following morning. The testicle was biopsied with a needle under local anesthesia and the diagnosis was recurrent leukemia. C.O. was treated with radiation to the testicle, the swelling went down, and he returned home. However, the specialist at the medical center had to tell the parents that the chance for cure was almost certainly lost. Two months later the pediatrician found on a blood count that the leukemia had returned. The family again returned to the medical center and intensive chemotherapy did produce another remission, but both parents knew the end was not far off.

C.O. had developed enough familiarity with the medical center and the other children with leukemia that he sensed his own impending death, and he talked to his parents about dying. He asked them questions such as what happens to children when they die. After agonizing for several months, his parents decided to have the tissue type of their daughter determined to find out if a bone marrow transplantation was possible. The daughter and C.O. were not closely matched. The parents felt both anguish and relief—anguish because the last hope for a cure for the child was gone and relief that they, and particularly their daughter, would not have to undergo the further burden of marrow transplantation. Six months after another relapse, and another remission, C.O. died.

Since the death of C.O., his parents have tried to reestablish some normalcy in their family. They have taken vacations and resumed activities they had all wanted to do but had foregone because of C.O.'s illness. Looking back, they are satisfied that they tried all that was possible and did the most to make C.O.'s last few years comfortable and enjoyable. However, they are still depressed. Both parents are back into many of their old activities but they still think of and often cry for their dead child.

Many cases of ALL end differently. C.O.'s case could have ended differently with the same treatment. He could now be off of treatment for several years, be entirely well, and almost certainly be cured.

MALIGNANT LYMPHOMAS

Hodgkin's disease and Hodgkin's lymphoma are not discussed in this chapter because they are discussed in chapter 18, "Cancers of the Blood Cells and Lymph Glands."

TUMORS OF THE CENTRAL NERVOUS SYSTEM

Tumors of the central nervous system are not discussed in this chapter because they are described in chapter 17, "Brain Tumors."

Complications of Therapy

Perhaps a word is also warranted about the long-term complications of treatment. There are long-term side effects for all people who take chemotherapy or radiation. For children, however, these side effects can be especially upsetting. For example, radiation will affect bone growth in the areas radiated. Therefore, if an extremity is radiated in a young child, it may be shorter than the other one; if the spine is radiated, the child may not grow as tall as he otherwise would. Radiation to the head occasionally results in cataracts, which may require eye surgery later. Radiation to the testes or ovaries will cause damage, leading to infertility and, in women, a lack of normal hormones. If this occurs, the child needs hormone shots as a teenager to develop normal breasts and pubic hair.

Chemotherapy can cause similar problems. Any child who receives long-term therapy may never be able to father or give birth to a child and may need hormone shots to develop sexually. However, some males and females who had chemotherapy as children have had normal children.

In addition, both radiation and chemotherapy are carcinogens. They can cause cancer and therefore children who are cured of one cancer have a somewhat increased risk to develop another.

Doctors treating children with cancer are well aware of these side effects and try to minimize them. Because these drugs have very undesirable long-term side effects, studies are going on at cancer centers and children's hospitals, trying not only to improve the cure rate in childhood cancers but also to do so with as little therapy as possible.

Parents of children with cancer will often be asked to place their children into clinical trials that evaluate different approaches for a particular cancer. You, as a parent, should feel free to ask many questions about the studies and especially whether the doctor thinks that one treatment is probably better than another. Also feel free to ask what is being done at other centers in the country. As a general rule, excellent treatment is available at most large children's cancer hospitals but you, the parent, must feel comfortable with the treatment.

SUMMARY

1. Cancer is the second leading cause of death in children.

2. Most childhood cancers are extremely malignant and will be rapidly fatal unless controlled by therapy.

3. If your child develops cancer, he or she should be taken to a large children's hospital or major cancer center. These centers have the specialists with the training and experience to deliver the best modern treatment. They also have available personnel to help support the family and child emotionally.

4. The treatment of most childhood cancers, including Wilms' tumor, rhabdomyosarcoma, Ewing's sarcoma, osteogenic sarcoma, and malignant lymphomas, often include surgery and/or radiation to treat the original site of tumor and chemotherapy to treat the disease that has spread to other parts of the body. Such intensive treatment is necessary to cure as many children as possible.

5. It is impossible to hide obvious truth from older children. Even if they are not told, they are aware of the gravity of their illness. If they are going to die, they will know it. Children deserve the same degree of honesty as do adults, both from their physicians and from their families.

6. Families must participate in the treatment decisions made for their children. This participation may take the form of deciding whether or not your child should get experimental treatment for his cancer or deciding whether or not to employ heroic measures such as bone marrow transplantation. The greater the degree of family participation in decisions, the less powerless the family feels and the better it will feel whether the child is cured or not.

24

Experimental Treatment for Cancer

The improvement in the treatment for cancer over the past three decades has resulted from research. New, more active anticancer drugs and better radiation therapy machines have been developed. Newer antibiotics and the wide availability of blood products such as platelets allow doctors to use more toxic therapy. All new treatments had to be tested on people with cancer. What was experimental and unproven treatment ten years ago has become accepted or standard treatment now. The aim of this chapter is not to explain or justify cancer research. Rather, it is to acquaint you with the kinds of experimental treatment currently under study. We want you to understand the possible benefits and risks of experimental therapy.

What Is Experimental Therapy?

Experimental therapy is unproven therapy. It may involve the use of new drugs whose efficacy and toxicity are not yet well established. These drugs have not been approved by the Food and Drug Administration and are not generally available to practicing physicians. Experimental therapy may involve the use of a new type of radiation machine such as neutron or pi meson radiation. It is also considered experimental to use "standard" drugs to treat a cancer for which their effectiveness is unproven or to use standard drugs in new combinations or in new ways. The comparison of two treatments, each of which is effective against a cancer, to see which is best is also experimental. It is obvious that all these situations offer different benefits and risks. The use of a new drug in people for the first time can be dangerous. In contrast, a study to see which of two effective treatments is best is less risky. If both treatments are effective, the patient will benefit no matter which one is taken. You need to find out the risks and the benefits if you are offered or ask for experimental therapy.

Not All Experimental Treatment Is Unproven

The Food and Drug Administration (FDA) is very conservative about approving drugs for use in humans. It requires several years or more of experience with the drug. The FDA wants to be sure that the drug is really beneficial and that the side effects are well known. In general, this is a good approach; there are too many drugs on the market, and many have limited usefulness. However, the FDA has delayed approving anticancer drugs that are of proven benefit. Some, in fact, are standard treatment for certain cancers. However, they are still classed as investigational or experimental drugs. For example, daunomycin is one of the most effective drugs to treat acute nonlymphocytic leukemia. Although it has been available since 1970, the FDA still considers it experimental. Likewise, although cis-platinum has been known since 1976 to be the best single drug for testicular cancer, it was considered experimental by the FDA until late in 1978. Even prior to its approval, not to use cis-platinum in a chemotherapy program for a patient with testicular cancer would be to deny the best available treatment. Adriamycin, a major cancer drug, is on the market now. However, it was approved several years after it was known to be very effective for a variety of common cancers.

For you, the person with cancer, this means that taking an investigational or experimental drug that requires a consent form does not mean you are necessarily taking unproven treatment. Most medical oncologists will explain this to you. These drugs may have completed phase 3 trials, be of known benefit, and be the standard treatment for a cancer, but the FDA has not yet approved them. You should not hesitate to take drugs in this category.

Clinical Trials Comparing Two Proven Treatments

When two or more different treatments are compared to see which is best, the treatment is considered experimental. Your doctor must explain the treatment choices and the reasons why a comparison is needed. You will be asked to sign a consent form. In some trials, all the treatment alternatives are proven. For example, several drugs are active against breast cancer. These drugs were tested with different schedules and combinations. A woman who agreed to enter these studies had to sign a consent form for experimental therapy, though, in fact, she was taking proven treatment for breast cancer. There were very few risks. The aim of the study was to see if one treatment was slightly better than the other.

Informed Consent

Every patient who participates in experimental therapy must sign an "informed" consent form. The form explains why the study is being done, the possible benefits and risks, and alternative treatment. It also tells you that you can withdraw from the study at any time. The aim is to insure that your participation is voluntary and that you understand that you are getting experimental treatment. Your physician should explain the treatment and give you and your family ample time to ask questions and think about it. The doctor must tell you that you can refuse to enter the study or discontinue it at any time without endangering your relationship with your physician.

All hospitals that conduct experimental studies on cancer have a Human Subjects Review Committee. This committee is charged with insuring that experimental therapy is well designed and "ethical." The committee is very concerned that you understand the possible benefits, risks, and alternatives to an experimental form of treatment. The committee of doctors, scientists, lay people, and students reviews all studies and "informed" consent forms. The committee tries to decide if the form gives the patient sufficient information. Does it state all the possible side effects? Does it tell the patient about alternative treatments? Does it tell the patient that he or she may withdraw from the study at any time? Only after a study has been approved by the Human Subjects Review Committee can an ethical cancer investigator offer experimental treatment to a patient.

Despite controls such as Human Subjects Review Committees and research funding review, there are many clinical trials where the benefits are quite small and the risks are substantial. We urge you to ask questions and be cautious about taking truly experimental, unproven treatment. Merely because experimental treatment has the approval of a committee and is offered to you at a cancer center is no reason to accept it.

We will devote most of this chapter to an explanation of the current practices in experimental chemotherapy. Most experimental therapy in cancer uses chemotherapy. We will also briefly review immunotherapy, thermal or heat therapy, and bone marrow transplantation.

We hope that you will get from this chapter at least a healthy skepticism about new miracle drugs. We want you to learn the important questions to ask if you are offered experimental therapy: What are the possible benefits? What are the risks? What is known about the treatment? Has the drug helped anyone with cancer? Has it helped people with my cancer? Has it hurt anyone? Has it killed anyone? You should also ask your cancer doctor's opinion as to whether the treatment is promising.

There are many ongoing clinical trials. Although no one can be completely sure until the results of the trials are in, most cancer specialists know the odds. For some cancers there are no promising drugs, and experimental therapy is almost bound to fail. For others there is promising therapy, and it may well pay to take the chance and try it.

No matter how grim the picture, some people decide to take experimental therapy. Americans are optimistic and think there is always a way out. Many people feel guilty for not trying all treatments available, including experimental therapy. It is difficult to accept that no effective treatment is available for your cancer. Experimental therapy may help you emotionally even if it offers no concrete medical hope. However, we have seen too many people take experimental therapy when it had almost no chance of working. The treatment may make you sick, may cause hospitalization, and/or may mean traveling far from your home and being away from your family and friends. It may even kill you.

Another reason some people take experimental therapy is to help future cancer victims. Although a person may not benefit personally from undergoing experimental therapy, he or she may help others by contributing to knowledge of how best to treat cancer. Even participating in a very early experimental trial in which a person has only a small chance to be helped may make it possible for others in the future to benefit from new treatments. To many cancer victims, this is an important motivation for trying new and experimental treatment.

Experimental Chemotherapy: How New Drugs Are Tested

The development of anticancer drugs is a slow process. Thousands of chemicals are tested against animal cancers each year. Only occasionally is one found that proves useful in human cancer.

Should you take experimental chemotherapy? We advise you to find out about its relative benefits and risks and if there are any alternative treatments for your cancer. Find out if the drug or drugs you are taking are in phase 1, 2, or 3 trials. Phase 1 trials are very risky and the chances for benefit are small. Although phase 2 trials are less risky, the benefit is still small. In phase 3 trials, the benefits far outweigh the risks. By the time a treatment has reached phase 3, much is known about it. Researchers only design phase 3 trials if they think a drug is effective against a cancer.

Animal Trials   Each year thousands of chemical are screened in mice with transplanted or induced cancers. If a drug slows the growth of mouse cancers it then undergoes further testing. First it is tested in rodents and larger animals including dogs and monkeys to find out how toxic it is. Tests to see what doses are tolerable are also done. After these toxicity and dosage studies have been completed, the drug must be tested in humans in a phase 1 trial.

Phase 1 Trial   The phase 1 trial is a toxicity study in man; this is the first time a new drug is used on people. Phase 1 drugs are used in people for whom no standard anticancer therapy is known to be effective. These people are at "the end of the road": they have had all the treatment that might be of help but are getting worse. The major aim of a phase 1 trial is to find out the answers to two questions about a new drug: What are the side effects? What dose is tolerable? Phase 1 drugs are started at low doses, then the dosage is increased until severe side effects occur. Since there is no prior experience in man, unexpected side effects are quite common. Some people die from these drugs.

Phase 1 drug trials are hazardous for patients. The chance of benefit is very slim. The consent form for phase 1 studies usually states that the side effects include the possibility of death and that the chance that the drug will help is slight. Despite ethical questions about these studies, there is no substitute for the human phase 1 trial. Every effective drug now in use had to go through such a trial.

We urge that you carefully consider whether you want to enter a phase 1 trial. We definitely do not feel it is worthwhile for you to travel to a medical center not in your community to receive a phase 1 drug. If the drug is available in your community, there are only two reasons for trying it: it offers hope and it may help others with cancer.

Phase 2 Trial   After phase 1 trials have been completed, a drug enters phase 2 trials. At this stage, doctors know many of the side effects of the drug and what doses to use. Although the risks with a phase 2 drug are less, the benefits are still minimal. Your chances for responding to a phase 2 drug are small. Phase 2 trials are done to see if a new drug is useful against any human cancer. People are asked to enter phase 2 trials after standard treatment no longer helps or if there is no standard treatment available for their cancer. Most phase 2 drugs do not prove useful to treat human cancers. However, every few years, a new drug is tested that represents a breakthrough. For example, when one anticancer drug, Adriamycin, was tested in phase 2 trials, tumor shrinkage was observed in people with lung cancer, ovarian cancer, breast cancer, leukemia, lymphomas, sarcomas, and cervical cancer. Adriamycin was a major addition to cancer chemotherapy. Those people who volunteered to take Adriamycin as part of phase 2 trials were helped. Since the drug was experimental, it was not available except in phase 2 trials.

If you are thinking about entering a phase 2 trial, you should find out what is known about the drug. Perhaps the drug is almost finishing its phase 2 trial and much is known about it. Find out whether the drug has helped other people with cancer. Ask specifically whether it has shown any effect on your type of cancer. If fifteen people with your cancer have been given the drug and no one has responded, you probably will not respond.

Phase 3 Trial   Phase 3 trials test new drugs against only those cancers that appeared to be helped in phase 2 trials. For example, if drug X was effective against Hodgkin's disease, non-Hodgkin's lymphoma, and acute leukemia but not against other cancers, it would be tested in phase 3 trials against only those three cancers. Therefore, if you enter a phase 3 trial, your chances of benefiting are quite good. The drug has already been proven effective against your cancer. Also, the risks are low. There is already extensive toxicity experience. Phase 3 trials are generally worth entering. Most drugs never reach phase 3. Those that do often become standard treatment for some cancers.

Where Can You Receive Experimental Chemotherapy? The answer to this question depends on what type of cancer you have and how experimental the chemotherapy is. Some types of experimental therapy are available only at major cancer centers or university hospitals with an interest in experimental cancer treatment. Others, however, are available at community medical centers and in the offices of board-certified medical oncologists and board-certified hematologists in private practice. Many practicing cancer specialists are members of cooperative groups that test new types of chemotherapy. You will have to find out from your oncologist where experimental therapy is available. For example, phase 3 trials are done anywhere in the country where interested cancer specialists are available. On the other hand, treatment such as bone marrow transplantation involving either major new radiation equipment or large teams of physicians is available only in a few centers.

What Does the Cancer Center Offer?

We cannot make any general recommendations as to whether you should seek experimental therapy at a cancer center. You should read about the treatment for your cancer in the chapter on that cancer in this book. Most people can receive the best standard or even good experimental treatment without going to a large cancer center. However, there are promising treatments for several cancers that are available only at large cancer centers or specialized centers. For example, bone marrow transplantation is only done well at a few centers in the United States. It offers a chance for cure to the person with acute leukemia who has relapsed on chemotherapy. Some people with end-stage leukemia who had a bone marrow transplant are alive, well, and probably cured. You must ask your cancer specialist and read about your cancer in this book to find out whether it pays to go to a cancer center for experimental treatment. You must also decide whether you want to search out even a slim chance for a longer life. Remember, most people will get sick and only a few will be helped.

Immunotherapy

Immunotherapy is experimental and unproven therapy for cancer. It has received wide attention in magazines, newspapers, and medical journals over the past five or ten years. Immunotherapy attempts to bolster the body's own immune system to fight a cancer. It is most effective in animal studies when it is given before the animal is given cancer cells. For example, animals given immunotherapy fight off larger numbers of transplanted cancer cells. However, there are only a few animal studies that show that immunotherapy helps an already established cancer. Therefore, there is little animal data supporting the use of immunotherapy in people with cancer. Furthermore, after many clinical trials with different forms of immunotherapy, there is no cancer for which immunotherapy is standard or proven treatment. Immunotherapy appeals to the public and physicians alike because it offers a way of treating cancer without toxic drugs. Unfortunately, at the present time there is little solid scientific evidence that it works. We advise against traveling out of your community for immunotherapy, because we do not think present approaches to immunotherapy are promising. There are oncologists who disagree with our point of view. Immunotherapy is still controversial.

Immunotherapy has side effects, although it is not as toxic as chemotherapy. If you are offered immunotherapy to treat your cancer, find out how effective it has been in the past and what the side effects are. Be sure there is no proven treatment such as radiation or chemotherapy that is more likely to help you.

BCG   BCG is an attenuated bacterium similar to the bacteria that cause tuberculosis. It has been widely used in Europe as an antituberculosis vaccine. BCG vaccinations are given to people with cancer to bolster their immune system nonspecifically. In animals, BCG helps fight small numbers of cancerous cells. In humans it is either injected under the skin or the skin is scratched and BCG is placed upon it in a process called "scarification." This causes a local infection similar to a smallpox vaccination and leaves scars. For cosmetic reasons, it is usually given on the thigh. BCG has several toxicities, including fever, chills, and fatigue. Rarely an easily treatable systemic infection similar to tuberculosis occurs. A few people have died from severe allergic-type reactions to BCG.

Levamisole   Levamisole is a drug that is being used to treat intestinal worm infestations in Third World countries. It bolsters the immune system only if the system is depressed. Levamisole is being tested in people with a variety of tumors. It is fairly nontoxic but has not yet been proven to be of value in cancer treatment.

Vaccination of Tumor Cells   There are trials in progress using injections of either killed or live tumor cells to "vaccinate" a person to resist his cancer. After an injection of cells, scientists hope the body will develop antibodies, or "killer lymphocytes," against tumor antigens and attack the cancer. At present the use of tumor cell vaccination is entirely experimental. It is possible that if the tumor cells are not killed, they can grow, metastasize, and add to the body's tumor burden.

Heat, or Hyperthermia

It was observed in the latter part of the nineteenth century that some cancers were very sensitive to hyperthermia. Dr. Cole of Memorial Hospital in New York injected extracts of dead streptococcus called "Cole's toxin" in the latter part of the century to produce high fevers. Some of his patients with widespread cancer responded and some even seemed to be cured. However, it never took hold as a form of treatment because it was very dangerous. Many people became extremely sick and some died from the high fevers.

Now, after almost seventy years, hyperthermia is again under investigation as a form of treatment. Several centers are conducting preliminary trials of hyperthermia. Patients under general anesthesia have their body temperature elevated to 107° by hot baths and warming their blood. There have been some responses but even now, hyperthermia is very dangerous. Possibly in the next few years, it may play a role in the treatment for some cancers. At the present hyperthermia is merely an interesting but dangerous approach still in its infancy.

Bone Marrow Transplantation

The amount of chemotherapy and radiation used to treat cancer is limited by the bone marrow. With too much treatment, the bone marrow is suppressed and problems with bleeding and infection that can be fatal occur. Bone marrow transplantation rescues the patient by transplanting normal marrow from a brother or sister after very high doses of chemotherapy and radiation have been given. This allows a person to withstand otherwise lethal amounts of treatment. Even resistant leukemia can sometimes be cured in this way. The transfused marrow grows in the patient and produces the needed blood cells. However, unless the donor is an identical twin, these cells differ from those of the recipient. They can recognize the patient as foreign and cause a disease called graft-versus-host disease, which damages organs such as the skin, the liver, and the gastrointestinal tract and can be fatal. Bone marrow transplantation is a hazardous procedure.

Bone marrow transplantation has been used to treat and cure acute leukemia. Some adults and children with acute leukemia unresponsive to chemotherapy have been treated with bone marrow transplantation and are alive and well years later. They have probably been cured. Because bone marrow transplantation can cure leukemia, it is now being tested in acute nonlymphocytic leukemia before people become refractory to drugs. Researchers want to see if it can cure more people. If you or your child has acute leukemia, you should ask your physician about the possibility of a bone marrow transplant. He or she will need to see if any of your brothers or sisters are "matched" with you. Bone marrow transplants are only done between identical twins or between brothers and sisters whose tissue types are closely matched. Physicians who do transplants hope that they will be able to cure 40–50 percent of people with acute nonlymphocytic leukemia by performing transplants early in the first remission. It is important, however, to remember that almost 40 percent of people will die from the transplant or from complications of graft-versus-host disease. Thus, you must weigh your chance for cure against your chance for an earlier death. Transplants after relapse have occurred are far less likely to be successful.

SUMMARY

1. Experimental therapy is unproven treatment. Most experimental therapy for cancer is experimental chemotherapy.

2. Drugs that show effectiveness against animal tumors enter trials in humans with cancer. A phase 1 trial is the first time a drug is used in humans. Little is known about the side effects in man. The main aim of the trial is to find out how to use the drug and what its side effects are. The chances of benefit are very small and the risks are high. However, this type of trial is necessary if new and effective treatments for cancer are to be found. Even if you do not benefit, you may help others.

3. A phase 2 trial is used to find out if a drug is effective against human cancers. The chances of responding are still small but the risks are lower because the side effects and dosage were defined in the phase 1 trial.

4. Phase 3 trials test the new drugs against cancers for which they have already shown some promise. The chances of benefiting are quite good and the risks are small.

5. Immunotherapy is still entirely experimental treatment. It has no proven benefit and is not the standard treatment for any human cancer.

6. Heat, or hyperthermia, is being evaluated at a few centers in the United States. It has shown some promise but is very toxic.

7. Bone marrow transplantation currently offers promise or hope to some people with acute leukemia, but it is only available in a few centers. Bone marrow transplantation can cure some people with leukemia who no longer respond to chemotherapy.

8. Experimental therapy is available at cancer centers, large medical centers, small medical centers, and from medical oncologists in private practice. You have to find out from your cancer specialist what kind of experimental therapy is available for your cancer. Many experimental drugs are available to medical oncologists who practice in small communities.

9. We urge caution in entering experimental trials. Find out what is

known about a drug or a treatment. Ask your specialist what he or she really thinks about it. Experimental therapy hurts more people than it helps. Yet only by having people enter into experimental trials can progress be made. You may decide to take experimental chemotherapy not solely for the slim chance that you may be helped, but for the opportunity to help future cancer victims. If you have a cancer for which good treatment exists, remember that the treatment was developed through sacrifice by people like you who decided to take a chance on what was then "experimental" treatment.

Epilogue

We have tried to give a fair, neither overly optimistic nor pessimistic view of the current state of knowledge about cancer. Progress in cancer medicine is slow. Although dramatic breakthroughs may occur at any time, they are not likely to help many people currently suffering from cancer. Truly amazing progress has been made in caring for some cancers; people with diseases such as Hodgkin's disease, childhood leukemia, and testicular cancer are now cured with regularity, whereas years ago most died shortly after diagnosis. Unfortunately, there has not been enough progress made to help many of the people who get such common cancers as cancer of the lung, colon, and pancreas. There has been essentially no improvement in the cure rate for these tumors over the past twenty years.

What can we expect from future progress in cancer research? To us, it seems likely that major strides will be made in the areas of early diagnosis of some tumors such as colon cancer and possibly even lung cancer, as well as identification and elimination of some of the agents that cause these diseases. For example, agents may be added to the diet to decrease the effect of carcinogens in foods and thus may protect us from developing gastrointestinal cancer. Although this remains speculative, it is not far-fetched. It may become possible to remove carcinogens from cigarettes and thus decrease the incidence of lung cancer. Rigorous controls over substances such as asbestos may protect future generations.

We hope you now believe that early cancer detection is worthwhile. Thousands of lives could be saved if women examined their breasts themselves, if doctors routinely checked stools for blood, and if people at high risk to develop some cancers were properly and regularly checked. Part of the responsibility of decreasing your risk of dying from cancer is yours. You must insure that you get diagnosed early, receive adequate health care, and protect yourself from as many known cancer-causing agents as possible.

Future advances in cancer prevention are most likely going to help our children and our children's children rather than us. Our best hope of saving our own lives lies with early detection of cancer through regular checkups and getting the best possible treatment. If this book helps our readers accomplish those objectives, we will be assured that we have done a greater service than we could by spending our lifetimes taking care of patients with advanced cancer.

Glossary

Adjuvant chemotherapy. The use of chemotherapy in combination with surgery and/or radiation to treat apparently localized cancers when the odds are high that microscopic nests of cancer cells are present in distant organs

Alopecia. Partial or complete baldness, which can result from radiation or chemotherapy

Angiosarcoma. A cancer arising from blood vessels. Angiosarcomas of the liver are caused by polyvinyl chloride, a commonly used plastic

Astrocytoma. The most common malignant brain tumor in adults

Asymptomatic. Without obvious symptoms of disease

BCG. A bacterium similar to the bacteria that cause tuberculosis. It is used as a vaccine to bolster the immune system to help fight cancer. This form of therapy is still experimental.

Benign. Not usually harmful; not malignant

Biopsy. Surgical removal of tissue, which is then examined under a microscope by a pathologist to determine whether a suspicious lump is cancerous or benign

Board-certified specialist. A physician who has received formal training and has passed an examination in a particular area of medicine.

Bone marrow. The spongy tissue in the center of the bones where blood cells are made

Bone marrow biopsy and aspiration. A procedure whereby bone marrow is obtained so it can be examined under the microscope. This is done by inserting a needle into the center of a bone, usually the hip bone or the breast bone (sternum).

Brain scan. A method of detecting brain tumors. Radioactive material is injected into an arm vein and a camera records the radioactivity of the brain. Tumors can thus be detected, because they accumulate more radioactivity than normal brain tissue.

Bronchoscopy. An examination of the breathing passages (bronchi) with a

389

flexible instrument called a bronchoscope, which is passed through the mouth or nose

Cancer. An uncontrolled growth of cells that, if unchecked, will eventually cause death

Carcinogen. A substance that causes or promotes the development of cancer

Carcinoma. A cancer arising from epithelial cells, cells of the gastrointestinal tract, the genitourinary tract, the skin, the lungs, or the glands

CAT (Computerized Axial Tomography) Scan. A newly developed computerized x-ray process that gives very detailed pictures of the body. It has proven highly useful in evaluating patients with cancer.

Chemotherapy. The use of drugs or chemicals to treat cancer

Cobalt therapy. Radiation therapy using radioactive cobalt as the source of the ray. This is the most commonly used modern source. It delivers more radiation to the cancer and less to the skin and normal surrounding tissues than the older, orthovoltage machines.

Colonoscopy. A visual examination of the entire colon using a flexible instrument called a fibrooptic colonoscope

Colostomy. A connection between the colon and the abdominal wall so that fecal material will pass into a collecting bag attached to the abdomen

Colposcopy. An examination of the vagina and cervix using a magnifying instrument that is inserted into the vagina

Combination chemotherapy. The use of two or more drugs together to treat a cancer more effectively than a single drug

Cordotomy. The cutting by a neurosurgeon of the section of the spinal cord that carries pain impulses, to relieve severe pain

Craniopharyngioma. A tumor that arises from the pituitary gland, which is located at the base of the brain. It is most common in children.

Cystoscopy. A visual examination of the bladder with an instrument called a cystoscope, which is inserted into the bladder through the body's natural passage, the urethra

Endometrium. The tissue lining the inner portion of the uterus, or womb

Endoscopy. The use of a hollow, tubelike instrument to visualize and biopsy otherwise inaccessible areas of the body, such as the stomach, colon, or bladder

Esophagoscopy. A visual examination of the esophagus, or swallowing tube, with a flexible, tubelike instrument called an esophagoscope or gastroscope

Gastroenterologist. An internist who is trained in and who restricts his practice to the diagnosis and nonsurgical treatment of diseases of the gastrointestinal tract

Gastroscopy. A visual examination of the stomach with a fiberoptic gastroscope, a flexible, tubelike instrument that is swallowed

Gingiva. The gums; the structure surrounding the teeth

Glioblastoma. A highly malignant type of brain tumor of adults

Glioma. The most common type of brain tumor. Gliomas are further subdivided into astrocytomas, oligodendrogliomas, and ependymomas.

Goiter. An enlarged thyroid gland due to noncancerous conditions

Granulocytes. The cells that circulate in the blood and protect against bacterial infection

Gynecologist. A physician who is trained in and who restricts his practice to the diagnosis and therapy (both medical and surgical) of diseases of the female reproductive organs

Hematologist.   A physician who is trained in and who restricts his practice to the evaluation and treatment of blood disorders. He has been trained to treat hematologic malignancies, leukemias, malignant lymphomas, multiple myeloma, etc.

Hepatoma (hepatocellular carcinoma).   A malignant tumor originating from liver cells

Hospice.   An organization, which may include living facilities, that provides care and support for the terminally ill

Hyperalimentation.   The administration of nutrients into a vein or a tube

Hypernephroma (renal cell cancer).   A cancer originating in the kidney

Hyperthermia.   The experimental treatment of cancer using heat either to the entire body or to just the portion of the body containing the tumor

Hyperthyroidism.   A disease caused by overproduction of thyroid hormone, characterized by weight loss, nervousness, weakness, and heart problems

Hypoparathyroidism.   A condition characterized by muscle twitching and low blood calcium, caused by an inadequate supply of parathyroid hormone

Hysterectomy.   Surgical removal of the uterus

Ileostomy.   An artificial opening between the small bowel (the ileum) and the abdominal wall so that fecal material will pass into a collecting bag attached to the abdomen

Immunotherapy.   The still-experimental attempts to treat cancer by either boosting the person's own immune defense system, most commonly with BCG, or administering serum, or cells, to fight the cancer

In situ.   The term used to describe the earliest stage of a cancer, a tiny cancer localized to the immediate area where it started. *In situ* cancers are almost 100 percent curable.

Internist.   A physician who is specially trained in and who restricts his practice to the diagnosis and treatment of adult, nonsurgical illness

Laparotomy.   An exploratory abdominal operation performed either to make a diagnosis or to determine the extent of a disease in the abdomen

Laryngectomy.   The surgical removal of the voice box, which results in loss of the normal speech mechanism and also a permanent hole in the throat. A person can learn to speak again after this operation.

Laryngoscopy.   *Indirect:* An examination of the larynx using a mirror. *Direct:* An examination of the larynx using an instrument called a laryngoscope, which is passed through the mouth into the upper portion of the windpipe

Larynx.   The upper portion of the windpipe, which functions as the voice box

Leiomyoma.   A benign tumor arising in smooth muscle, the type of muscle lining the gastrointestinal tract, the bladder, and the uterus

Leukoplakia.   A premalignant disease of the mouth and gums characterized by the development of white plaques

Linear accelerator.   A relatively new machine that is used as an alternative to radioactive cobalt to deliver radiation therapy. Both these types of radiation deliver more radiation to the cancer and less to the skin and normal surrounding tissues; therefore, the cancer cells are damaged and the patient has fewer side effects.

Lymphangiogram.   A method of visualizing the lymph glands deep in the abdomen. Radiopaque dye is injected into small lymphatics in the feet; it then spreads into the lymph glands in the abdomen.

Lymphocytes.   Cells that help fight infection by producing antibodies

Lymphoma.   A cancer arising in the lymph glands

Mammography.   X-rays of the breast, which can detect very small (early) breast cancers

Mastectomy.   The surgical removal of a breast. A "simple" mastectomy is the removal of just the breast. A modified or "radical" mastectomy also involves the removal of the underlying muscle and draining lymph nodes under the arm.

Medical oncologist.   A physician who is trained in and who restricts his practice to the use of drugs to treat cancer

Megavoltage therapy.   A measure of radiation beam energy. Both cobalt and linear accelerator sources are in the megavoltage range. This means the beam energy is high and they deliver more of the energy to the tumor and less to the normal tissues surrounding the cancer and the skin. Thus, they cause more damage to the cancer and less to normal tissues.

Melanoma.   A pigmented, highly malignant skin cancer

Meningioma.   A common, benign brain tumor that starts in the tissues lining the brain (the meninges)

Mesothelioma.   A tumor of the lining of the lung (pleura) or abdominal cavity (peritoneum) that is caused by asbestos

Metastasis.   The spread of a tumor from one site to another. The result is one or more new foci of cancer in organs distant from the original site.

Mucositis.   Sores in the mouth caused by radiation or chemotherapy

Neuroma.   A benign tumor made up of nerve cells and/or nerve fibers

Neurosurgeon.   A physician who has received special training in and who restricts his practice to the diagnosis of and use of surgery to treat diseases of the nervous system (brain, spinal cord, and nerves)

Oncologist.   A physician who specializes in cancer treatment. A *radiation oncologist* is trained in the use of radiation to treat cancer. A *medical oncologist* specializes in the use of drugs for cancer treatment. A *pediatric oncologist* is a pediatrician (a children's specialist) who is trained in the drug treatment of childhood cancer. A *gynecologic oncologist* is a gynecologist who specializes in treating cancers of the female reproductive tract. For these specialties, there are formal training programs and board-certification examinations. At the present time there are no formal training programs and therefore no board-certification examinations in surgical oncology.

Oophorectomy.   Surgical removal of the ovaries

Orthopedic surgeon.   A physician who is trained in and who restricts his practice to the diagnosis and surgical treatment of diseases of the bones and joints

Orthovoltage.   Radiation therapy, now rarely used, that has a lower beam energy than megavoltage equipment and thus has more side effects. However, it is still useful and as efficacious as megavoltage machines in certain situations.

Ostomy.   An artificial opening between an organ and the abdominal wall for the excretion of intestinal contents (colostomy or ileostomy) or urine

Otolaryngologist.   A physician who has been trained in and who restricts his practice to the evaluation and treatment of diseases of the ear, nose, mouth, and throat

Palliation.   Treatment that makes a person feel better, such as relieving pain, but that is not curative

Pap(inicolau) smear.   The collection of cells obtained by scraping the uterine cervix, for examination under the microscope to diagnose early cancer

Pediatric oncologist-hematologist. A pediatrician who is trained in and who restricts his practice to the use of drugs to treat cancer

Peritoneum. The membranous lining that covers the abdominal organs

Platelets. Small cell fragments that circulate in the blood and protect against bleeding

Pleura. The membranous lining around the lung

Polyp. A benign protruding growth from a mucous membrane, such as colon polyps, nasal polyps, etc.

Polyposis. The development of multiple polyps on the surface of a mucous membrane. Although polyps are not cancerous themselves, some types (for example, familial polyposis of the colon) may develop into cancer.

Precancerous (premalignant) lesion. A lesion that is benign but that may develop into cancer, such as leukoplakia of the mouth, villous adenoma of the colon, etc.

Prognosis. A prediction regarding what will occur based upon the usual course of a disease. This is the result of many cases; therefore, it does not exactly predict the outcomes for any given individual.

Pylorus. The valvelike lower portion of the stomach

Quackery. The use of unproven or unorthodox methods to treat cancer victims for financial gain

Radiation. A process of delivering energy to cells that absorb it and are thereby damaged or killed by it

Radiation oncologist. A physician who is trained in and who restricts his practice to the use of radiation to treat cancer

Radioactive implants. The application of radioactive material in the form of a wire, a needle, or small capsules to an area of cancer. This delivers a high dose of radiation to the cancer and a minimal amount to surrounding normal tissues.

Radiocurable. A cancer that may be cured by the use of radiation therapy alone

Radioisotopic scans. The administration of small amounts of radioactive isotopes followed by the imaging of various organs using a special camera sensitive to radioactivity. Abnormalities may show up as areas of increased or decreased radioactivity. Commonly scanned organs include the liver, spleen, bone, brain, and thyroid.

Radiologist. A physician who is trained in and who restricts his practice to the use of x-rays for diagnosis. Some radiologists also administer radiation to treat cancer.

Radioresistant. A cancer that does not usually respond, or shrink, when treated with tolerable doses of radiation

Radiosensitive. A cancer that can be eradicated by irradiation in doses that are tolerated by the normal surrounding tissues; a cancer that usually responds, or shrinks, with radiation treatment

Regional perfusion. The administration of an anticancer drug by injection into the artery feeding the cancer. The aim is to destroy more cancer cells with fewer side effects.

Relapse. This term refers to the regrowth of the cancer after its improvement or shrinkage with therapy.

Remission. Shrinkage of the cancer accompanied by feeling better, usually in response to therapy. *Partial remission:* Shrinkage of the cancer. *Complete remission:* All evidence of the cancer disappears. This does not mean cure, but rather that all visible disease has disappeared.

Rhizotomy. Cutting nerve tracts outside the spinal cord to relieve pain

Sarcoma. A cancer that arises in the cells located between the organs and the skin that form the body's supportive tissues, such as bone, cartilage, fibrous tissue, fat, or muscle

Sigmoidoscopy. A visual examination of the lower portion of the colon with an instrument called a sigmoidoscope, which is passed through the rectum

Specialist. A physician who is trained in and who restricts his practice to a limited area of medicine; for example, a radiation oncologist, a physician who uses radiation to treat cancer

Spinal tap. The introduction of a small needle into the spinal canal either to obtain fluid or to administer a drug. This is done by numbing the area and then inserting a needle between the vertebrae (back bones) into the canal.

Staging. The process of determining if and how far a cancer has spread. This is accomplished by a careful physical examination and tests such as x-rays and scans.

Telangiectasia. A dilatation of the capillary vessels and minute arteries under the skin forming an angioma, a benign tumor

Tomograms. X-rays of selected layers of the body. This method can detect small tumors and other abnormalities not detectable with the usual x-ray picture.

Tumor. A swelling or lump, which may be benign or cancerous

Tumor board. An official hospital committee composed of physicians who either specialize or have a special interest in cancer medicine. It should consist of at least a pathologist, a radiation oncologist, a surgeon, and a medical oncologist. The tumor board's function is to review the cases of cancer in the hospital and to make recommendations concerning evaluation and therapy.

Ulcer. An erosion through the surface of the skin or membranes that line the inner surfaces (gastrointestinal tract, respiratory tract) of the body

Ultrasound examination. A test performed using a probe that transmits sound waves and records their echoes. It is useful for detecting masses or lumps and also to determine whether a mass is solid or cystic (fluid filled).

Upper gastrointestinal x-rays. An x-ray examination in which a white liquid (barium) is swallowed that outlines the esophagus and the stomach

Urologist. A physician who has been trained in and who restricts his practice to the diagnosis and surgical treatment of diseases of the genitourinary system

Xerography. X-rays of the breast that can detect very small (early) breast cancers

Further Sources of Information

INFORMATION ABOUT YOUR PHYSICIAN

There are three books that can help you assess a doctor's qualification as a cancer specialist, and thereby help you find a qualified doctor or doctors to treat you. These books are available in some large public libraries and are generally available in medical school libraries, at county medical society offices, or at American Cancer Society offices. The *Directory of Medical Specialists* is extremely valuable, as it lists board-certified specialists. Here you can find out if your doctor is a board-certified oncologist, etc. The American Medical Association's *Directory of Physicians* lists all the doctors in the United States by alphabetical order and by geographic region but does not give any information about board certification in cancer specialties. The third book, the *Directory of Members of the American Federation of Clinical Societies*, lists the members of several medical societies concerned with the treatment of cancer. Members of these societies usually are well trained, interested, and experienced in the evaluation and treatment of cancer.

Directory of Medical Specialists, 18th edition, 2 volumes (Chicago: A. N. Marquis Co., 1977–78)
 A listing of board-certified physicians by state, city, and town. Look in this book to see if your doctor is a board-certified oncologist, hematologist, radiation oncologist, general surgeon, or surgical subspecialist (e.g., urologist).

American Medical Association Directory of Physicians in the United States, 27th edition, 5 volumes (Chicago: American Medical Association, 1979)
 A listing of all physicians in this country by alphabetical order and geographic region. Doctors furnish information themselves about areas of special interest. Therefore, a designation of "medical oncologist," for example, in this book

does not guarantee formal training, board qualification, or certification as in the previous book.

Directory of Members: American Federation of Clinical Oncologic Societies (New York: American Federation of Clinical Societies, 1977–78)
A listing of physicians who are members of several societies concerned with the treatment of cancer. Members of these societies have been well trained and are interested and experienced in the treatment of people with cancer. This book lists members of the Society of Surgical Oncology (Ewing Society), surgeons who are trained and experienced in cancer surgery; the American Society for Head and Neck Surgery and the Society of Head and Neck Surgeons, board-certified otolaryngologists, general surgeons, or plastic surgeons who are experienced in surgery for head and neck cancers; the Society of Gynecologic Oncologists, board-certified obstetrician-gynecologists with three years of additional training in cancer of the female reproductive organs; and the American Society of Therapeutic Radiologists, board-certified radiologists who do radiation therapy full time.

THE AMERICAN CANCER SOCIETY

The American Cancer Society offers several important services to people with cancer. These vary from community to community. Some common services are: transportation service to and from the physician's office; cancer detection programs; educational services such as pamphlets, films, and speakers; equipment such as hospital beds, walkers, and crutches; nursing and homemaker services; and rehabilitation programs for people with a laryngectomy, mastectomy, or ostomy. Call the nearest chapter for help. There are almost 3,000 local chapters.

Central Office   777 Third Avenue, New York, New York 10017   *(212) 371–2900*

State Divisions

Alabama Division, Inc.   2926 Central Avenue, Birmingham, Alabama 35209 *(205) 879–2242*
Alaska Division, Inc.   1343 G Street, Anchorage, Alaska 99501   *(907) 277–8696*
Arizona Division, Inc.   634 West Indian School Road, Phoenix, Arizona 85011 *(602) 264–5861*
Arkansas Division, Inc.   5520 West Markham Street, Little Rock, Arkansas 72203 *(501) 664–3480–1–2*
California Division, Inc.   731 Market Street, San Francisco, California 94103 *(415) 777–1800*
Colorado Division, Inc.   1809 East 18th Avenue, Denver, Colorado 80218   *(303) 321–2464*
Connecticut Division, Inc.   Professional Center, 270 Amity Road, Woodbridge, Connecticut 06525   *(203) 389–4571*
Delaware Division, Inc.   Academy of Medicine Building, 1925 Lovering Avenue, Wilmington, Delaware 19806   *(302) 654–6267*
District of Columbia Division, Inc.   Universal Building, South, 1825 Connecticut Avenue, N.W., Washington, D.C. 20009   *(202) 483–2600*

Florida Division, Inc.   1001 South MacDill Avenue, Tampa, Florida 33609   *(813)* *253–0541*

Georgia Division, Inc.   2025 Peachtree Road, N.E., Suite 14, Atlanta, Georgia 30309   *(404) 351–3650–1–2*

Hawaii Division, Inc.   Community Services Center Building, 200 North Vineyard Boulevard, Honolulu, Hawaii 96817   *(808) 531–1662–3–4–5*

Idaho Division, Inc.   P.O. Box 5386, 1609 Abbs Street, Boise, Idaho 83705   *(208)* *343–4609*

Illinois Division, Inc.   37 South Wabash Avenue, Chicago, Illinois 60603   *(312)* *372–0472*

Indiana Division, Inc.   2702 East 55th Place, Indianapolis, Indiana 46220   *(317)* *257–5326*

Iowa Division, Inc.   P.O. Box 980, Mason City, Iowa 50401   *(515) 423–0712*

Kansas Division, Inc.   3003 Van Buren, Topeka, Kansas 66611   *(913) 267–0131*

Kentucky Division, Inc.   Medical Arts Building, 1169 Eastern Parkway, Louisville, Kentucky 40217   *(502) 452–2676*

Louisiana Division, Inc.   Masonic Temple Building, Room 810, 333 St. Charles Avenue, New Orleans, Louisiana 70130   *(504) 523–2029*

Maine Division, Inc.   Federal and Greene Streets, Brunswick, Maine 04011   *(207)* *729–3339*

Maryland Division, Inc.   200 East Joppa Road, Towson, Maryland 21204   *(301)* *828–8890*

Massachusetts Division, Inc.   247 Commonwealth Avenue, Boston, Massachusetts 02116   *(617) 267–2650*

Michigan Division, Inc.   1205 East Saginaw Street, Lansing, Michigan 48906   *(517) 371–2920*

Minnesota Division, Inc.   2750 Park Avenue, Minneapolis, Minnesota 55407   *(612) 871–2111*

Mississippi Division, Inc.   345 North Mart Plaza, Jackson, Mississippi 39206   *(601) 362–8874*

Missouri Division, Inc.   P.O. Box 1066, 715 Jefferson Street, Jefferson City, Missouri 65101   *(314) 636–3195*

Montana Division, Inc.   2115 Second Avenue North, Billings, Montana 51901   *(406) 252–7111*

Nebraska Division, Inc.   6910 Pacific Street, Suite 210, Omaha, Nebraska 68106   *(402) 551–2422*

Nevada Division, Inc.   4220 Maryland Parkway, Suite 105, Las Vegas, Nevada 89109   *(702) 736–2999*

New Hampshire Division, Inc.   22 Bridge Street, Manchester, New Hampshire 03101   *(603) 669–3270*

New Jersey Division, Inc.   2700 Route 22, P.O. Box 1220, Union, New Jersey 07083   *(201) 687–2100*

New Mexico Division, Inc.   205 San Pedro, N.E., Albuquerque, New Mexico 87108   *(505) 268–4501*

New York State Division, Inc.   6725 Lyons Street, East Syracuse, New York 13057   *(315) 437–7025*

Long Island Division, Inc.   535 Broad Hollow Road (Route 110), Melville, New York 11746   *(516) 420–1111*

New York City Division, Inc.   19 West 56th Street, New York, New York 10019   *(212) 586–8700*

Queens Division, Inc.   111-15 Queens Boulevard, Forest Hills, New York 11375 *(212) 263–2224*

Westchester Division, Inc.   107 Lake Avenue, Tuckahoe, New York 10707   *(914) 793–3100*

North Carolina Division, Inc.   P.O. Box 27624, 222 North Person Street, Raleigh, North Carolina 27611   *(919) 834–8463*

North Dakota Division, Inc.   P.O. Box 426, Hotel Graver Annex Building, 115 Roberts Street, Fargo, North Dakota 58102   *(701) 232–1385*

Ohio Division, Inc.   453 Lincoln Building, 1367 East Sixth Street, Cleveland, Ohio 44114   *(216) 771–6700*

Oklahoma Division, Inc.   1312 Northwest 24th Street, Oklahoma City, Oklahoma 73106   *(405) 525–3515*

Oregon Division, Inc.   1530 S.W. Taylor Street, Portland, Oregon 97205   *(503) 228–8331*

Pennsylvania Division, Inc.   P.O. Box 4175, Harrisburg, Pennsylvania 17111 *(717) 545–4215*

Philadelphia Division, Inc.   21 South 12th Street, Philadelphia, Pennsylvania 19107   *(215) 567–0559*

Puerto Rico Division, Inc.   GPO Box 6004, San Juan, Puerto Rico 00936   *(809) 764–2295*

Rhode Island Division, Inc.   333 Grotto Avenue, Providence, Rhode Island 02906 *(401) 831–6970*

South Carolina Division, Inc.   4482 Fort Jackson Boulevard, Columbia, South Carolina 29209   *(803) 787–5624*

South Dakota Division, Inc.   700 South 4th Avenue, Sioux Falls, South Dakota 57104   *(605) 336–0897*

Tennessee Division, Inc.   2519 White Avenue, Nashville, Tennessee 37204   *(615) 383–1710*

Texas Division, Inc.   P.O. Box 9863, Austin, Texas 78766   *(512) 345–4560*

Utah Division, Inc.   610 East South Temple, Salt Lake City, Utah 84102   *(801) 322–0431*

Vermont Division, Inc.   13 Loomis Street, Drawer G, Montpelier, Vermont 05602 *(802) 223–2348*

Virginia Division, Inc.   3218 West Cary Street, P.O. Box 7288, Richmond, Virginia 23221   *(804) 359–0208*

Washington Division, Inc.   323 First Avenue West, Seattle, Washington 98119 *(206) 284–8390*

West Virginia Division, Inc.   325 Professional Building, Charleston, West Virginia 25301   *(304) 344–3611*

Wisconsin Division, Inc.   P.O. Box 1626, Madison, Wisconsin 53701   *(608) 249–0487*

Milwaukee Division, Inc.   6401 West Capitol Drive, Milwaukee, Wisconsin 53216 *(414) 461–1100*

Wyoming Division, Inc.   1118 Logan Avenue, Cheyenne, Wyoming 82001   *(307) 638–3331*

Canadian Cancer Society

Central Office   Suite 401, 77 Bloor Street West, Toronto, Ontario M5S 2V7   *(416) 961–7223*

By Province

Quebec Division   Canadian Cancer Society, 1118 St. Catherine Street West, Montréal, Quebec   *(514) 866–2613*

Manitoba Division   Canadian Cancer Society, 960 Portage Avenue, Winnipeg, Manitoba R3G 0R4   *(204) 775–4449*

British Columbia & Yukon Division   Canadian Cancer Society, 1926 West Broadway, Vancouver, British Columbia V6J 1Z2   *(604) 736–1211*

New Brunswick Division   Canadian Cancer Society, Post Office Box 2089 (61 Union Street, E2L 1A2—parcels), Saint John, New Brunswick E2L 3T5   *(506) 652–7600*

Nova Scotia Division   Canadian Cancer Society, 1485 South Park Street, Halifax, Nova Scotia B3J 2L1   *(902) 423–6550*

Newfoundland Division   Canadian Cancer Society, 3rd Floor, Philip Place, St. John's, Newfoundland A1A 2Y4   *(709) 753–6520*

Ontario Division   Canadian Cancer Society, 185 Bloor Street East, 6th Floor, Toronto, Ontario M4W 3G5   *(416) 923–7474*

Alberta Division   Canadian Cancer Society, Main Floor, 1134 — 8th Avenue South West, Calgary, Alberta T2P 1J5   *(403) 263–3120*

Saskatchewan Division   Canadian Cancer Society, 1501 — 11th Avenue, Regina, Saskatchewan S4P 0H3   *(306) 522–6320*

Prince Edward Island Division   Canadian Cancer Society, 51 University Avenue, 3rd Floor, Charlottetown, Prince Edward Island   *(709) 753–6520*

REHABILITATION PROGRAMS

Contact the local or state chapters of the American Cancer Society for information on rehabilitation programs. Reach to Recovery helps victims of breast cancer. The International Association of Laryngectomies and the Lost Chord, Anamilo, and New Voice clubs help people with larynx cancers. The American Cancer Society Ostomy Rehabilitation Program helps people with colon, rectal, or bladder cancer. You may also call or write:

International Association of Laryngectomies, American Cancer Society   777 Third Avenue, New York, New York 10017

United Ostomy Association, Inc.   111 Wilshire Boulevard, Los Angeles, California 90017

THE LEUKEMIA SOCIETY OF AMERICA, INC.

The Leukemia Society of America supports patients with leukemia or lymphomas (Hodgkin's disease and non-Hodgkin's lymphomas). Information is available from national headquarters and from the local offices. Assistance is available to qualified patients to cover payment for: drugs used in the care, treatment, or control of leukemia and lymphomas; blood transfusions; transportation to and from a doctor's office, hospital, or treatment center; and x-ray therapy for patients with malignant lymphomas.

Leukemia Society of America, Inc.   211 East 43rd Street, New York, New York 10017   *(212) 573–8484*

THE NATIONAL CANCER INSTITUTE

The National Cancer Institute provides information and educational materials. It has designated eighteen medical institutions as "comprehensive cancer centers." These centers will either provide care directly or help patients and/or doctors find qualified cancer specialists. They are listed by states below. Contact:

Office of Cancer Communications, National Cancer Institute   Building 31, Room 10 A 30, Bethesda, Maryland 20014   *(301) 496–6631*

Alabama

University of Alabama Hospitals and Clinics   619 South 19th Street, Birmingham, Alabama 35233   *(205) 934–5077*

Director, Cancer Communications Office   205 Mortimer Jordan Hall, University of Alabama in Birmingham, Birmingham, Alabama 35294   *(205) 934–2651* or *934–2671*

California

Los Angeles County University of Southern California, Cancer Center School of Medicine   2025 Zonal Avenue, Los Angeles, California 90033   *(213) 226–2008*

Los Angeles County, University of Southern California, Director, Office of Cancer Communications   1721 Griffin Avenue, Los Angeles, California 90031 *(213) 226–4043* or *226–4044*

Colorado

Director of Education and Information   Colorado Regional Cancer Center, Inc., 165 Cook Street, Denver, Colorado 80206   *(303) 320–5921*   *(800) 332–1850*

Connecticut

Yale Comprehensive Cancer Center, Yale University School of Medicine   333 Cedar Street, New Haven, Connecticut 06510   *(203) 432–4122*

Communications Program Manager, Yale Comprehensive Cancer Center, Yale University School of Medicine   333 Cedar Street, Room 1HR-E19, New Haven, Connecticut 06510   *(203) 436–3779* or *436–0517*   *(800) 922–0824*

District of Columbia

Howard University with Georgetown University, Howard University Hospital   2041 Georgia Avenue, N.W., Washington, D.C. 20060   *(202) 745–1406* or *462–8488*

Lombardi Cancer Research Center   Georgetown University, 3800 Reservoir Road, N.W., Washington, D.C. 20007   *(202) 625–7066*

Communications Officer, Cancer Communications for Metropolitan Washington Suite 218, 1825 Connecticut Avenue, N.W., Washington, D.C. 20009 *(202) 797–8876* or *797–8893*

Florida

Comprehensive Cancer Center for the State of Florida University of Miami School of Medicine, Jackson Memorial Medical Center, P.O. Box 520875, Biscayne Annex, Miami, Florida 33152 *(305) 547–6096*

Cancer Information Service, Comprehensive Cancer Center for the State of Florida 2 S.E. 13th Street, Miami, Florida 33131 *(305) 547–6920* *(800) 432–5953*

Illinois

Communications Specialist, Illinois Cancer Council 37 South Wabash, Suite 507, Chicago, Illinois 60603 *(312) 346–9813* *(800) 972–0586*

Maryland

The Johns Hopkins Medical Institutions *(301) 955–3300*

Communications Director, The Johns Hopkins Cancer Center 550 N. Broadway, Suite 503, Baltimore, Maryland 21205 *(301) 955–3636*

Massachusetts

Sidney Farber Cancer Center 44 Binney Street, Boston, Massachusetts 02115 *(617) 739–1100*

Communications Officer, Cancer Control Program 35 Binney Street, Boston Massachusetts 02115 *(617) 734–7950* *(800) 952–7420*

Minnesota

Mayo Comprehensive Cancer Center, Mayo Clinic Rochester, Minnesota 55901 *(507) 282–2511* Communications Specialist *(507) 282–2511, Ext. 8377* *(800) 582–5262*

New York City

Memorial Sloan-Kettering Cancer Center 1275 York Avenue, New York, New York 10021   Director of Cancer Communications *(212) 794–7982*

New York State

Cancer Control Communications Officer, Research Study Center, Rosewell Park Memorial Institute 666 Elm Street, Buffalo, New York 14263 *(716) 845–4402*

North Carolina

Duke University Comprehensive Cancer Center   Duke University Medical Center, Box 3814, Durham, North Carolina 27710   *(919) 684–2282*

Coordinator, Cancer Information Services   200 Atlas Street, Durham, North Carolina 27705   *(919) 286–2214*   *(800) 672–0943*

Ohio

Communications Office, Ohio State University Cancer Research Center   1580 Cannon Drive, Columbus, Ohio 43210   *(614) 422–5022*

Pennsylvania

Fox Chase and University of Pennsylvania Cancer Center Program   7701 Burholme Avenue-Fox Chase, Philadelphia, Pennsylvania 19111   Communications Coordinator   *(215) 342–1000, Ext. 498*   *(800) 822–2963*

Texas

The University of Texas System Cancer Center   M. D. Anderson Hospital and Tumor Institute, 6723 Bertner Avenue, Houston, Texas 77030   Program Administrator   *(713) 792–3363*   *(800) 392–2040*

Washington

Fred Hutchinson Cancer Research Center   1124 Columbia Street, Seattle, Washington 98104   Communications Officer   *(206) 292–6301*

LARGE CHILDREN'S HOSPITALS

This list is not complete. It does not include every children's hospital with a qualified team of children's cancer specialists. It does, however, include most of these hospitals in the United States.

If you do not live near one of these institutions, we recommend calling the closest one to see if a hospital nearer your community can offer your child care for cancer.

Alabama

Children's Hospital, Birmingham

Arizona

Department of Pediatrics, University of Arizona Medical School, Tucson

Arkansas

Arkansas Children's Hospital, Little Rock

California

Children's Hospital of Los Angeles, Los Angeles
Harbor General Hospital in Torrance, Los Angeles
UCLA University Hospital, Los Angeles
Department of Pediatrics, School of Medicine, University of Southern California, Los Angeles
Children's Hospital and Medical Center of Northern California, Oakland
Department of Pediatrics, University Hospital, San Diego
Department of Pediatrics, Stanford Medical Center, San Francisco
Department of Pediatrics, School of Medicine, University of California at San Francisco, San Francisco

Colorado

Denver Children's Hospital, Denver

Connecticut

Department of Pediatrics, Yale University School of Medicine, New Haven

District of Columbia

Children's Hospital and National Medical Center
Department of Pediatrics, Georgetown University Hospital
Department of Pediatrics, Walter Reed Army Medical Center

Florida

Department of Pediatrics, University of Florida College of Medicine, Gainesville
Department of Pediatrics, University of Miami, Miami
Department of Pediatrics, University of South Florida, Tampa

Georgia

Department of Pediatrics, Emory University School of Medicine, Atlanta
Henrietta Egleston Hospital for Children, Atlanta

Illinois

Children's Memorial Hospital, Chicago

Indiana

James Whitcomb Riley Hospital for Children, Indianapolis

Kansas

Department of Pediatrics, University of Kansas Medical Center, Kansas City

Kentucky

Children's Hospital of Louisville, Louisville

Louisiana

Department of Pediatrics, Tulane School of Medicine, New Orleans

Maryland

Department of Pediatrics, The Johns Hopkins Medical Center, Baltimore
Department of Pediatrics, University of Maryland School of Medicine, Baltimore
Department of Pediatrics, National Cancer Institute, Bethesda

Massachusetts

Department of Pediatrics, Massachusetts General Hospital, Boston
Sidney Farber Cancer Center, Boston
New England Medical Center, Tufts University, Boston

Michigan

Department of Pediatrics, University Hospital, University of Michigan, Ann Arbor
Children's Hospital, Wayne State School of Medicine, Detroit

Minnesota

Department of Pediatrics, University of Minnesota Medical School, Minneapolis
Department of Pediatrics, Mayo Clinic, Rochester

Mississippi

The Children's Hospital, Jackson

Missouri

Department of Pediatrics, University of Missouri, Columbia
St. Louis Children's Hospital, Washington University School of Medicine, St. Louis

New Hampshire

Department of Pediatrics, Hickock Clinic, Hanover

New York

Department of Pediatrics, Roswell Park Memorial Hospital, Buffalo
Department of Pediatrics, Northshore University Hospital, Manhasset
Department of Pediatrics, Long Island Jewish Medical Center, New Hyde Park
Babies Hospital, Columbia Medical School, New York City
Department of Pediatrics, Memorial Sloan-Kettering Cancer Center, New York City
Department of Pediatrics, Cornell Medical Center, New York Hospital, New York City
Department of Pediatrics, Strong Memorial Hospital, Rochester
Department of Pediatrics, Upstate Medical Center, Syracuse

New Jersey

Department of Pediatrics, New Jersey College of Medicine & Dentistry, Newark

North Carolina

Department of Pediatrics, University of North Carolina School of Medicine, Chapel Hill
Department of Pediatrics, Duke University Medical Center, Durham
Department of Pediatrics, Bowman Gray School of Medicine, Winston-Salem

Ohio

Children's Hospital, Cincinnati
Department of Pediatrics, Cleveland Clinic, Cleveland
Rainbow Babies and Children's Hospital, Cleveland
Children's Hospital of Columbus, Columbus

Oklahoma

Oklahoma Children's Memorial Ward, Oklahoma City

Oregon

Doernbecher Memorial Hospital for Children, Portland

Pennsylvania

Cardoza Foundation, Philadelphia
Children's Hospital of Philadelphia, Philadelphia
St. Christopher's Hospital, Philadelphia
Children's Hospital of Pittsburgh, Pittsburgh

Rhode Island

Department of Pediatrics, Rhode Island Hospital, Providence

South Carolina

Department of Pediatrics, Medical University of South Carolina, Charleston

Tennessee

St. Jude Children's Hospital, Memphis
Department of Pediatrics, Vanderbilt University School of Medicine, Nashville

Texas

Department of Pediatrics, M. D. Anderson Cancer Center, Houston
Texas Children's Hospital, Houston
Department of Pediatrics, Health Science Center, University of Texas, San Antonio

Utah

Department of Pediatrics, University of Utah Medical Center, Salt Lake City

Vermont

Department of Pediatrics, University of Vermont, Burlington

Virginia

Department of Pediatrics, University of Virginia School of Medicine, Charlottesville
Department of Pediatrics, Medical College of Virginia, Commonwealth University, Richmond

West Virginia

Charleston Area Medical Center, Charleston
Department of Pediatrics, West Virginia School of Medicine, Morgantown

Washington

Children's Orthopedic Hospital, Seattle

Wisconsin

Department of Pediatrics, University of Wisconsin School of Medicine, Madison
Children's Hospital of Milwaukee, Milwaukee

Index

The Johns Hopkins University Press

This book was composed in Optima text and display type by The Maryland Linotype Composition Co., Inc., from a design by Alan Carter. It was printed on 50-lb. Publishers Eggshell Offset Cream and bound in an impregnated cloth by Universal Lithographers, Inc.

Library of Congress Cataloging in Publication Data

Glucksberg, Harold.
  Cancer care.

  Bibliography: p. 395
  Includes index.
    1. Cancer.   2. Cancer—Psychological aspects.
3. Cancer—Social aspects.   I. Singer, Jack W.,
joint author.   II. Title.
RC263.G58   616.9′94   79–16930
ISBN 0–8018–2255–6